Diabetes
For Canadians
FOR
DUMMIES®
2ND EDITION

Vit. D
Injectable Glucagon

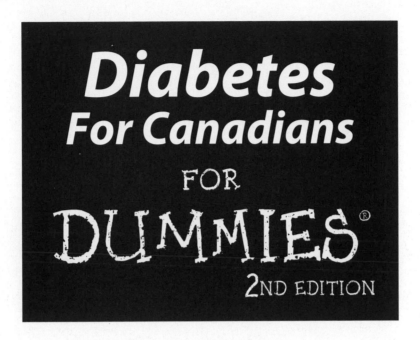

Diabetes
For Canadians
FOR DUMMIES®
2ND EDITION

by Ian Blumer, MD, FRCPC
Alan L. Rubin, MD

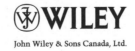

John Wiley & Sons Canada, Ltd.

Diabetes For Canadians For Dummies, 2nd Edition

Published by
John Wiley & Sons Canada, Ltd.
6045 Freemont Blvd.
Mississauga, ON L5R 4J3

www.wiley.com

For general information on John Wiley & Sons Canada, Ltd., including all books published by Wiley Publishing Inc., please call our warehouse, Tel. 1-800-567-4797. For reseller information, including discounts and premium sales, please call our sales department, Tel. 416-646-7992. For press review copies, author interviews, or other publicity information, please contact our publicity department, Tel. 416-646-4582, Fax 416-236-4448.

Library and Archives Canada Cataloguing in Publication Data

Blumer, Ian
    Diabetes for Canadians for dummies / Ian Blumer, Alan L. Rubin. — 2nd ed.

Includes index.
ISBN 978-0-470-15677-3

    1. Diabetes—Popular works. I. Rubin, Alan L II. Title.

RA645.D5B48 2009   616.4'62   C2008-907809-8

Printed in the United States

13 12 11 10 9 8 7 6 5 4 3 2

WILEY

About the Authors

Ian Blumer, MD, FRCPC, is a diabetes specialist in the Greater Toronto Area of Ontario. He has a teaching appointment with the University of Toronto, is the medical advisor to the adult program of the Charles H. Best Diabetes Centre in Whitby, Ontario, and is actively involved in diabetes research. An enthusiastic lecturer, he has spoken about diabetes to numerous professional and lay audiences and has appeared regularly in the Canadian media.

Dr. Blumer is a member of the Clinical and Scientific Section of the Canadian Diabetes Association (CDA), where he currently serves as Chair of the Dissemination and Implementation Committee for the 2008 CDA Clinical Practice Guidelines. He is also a member of the American Diabetes Association, and the European Association for the Study of Diabetes.

Dr. Blumer is the author of *What Your Doctor Really Thinks* (Dundurn, 1999), and co-author of *Understanding Prescription Drugs For Canadians For Dummies* (co-written with Dr. Heather McDonald-Blumer). His Web site (www.our diabetes.com) offers practical advice on how to manage diabetes. Ian welcomes your comments about this book at diabetes@ianblumer.com.

Alan L. Rubin, MD, is one of America's foremost experts on diabetes. He is a professional member of the American Diabetes Association and the Endocrine Society and has been in private practice specializing in diabetes and thyroid disease for more than 30 years. Dr. Rubin was Assistant Clinical Professor of Medicine at University of California Medical Center in San Francisco for 20 years. He has spoken about diabetes to professional medical audiences and non-medical audiences around the world. He has been a consultant to many pharmaceutical companies and companies that make diabetes products.

Dr. Rubin was one of the first specialists in his field to recognize the significance of patient self-testing of blood glucose, the major advance in diabetes care since the advent of insulin. As a result, he has been on numerous radio and television programs, talking about the cause, the prevention, and the treatment of diabetes and its complications.

Since publishing *Diabetes For Dummies*, Dr. Rubin has had four other bestselling *For Dummies* books — *Diabetes Cookbook For Dummies, Thyroid For Dummies, High Blood Pressure For Dummies,* and *Type 1 Diabetes For Dummies* — all published by Wiley Publishing. His five books cover the medical problems of 100 million Americans.

Dedication

Ian: This 2nd edition of *Diabetes For Canadians For Dummies* is dedicated to diabetes educators from coast to coast to coast. Not a day passes when Ian doesn't thank his lucky stars that he and his fellow physicians have such a dedicated group of caring individuals working together as part of a team striving to keep people living with diabetes healthy.

Alan: This book is dedicated to Alan's wife Enid and their children, Renee and Larry. Their patience, enthusiasm, and encouragement helped to make the writing a real pleasure. This book is also dedicated to the thousands of people with diabetes who have written to thank Alan for helping them to understand what they are dealing with and for telling him where he needs to provide more information and emphasis to make this an even better book.

Authors' Acknowledgements

Ian: I cannot imagine there exists a nicer, more mentoring, and more thoughtful editor than Robert Hickey. Robert; thank you (again!). I would also like to thank Lisa Berland whose skilled review of my manuscript has saved me from committing egregious (and embarrassing) grammatical errors and has kept a potentially disparate several hundred pages from being, well, disparate. Thanks also to Lindsay Humphreys who has so ably overseen this project.

I would like to thank Bin Chin, who has once again educated me on the nuances of nutrition and to Marian Barltrop, who helped research the first edition of this book and who continues to be such a wonderful partner in both clinical work and scientific research. It will never be possible for me to express my degree of respect and admiration for Marlene Grass, the epitome of selfless dedication and a pioneer in childhood and young adult diabetes education. Marlene has improved the lives of thousands of people with diabetes. It was Marlene who brought me into the diabetes fold; how very lucky I am that she did so!

Thanks to those who have provided helpful tips for this book including Keith Bowering, Jeannette Goguen, Henry Halapy, Robin Ingle, Claire Lightfoot, Jill Milliken, Paul Oh, Ron Sigal, and Karyn Thompson. And a special thanks to Maureen Clement, a physician of immense knowledge and caring who has contributed enormously to the improvement of diabetes care in Canada and who, on a personal level, has been kind enough to review this manuscript.

Thanks to those readers of the first edition of this book who sent me such kind emails. I cannot tell you how much these have meant to me. And to my patients I extend my profound appreciation for giving me the honour of assisting you with your health care and my great thanks for the lessons I learn from you.

Last, but heavens, not least, I would like to thank my wonderful wife Heather whose love, companionship, partnership, encouragement, and support have brought me nothing but joy for almost twenty-five years now. Everyone — including our kids! — tells me I'm the most fortunate husband alive. They're right.

Alan: For this edition, acquisitions editor Michael Lewis deserves major thanks. I have had the pleasure of working with him for several years. He is supportive, encouraging, and fun and I look forward to a long association with him. I am also blessed with another great project editor, Jennifer Connolly, who not only made sure that everything was readable and understandable, but offered excellent suggestions to improve the information. My thanks also to Dr. Seymour Levin for reviewing the book for scientific accuracy.

Ronnie and Michael Goldfield should definitely be considered the godparents of this book.

My friends in the Dawn Patrol, a group of guys with whom I play squash and solve the problems of the world thereafter, kept me laughing throughout the production of this book. Their willingness to follow me convinced me that others would be willing to read what I wrote.

My teachers are too numerous to mention, but one group deserves special attention. They are my patients over the last 35 years, the people whose trials and tribulations caused me to seek the knowledge that you will find in this book.

This book is written on the shoulders of thousands of men and women who made the discoveries and held the committee meetings. Their accomplishments cannot possibly be given adequate acclaim. We owe them big-time.

Publisher's Acknowledgements

We're proud of this book; please send us your comments through our Dummies online registration form located at www.dummies.com/register/.

Some of the people who helped bring this book to market include the following:

Acquisitions, Editorial, and Media Development

Editor: Robert Hickey

    Editor, previous edition:
    Michelle Marchetti

Project Manager: Elizabeth McCurdy

Project Editor: Lindsay Humphreys

Copy Editor: Lisa Berland

Cover photo: Mauritius Images/PhotoLibrary

Cartoons: Rich Tennant
(www.the5thwave.com)

Composition Services

Vice-President Publishing Services:
Karen Bryan

Project Coordinator: Lynsey Stanford

Layout and Graphics: Samantha K. Allen, Reuben W. Davis

Proofreaders: Laura Albert, Laura L. Bowman, Dwight Ramsey

Indexer: Potomac Indexing, LLC

John Wiley & Sons Canada, Ltd.

    Bill Zerter, Chief Operating Officer

    Jennifer Smith, Vice-President and Publisher, Professional and Trade Division

Publishing and Editorial for Consumer Dummies

    Diane Graves Steele, Vice President and Publisher, Consumer Dummies

    Kristin Ferguson-Wagstaffe, Product Development Director, Consumer Dummies

    Ensley Eikenburg, Associate Publisher, Travel

    Kelly Regan, Editorial Director, Travel

Publishing for Technology Dummies

    Andy Cummings, Vice-President and Publisher, Dummies Technology/General User

Composition Services

    Gerry Fahey, Vice-President of Production Services

    Debbie Stailey, Director of Composition Services

Contents at a Glance

Table of Contents

Introduction

A second edition: Wow, is it really necessary? You bet it is. So much has happened since the last edition. As the *2008 Canadian Diabetes Association Clinical Practice Guidelines* (upon which this book is based) reveal, doctors now know much more about diabetes. (And after reading this book, *you'll* know it too.) Best of all, the guidelines include increasingly effective ways of keeping people with diabetes healthy. We have new and better ways of using nutrition therapy; we have, thanks to Canadian researchers, more effective ways of using exercise; and we also have entirely new types of medicines available.

In 1985 there were 30 million people with diabetes in the world. By 2000 that number had risen to 150 million. By the year 2025 it's estimated that 380 million people will have diabetes. If you're like us, these numbers sound alarming but are so large they're hard to relate to. So, looking closer to home, a recent study found that from 1995 to 2005 the number of people in Ontario living with diabetes doubled, reaching 9 percent of the population, or 827,000 individuals. (It is quite likely that similar figures are present elsewhere in Canada, too.) Nine percent! Next time you're at a hockey game, look around the stands and just imagine that nearly one in ten people in the arena have diabetes. As we mention in Chapter 1, you surely are not alone in having diabetes.

Diabetes has become so prevalent and so important in its worldwide health (and, therefore, financial) implications that the United Nations has recently declared November 14 (the birthday of the co-discoverer of insulin, Frederick Banting) to be World Diabetes Day.

In a sense, a diagnosis of diabetes is both good news and bad news. It's bad news to be told you have a health problem you could do without, thank you very much. But it can be good news if you see it as an opportunity to have a look at your lifestyle and make those changes that may have been due anyhow. It's never too late to start leading a healthier life!

As for humour, at times you will feel like doing anything but laughing about your diabetes. But scientific studies are clear about the benefits of a positive attitude on a person's diabetes. In very few words: He who laughs, lasts. Also, people find out and remember more when humour is part of the process. Our goal isn't to trivialize human suffering by being comic about it, but to lighten the burden of a chronic disease by showing that it's not all doom and gloom.

About This Book

We've designed *Diabetes For Canadians For Dummies* so you don't have to read it cover to cover, but if you know nothing about diabetes, doing so may be a good approach. (Indeed, many readers of our first edition have told us this is exactly what they did!) We want this book to serve as a source for information about diabetes, what causes it, how it affects you, and, most importantly, how to effectively deal with diabetes so that you can achieve and maintain good health.

Canada has a long and proud history of being in the forefront of diabetes research and therapy. *Diabetes For Canadians For Dummies* looks at the special issues that Canadians with diabetes have to face (like Ian's patient who returned to his car one February morning after his son's hockey practice, only to find his insulin frozen solid!) and uses the most recent Canadian Diabetes Association recommendations *(2008 Clinical Practice Guidelines for the Prevention and Management of Diabetes in Canada)*. These guidelines are of such high quality that they're referred to and used around the world. (You can find the guidelines online at www.diabetes.ca/for-professionals/resources/2008-cpg).

In addition to discussing the latest facts about diabetes, this book tells you about the best sources you can access to discover any information that comes out after the publication of this edition. You'll find frequent references to Web sites that offer excellent information. If you don't have Internet access yourself, you can still get online at your neighbourhood library. As Internet addresses change frequently, if you find a recommended link to be non-functional, try going to the home page of the site and check their site map to find the new page.

Conventions Used in This Book

Diabetes, as you know, is associated with sugar problems. But sugars come in many types, so doctors avoid using the words *sugar* and *glucose* interchangeably. In this book, we use the word *glucose* rather than *sugar* (unless we're talking about things such as table sugar or sweets you have in your diet). As well, because it gets to be redundant to keep adding mmol/L (which is short for millimoles per litre) after every blood glucose value to which we refer, you can safely assume that when we say, for example, that a fasting blood glucose of 7 (or higher) is indicative of diabetes, we mean 7.0 mmol/L.

What You Don't Have to Read

We hope you'll enjoy reading everything in this book; however, throughout the book, you'll find shaded areas, which are called sidebars, that contain material that's interesting but not essential. We hereby give you permission to skip them if the material they cover is of no particular interest to you. You'll still understand everything else.

In addition, we've noted some paragraphs that have a more technical nature with the Technical Stuff icon (see the section "Icons Used in This Book," later in this Introduction for more information on icons). Although these paragraphs deepen your knowledge of diabetes, you can still understand the text without reading them. Our feelings won't get hurt if you don't read these paragraphs, but these technical tidbits may come in handy during a high-stakes trivia game, or at the very least can make you sound pretty smart in front of your doctor.

Foolish Assumptions

This book assumes that you know nothing about diabetes. You won't suddenly have to face a term you've never heard before that isn't explained. However, if you already know a lot about diabetes, you'll find more in-depth explanations. You can pick and choose how much you want to know about a subject. The key points are clearly marked.

How This Book Is Organized

This book is divided into six parts to help you find out all you can about the topic of diabetes.

Part 1: Dealing with the Diagnosis of Diabetes

To slay the dragon, you have to be able to identify it. This part sorts out the different types of diabetes and looks at how you get diabetes and how you can help protect your family from developing it.

In this part, you'll also find out how to deal with the emotional and psychological consequences of the diagnosis and what all those intimidating-looking polysyllabic words mean.

Part II: How Diabetes Can Affect Your Body

Diabetes may be associated with sugar, but to say that it's the same as sugar is like saying that a car is the same as a spark plug. Diabetes is far more than that and can affect every part of you. If you understand diabetes, you'll understand how your body works both when it's healthy and when it's not.

In this part, you find out what you need to know about both the acute and long-term problems that diabetes can cause. You also find out about sexual problems related to diabetes and about how diabetes can affect pregnancy.

Part III: Rule Your Diabetes: Don't Let It Rule You

In this part, you discover all the tools available to treat diabetes. You find out about the health care team that is there to assist you and about the ways that you can make effective use of good nutrition and exercise to keep yourself healthy. You also discover the medications that may assist you with controlling your blood glucose.

We also take a look at alternative and complementary therapies, including natural products that people with diabetes often take.

Part IV: Particular Patients and Special Circumstances

Diabetes affects people differently depending on their age group. In this part, you hear about those differences and how to manage them. You also find out about diabetes in Aboriginal peoples.

We look at employment and insurance difficulties that people with diabetes can face and how to address them. This part also discusses diabetes and driving and offers suggestions to help you maintain a driver's licence and to obtain a commercial licence. We also look at the implications of having diabetes on the ability to pilot an aircraft.

And so that you are always prepared, we discuss precautions you can take so that you can look after your diabetes in the event that a disaster strikes.

Part V: The Part of Tens

This part presents a concise summary of the most crucial stuff you need to know. Find out not only Ten Ways to Stay Healthy and Prevent Complications, but also Ten Frequently Asked Questions and Ten Ways to Get the Best Possible Health Care.

Part VI: Appendixes

This is where you'll find information on the Food Group System used in diabetes meal planning. We also look at some terrific diabetes-oriented Internet sites and, last, we present a glossary. (We define words as we go along, but in case you forget what a term means, you can quickly flip to the back of the book.)

Icons Used in This Book

The icons tell you what you must know, what you should know, and what you might find interesting but can live without.

This icon indicates a story about one of our patients. (The names and other identifiers have been changed to maintain confidentiality.)

This icon gives you technical information or terminology that may be helpful, but not necessary, to your understanding of the topic.

When you see this icon, it means the information is critical and is not to be missed.

This icon points out when you should contact your health care team (for example, if your blood glucose control is in need of improving or if you need a particular test done). Your health care team includes your family doctor, your diabetes specialist, your diabetes nurse educator, your dietitian, your eye doctor (optometrist or ophthalmologist), your pharmacist, and, when necessary, other specialists (such as a podiatrist, dentist, cardiologist, kidney specialist, neurologist, emergency room physician, and so forth). We'll let you know which member of your team you should contact. (Incidentally, the most important member of your health care team is *you*.)

This icon is used when we share a practical, timesaving piece of advice, sometimes providing some additional detail on an important point.

Part I
Dealing with the Diagnosis of Diabetes

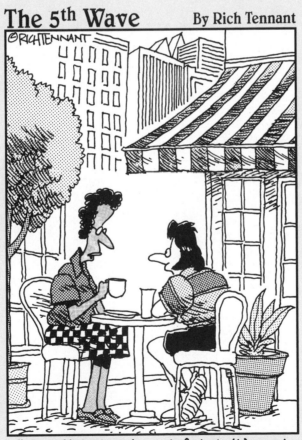

The 5th Wave   By Rich Tennant

"No, diabetes is not fatal, it's not contagious, and it doesn't mean you'll always get half my desserts."

In this part . . .

You have found out that you or a loved one has diabetes. What do you do now? This part looks at the cause of your diabetes and how it can make you feel — both mentally and physically.

Chapter 1

Membership in a Club You Didn't Ask to Join

As a person with diabetes, you already know that diabetes isn't "just a sugar problem." In fact, the moment you were told you had diabetes, many different thoughts may have run through your mind. You have feelings, and you have your own personal story. You're not the same person as your next-door neighbour or your sister or your friend, and your diabetes and the way that you respond to its challenges are unique to you.

And unless you live alone on a desert island, your diabetes doesn't affect just you. Your family, friends, and co-workers are influenced by your diabetes and by their desire to help you.

In this chapter we consider how you might feel after you first find out you have diabetes, and we also look at some coping strategies to help you deal with this unwelcome news.

Figuring Out What Diabetes Is

Because we spend so much time discussing diabetes in this book, we want to start by defining the condition. *Diabetes* is a *metabolic* disorder (a problem with the body's internal chemistry) characterized by the presence of high blood glucose because the pancreas is unable to make enough insulin hormone or because the insulin the pancreas makes is not working properly, or both. (We take a closer look at glucose in Chapter 2.)

That may be the technically correct definition of diabetes, but to leave it at that would be akin to defining Paris as "a city with a metal tower located in France." France does indeed have a metal tower — and diabetes does indeed have high blood glucose — but to limit your perspective to such simple definitions would be to miss out on so, so much. Diabetes isn't just a sugar problem; it's a whole body problem. To make this point, Ian made up his own definition of diabetes: "A disease that involves high blood glucose levels and an increased risk of damage to the body, much of which is preventable."

Diabetes is actually the short form for diabetes mellitus. The Romans noticed that the urine of certain people was *mellitus,* the Latin word for "sweet." The Greeks noticed that when people with sweet urine drank, fluids came out in the urine almost as fast as they went in the mouth, like a siphon. They called this by the Greek word for "siphon" — *diabetes.* Hence diabetes mellitus, but we think this is much better captured by the 17th-century definition of diabetes: "the pissing evil." Talk about calling it the way you see it!

You may have done some searching in books or on the Internet and come across another form of diabetes called *diabetes insipidus.* This term refers to an entirely different condition than diabetes mellitus. The only thing they have in common is a tendency to pass lots of urine. And now that we've clarified that, you won't see diabetes insipidus mentioned again in this book (unless you count the index at the back!).

You're Not Alone

Hardly a day goes by when a person with diabetes isn't in the news. Years ago, such appearances were often of heartbreak or loss. Nowadays it's more likely to celebrate an achievement. On May 25, 2008, Sebastien Sasseville (www.sebinspires.com) became the first Canadian with type 1 diabetes to reach the summit of Mount Everest. In 2007, Chris Jarvis (www.ichallenge diabetes.org), a resident of Victoria, B.C., won a rowing gold medal at the Commonwealth Games. And in that same year Scott Verplank, insulin pump and all, won the EDS Byron Nelson Championship (and the US$1,134,000 that went with it!).

Away from the sports arena, Ernest Hemingway, Thomas Edison, Jack Benny, Elizabeth Taylor, and — Ian's all-time favourite piece of diabetes lore — Elvis Presley all lived with diabetes.

You may not have spoken to Stephen Steele, but it is quite possible he has spoken to you. Stephen is a commercial pilot with a major Canadian airline. (You get to know Stephen better in Chapter 18.) And in the event that you had the bad luck to be in dire straits on some sinking vessel off the Atlantic coast, it is quite possible that the hero that plucked you from the ocean was none other than Major Chuck Grenkow, a Medal of Bravery–winning Canadian Forces pilot and aircraft commander performing search and rescue operations with the Canadian military. Oh, by the way, they both have diabetes.

Diabetes is a common disease, so it's bound to occur in some very uncommon people. But you don't have to be famous to be considered exceptional. Indeed, every day of the week in our practices we see special people, people who have diabetes yet look after families, work in automotive plants or office buildings, write exams, go to movies, and do their best to live life to the fullest — people, perhaps, just like you.

The point is, diabetes shouldn't define your life. You're the same person the day after you found out you had diabetes as you were the day before. It just happens that you've been given an additional issue to deal with. Diabetes shouldn't stop you from doing what you want to do with your life. Certainly, it does complicate things in some ways, but if you follow the principles of good diabetes care that we discuss in this book, you may actually be healthier than people without diabetes who smoke, overeat, underexercise, or engage in other unhealthy activities.

Handling the News

Do you remember what you were doing when you found out that you or a loved one had diabetes? Unless you were too young to understand, the news was likely quite a shock. Suddenly you had a condition from which people get sick and can die. The following sections describe the normal stages of reacting to a diagnosis of a major medical condition such as diabetes.

Experiencing denial

You may have begun by denying that you had diabetes, despite all the evidence to the contrary. You probably looked for any evidence that the whole thing was a mistake, and you may not have followed the advice you were given. But ultimately, you had to accept the diagnosis and begin to gather the information needed to start to help yourself.

Hopefully, you not only came to accept the diabetes diagnosis yourself, but also shared the news with your family and other people close to you. Having diabetes isn't something to be ashamed of, and it isn't something that you should have to hide from anyone.

Your diabetes isn't your fault. You didn't want to have diabetes. You didn't try to get diabetes. And no one can catch it from you. There are over 2 million Canadians living with diabetes. You have joined a very, very large club!

When you and others are accepting and open about having diabetes, you'll find that you're far from alone in your situation. (If you don't believe us, read the section "You're Not Alone" earlier in this chapter.) And you will likely find it comforting to know there are others you can relate to and draw support from. For example, a number of years ago, one of Ian's patients, newly diagnosed with diabetes, was buying her diabetes supplies at the pharmacy and mentioned to the person beside her in line how worried she was about her health. Turns out this other person also had diabetes and was able to provide lots of reassurance. Well, more than just reassurance as it turns out — they got married a year later!

Feeling anger

When you've passed the stage of denying that you have diabetes, you may become angry that you're saddled with this "terrible" diagnosis. But you'll quickly find that diabetes isn't so terrible and that you can't rid yourself of the disease. Anger only worsens your situation, and being angry about your diagnosis is detrimental in the following ways:

- ✔ If your anger becomes targeted at a person, he or she is hurt.
- ✔ You may feel guilty that your anger is harming you and those close to you.
- ✔ Anger can prevent you from successfully managing your diabetes.

As long as you're angry, you're not in a problem-solving mode. Diabetes requires your focus and attention. Use your energy positively to find creative ways to manage your diabetes. (For ways to manage your diabetes, see Part III.)

Bargaining for more time

The stage of anger often transitions into a stage when you become increasingly aware of your mortality and bargain for more time. Even though you probably realize that you have plenty of life ahead of you, you may feel overwhelmed by the talk of complications, blood tests, and pills or insulin. You may even experience depression, which makes good diabetes care all the more difficult.

Studies have shown that people with diabetes suffer from depression at a rate that is two to four times higher than the rate for the general population. Those with diabetes also experience anxiety at a rate three to five times higher than people without diabetes.

If you suffer from depression, you may feel that your diabetes situation creates problems for you that justify your being depressed. You may rationalize your depression by saying that it's caused by the following: You

✔ Don't have the freedom to eat whatever you want whenever you want.

✔ Have to adjust your leisure activities.

✔ May feel that you're too tired to overcome difficulties.

✔ May dread the future and possible diabetic complications.

✔ May feel that diabetes hinders you as you try to form new relationships.

✔ May feel annoyed over all the minor inconveniences of dealing with diabetes.

All of the preceding concerns are legitimate, but they also are all surmountable. How do you handle your many concerns and fend off depression? The following are a few important methods:

✔ Try to achieve excellent blood glucose control (see Chapter 9).

✔ Begin a regular exercise program (see Chapter 11).

✔ Tell a friend or relative how you are feeling; get it off your chest.

✔ Recognize that not every abnormal blip in your blood glucose is your fault (see Chapter 9).

Sometimes, in order to surmount these challenges, professional help is required. We look at this in the sidebar "When you're having trouble coping."

Moving on

If you can't overcome the depression brought on by your diabetes concerns, you may need to consider therapy. But you probably won't reach that point. You may experience the various stages of reacting to your diabetes in a different order than we describe in the previous sections. Some stages may be more prominent, and others may be hardly noticeable.

Almost everyone with diabetes goes through periods when they pay less attention to their health, do less blood glucose testing, fall off their lifestyle treatment program, and even start missing some of their medicines. That's a fact of diabetes life and you needn't feel guilty. By the time you recognize that this is happening to you, you will probably also discover that you are ready to get back on track. The trick is not to dwell on perceived "failure," but to refocus on future success. It's just like when driving: gazing too long in the rearview mirror distracts you from focusing on where you're heading.

Don't feel that any anger, denial, or sadness is wrong. These are natural coping mechanisms that serve a psychological purpose for a brief time. Allow yourself to have these feelings, but then drop them. Move on and learn to live normally with your diabetes. You'll be surprised how much more easily you can control your diabetes when your spirits improve.

Here are some key steps you can take to manage the emotional side of diabetes:

- **Focus on your successes.** Some things may go wrong as you find out all about managing your diabetes, but most things will go right. As you concentrate on your successes, you will realize that you can cope with diabetes and not let it overwhelm you.

- **Involve the whole family in your diabetes.** A diabetic diet is a healthy diet for everyone. And the exercise you do is good for the whole family too. By doing things together, you strengthen the family ties while everyone benefits from a healthier lifestyle. Also, should you need your family to help you, for instance, if your blood glucose level is severely low, their being aware of how to help you will both reassure them and benefit you. (We discuss low blood glucose and how to treat it in Chapter 5.)

- **Develop a positive attitude.** A positive attitude gives you a can-do mindset, whereas a negative attitude leads to low motivation, preventing you from doing all that is necessary to manage your diabetes.

- **Find a great team.** Don't try to be your own doctor, nurse, or dietitian. Rather, assemble a great team of supporting players like the family physician, the diabetes nurse educator, the dietitian, the eye doctor, and so forth; and work together with them. They can help you set realistic, doable goals and, more importantly, assist you to achieve them. (We discuss the members of the diabetes team in Chapter 8.)

- **Don't expect perfection.** Although you may feel that you're doing everything right, you may find that, at times, your blood glucose levels are off. This situation happens to every person with diabetes and isn't always readily explained. Simply put, it's likely not your fault. So don't beat yourself up over it. If this happens to you, contact your health care team (see Chapter 8) and they can work with you to improve things.

When you're having trouble coping

You wouldn't hesitate to seek help for your physical ailments associated with diabetes, but it's possible you may be reluctant to seek help when you can't adjust psychologically to diabetes. The problem is that sooner or later, if you can't adjust psychologically, it will prevent you from properly looking after your diabetes, and as a result your general health will suffer. The following symptoms are indicators that it's time for you to seek professional help:

- You can't sleep.
- You have no energy.
- You have no appetite.
- You can't think clearly.
- You can't find activities that interest or amuse you.
- You don't find humour in anything.
- You feel worthless.
- You have frequent thoughts of suicide.

If you recognize these symptoms in your daily life, you need to get some help. Your sense of hopelessness may include the feeling that no one else can help you — but that simply isn't true. Your family physician is the first person to go to for advice. He or she may help you to see the need for some short-term or long-term therapy. Well-trained therapists can see solutions that you can't see in your current state. You need to find a therapist whom you can trust, so that when you're feeling low you can talk to this person and feel assured that he or she is very interested in your welfare.

Your therapist may decide that your situation is appropriate for medication to treat your anxiety or depression. Currently, many drugs are available that have been proven safe and effective. Sometimes a brief period of medication is enough to help you cope with your difficulties.

You can also find help in a support group. In most support groups, participants share their stories and problems, which helps everyone involved to cope with their own feelings of isolation, futility, or depression. A good place to start is to contact a local chapter of the Canadian Diabetes Association (www.diabetes.ca). Another good place to seek out support is the online community. If you search online, you'll find many diabetes-oriented forums where people share their common concerns. The American Diabetes Association (www.diabetes.org) also has some excellent community forums. Just be aware that most diabetes forums or newsgroups don't have professional health care providers moderating them, so take any medical advice or information with some skepticism.

Chapter 2

You and Your Blood Glucose

*T*he ancient Greeks and Romans knew about diabetes. Fortunately, the way they tested for the condition — by tasting the urine — has gone by the wayside. (So has the other old way of testing for diabetes — urinating near an anthill and seeing if the ants came scurrying for takeout.)

For most people, diabetes is diagnosed when they have their blood glucose level measured either as part of a routine checkup with their family doctor, or for some other coincidental reason (such as when tests are taken for an insurance application or in preparation for surgery). Others have their diabetes discovered when they seek medical attention after they've started to feel unwell due to symptoms of high blood glucose (which we discuss later in this chapter).

In this chapter you discover how diabetes is diagnosed, how you may feel if your blood glucose is too high, and what you can do to bring things under control.

What Is Glucose?

The sweetness of the urine with which the ancients had first-hand experience comes from *glucose,* the body's predominant form of sugar. Glucose is the fuel that your body uses to provide instant energy so that muscles can move and important chemical reactions can take place. Glucose is a *carbohydrate,* one group of the three sources of energy in the body. The others are protein and fat, which we discuss in greater detail in Chapter 10.

Many different kinds of sugar exist, but the important one when it comes to diabetes is glucose. Unlike in high school chemistry class, here we let you off easy and, apart from our discussion about nutrition therapy, we don't talk about all the other sugars that are around. But just in case you're wondering, some examples of other sugars are *fructose* (the sugar found in fruits and vegetables) and *sucrose* (or table sugar, which is actually a combination of glucose and fructose).

Diagnosing Diabetes

Diagnosing diabetes should be simple. You likely know by now that you have diabetes when your glucose level is too high. But what, exactly, is too high? One way to think of "too high" is to think of the level of blood glucose that can cause damage to your body. The Canadian Diabetes Association considers people to have diabetes if they meet *any* one of the following three criteria:

- ✔ A **casual** blood glucose level (*casual* is defined as any time of day or night, without regard to how long it's been since the last time you ingested anything containing calories) equal to or greater than 11.1 millimoles per litre (mmol/L) with symptoms of high blood glucose (we discuss those symptoms in the next section).

- ✔ A **fasting** blood glucose level (*fasting* is defined as eight or more hours without calorie intake) equal to or greater than 7.0 mmol/L.

- ✔ A blood glucose level equal to or greater than 11.1 mmol/L, when tested two hours after ingesting 75 grams of glucose as part of what is called a **glucose tolerance test.** Doctors used to order this test quite often, but nowadays doctors have learned that it's usually unnecessary. Diabetes can generally be diagnosed more easily with one of the other two tests we mention just above.

Testing positive for one of the above criteria is typically not enough to result in a diagnosis of diabetes (although exceptions exist, which we discuss next). Any one of the tests must be positive on another day to establish the diagnosis. More than one patient has come to us with a diagnosis of diabetes after having been tested only once, and then when we retested their blood glucose it turned out to be normal. They didn't have diabetes after all.

The diagnosis of diabetes should be based on a blood sample taken *from a vein.* If you borrow your friend's blood glucose meter, prick your finger to get a blood glucose sample, and find your blood glucose level to be high, see your doctor to have a blood sample drawn from a vein at a laboratory. Don't diagnose yourself based on a glucose meter result.

Waiting for another day to have a second test performed after having an initial high blood glucose discovered is *not* required — and indeed, can be dangerous in two circumstances:

✔ If your blood glucose level is very high and you're clearly ill from it

✔ If your doctor thinks you may have type 1 diabetes (especially if you are a child)

In either of these circumstances, you need to start treatment *immediately.*

If you have visited U.S. Web sites, you may have noticed that in the United States (and nowhere else) they use different units — called milligrams per decilitre (abbreviated mg/dL). To convert mg/dL to mmol/L you divide mg/dL by 18. For example, 200 mg/dL divided by 18 equals 11.1 mmol/L.

How High Blood Glucose Makes You Feel

Knowing a bit about how your body normally handles blood glucose will help you understand the symptoms of high blood glucose. In this section we look at both these issues.

Understanding how your body handles blood glucose

The pancreas makes a hormone called *insulin.* (We talk more about the pancreas in Chapter 3.) A *hormone* is a chemical substance made in one part of the body that travels (usually through the bloodstream) to another part of the body where it performs its work. Insulin finely controls the level of glucose in your blood. Insulin acts like a key to open the outside lining of a cell so that glucose can enter the cell. If glucose can't enter the cell, it can't provide energy to the body.

Insulin is an amazing substance. Not only does it allow glucose to enter cells, but it also enables fat and muscle to form and allows the liver to store glucose (in a form called glycogen) for use when you may not be eating properly. No wonder this powerful hormone is sometimes called the Viagra of the cell!

Without insulin, the body's tissues start to break down. Perhaps you have seen a heart-rending photo of an ill-looking child with diabetes from before insulin was discovered, and the thrilling photo of that same child, now the picture of health, after starting insulin therapy. (We talk more about the discovery of insulin — and Canada's important contribution — in Chapter 3.)

The pancreas normally functions like a precision tool, releasing just the right amount of insulin to keep your body's blood glucose in a remarkably tight range of about 3.3 to 6.1 mmol/L. If the pancreas isn't able to produce the proper amount of insulin, or if the insulin it makes isn't working effectively, then your blood glucose level will start to rise. If it goes up just a bit, you won't have any symptoms, but if it reaches as high as 10.0 mmol/L or so, glucose begins to filter through the kidneys and spill into the urine. It's at that stage that you'll begin to experience symptoms (see the next section for more).

It's a shame that people don't get symptoms until the glucose level is almost twice the normal level, because by the time symptoms arise, damage may already have occurred to the body. We would be much better off if even slightly high glucose levels made our skin glow bright green; that way we would all know when there is a problem.

Examining symptoms caused by high blood glucose

The following list contains the most common symptoms of uncontrolled blood glucose. You may find that some of these remind you of what you were feeling when you first found out you had diabetes:

- **Frequent urination and thirst:** High blood glucose makes more urine form, and the more urine you make, the more fluid you lose from your body. The large quantity of urine makes you feel the need to urinate more frequently during the day and to get up at night to empty your bladder, which keeps filling up. As the amount of water in your blood declines, you feel thirsty and drink much more frequently. Many people with newly diagnosed diabetes believe that they are urinating more often because they are drinking more, but it is actually the other way around.

- **Blurred vision:** When the blood glucose level changes substantially, it causes the amount of fluid in the lens of the eye to change also. This alters the way that light passes through your eye, making it bend more than usual and making things around you look blurry. Have you ever noticed how a knife in a glass of water looks bent? The same sort of thing is going on in your eye.

In the same way that your eyesight can become blurry as your blood glucose rises, it can become blurry as your blood glucose falls. Many people with diabetes become understandably alarmed when their vision gets worse after they first start diabetes therapy, but in fact this is often a good sign, as it means their treatment program is working. The visual blurring in this setting is caused by a change in the way that light is bending as it goes through the eye, and is not a result of damage to the eye. Your vision will return to its usual state within a few weeks. Don't waste your hard-earned money on expensive glasses. Buy inexpensive over-the-counter glasses at your neighbourhood drugstore, and you'll likely find that within a month you can give them away.

✔ **Hunger:** Inability to get energy in the form of glucose into the muscle cells that need it leads to a feeling of hunger despite all the glucose that is floating in the blood stream.

✔ **Fatigue:** Because glucose can't enter most cells in the absence of insulin or with ineffective insulin (see Chapter 3 for more), if you have uncontrolled diabetes, glucose can't be used as a fuel to move muscles and help other tissues function properly. And just like when you try to pedal a bike with deflated tires, you get tired awfully quickly.

✔ **Weight loss:** Because you can't nourish your cells without sufficient or effective insulin (see the preceding bullets), weight loss is common among people with newly diagnosed diabetes (especially if you have type 1 diabetes, as we discuss in Chapter 4). You lose muscle tissue. You lose fat tissue. And as these tissues are lost, the body wastes away (again, this is especially true of type 1 diabetes). Your blood glucose level is high, but the glucose just can't work. It's as if your car has a full gas tank but the fuel line is blocked. The gauge reads "full" but the car stalls anyhow.

✔ **Persistent vaginal infections:** When blood glucose rises, it rises in all the fluids in your body. For women, this means higher glucose levels in their vaginal secretions. Yeast organisms thrive in a high-glucose environment, and as a result, women with elevated glucose levels are prone to vaginal yeast infections. Symptoms include vaginal itching or burning, an abnormal discharge from the vagina, and sometimes an odour.

Although people with high blood glucose commonly experience the symptoms in this list, many people with undiagnosed diabetes don't have these symptoms. It's no wonder, therefore, that the diagnosis of diabetes can be especially surprising to them.

Doctor, my eyes!

Sam O'Reilly was a 60-year-old man who had just been diagnosed with diabetes. This was discovered shortly after he developed bothersome thirst and frequent urination and had gone to the hospital to get checked out. His blood glucose level was found to be 25 mmol/L. He was immediately started on pills to reduce his glucose level, and an appointment was arranged to see Ian two weeks thereafter.

About five days before his appointment, Mr. O'Reilly called Ian's office in a near panic. He was sure he was going blind. Days after starting his new pills, his thirst and urine problems had improved, but now he could no longer read his daily newspaper or even see the television; everything had become one big blur. Ian had him come to the office right away, not because he was worried about Mr. O'Reilly but to reassure him. The only additional prescription Mr. O'Reilly needed turned out to be "tincture of time," and this worked perfectly. Indeed, within a week or so, Mr. O'Reilly's eyesight was back to normal.

Controlling Your Blood Glucose

Although there may never be a good time to have diabetes, far better to have it now than 100 years ago, when almost no therapy was available. Until insulin was discovered in the 1920s, little could be done to help people with diabetes. For years after that, insulin was the mainstay of therapy, but in the middle years of the last century, a number of different drugs were discovered that combat high blood glucose (also called *hyperglycemia*). In recent years, further discoveries have made several entirely new types of medicine available. As Ian likes to say, it was about time that diabetes specialists were given more tools; we were getting very jealous of cardiologists who seemed to be getting all the neat drugs. Nowadays virtually anyone with diabetes can have excellent blood glucose control. It may not always be easy to achieve, but it can be achieved and must be achieved if you are going to keep healthy.

Treatment is not just a matter of taking medicine, of course. In fact, medicine is often the least important of the diabetes treatments. The three key therapies are

   ✔ Diet (more aptly called nutrition therapy; see Chapter 10)

✔ Exercise (see Chapter 11)

✔ Medication (see Chapters 12 and 13)

Most people with diabetes require a combination of all three of these strategies.

What You Can Do If You Lose Control of Your Blood Glucose

You will find that when you improve your blood glucose control, you will feel better. You won't be running to the bathroom around the clock, your energy level will improve, and you'll have a better sense of well-being. At times, however, your blood glucose control may worsen and some of your symptoms may start to return. You may find that your blood glucose levels go up if you're under greater stress, or if you've gotten off track with your nutrition plan, or if there's been yet another February blizzard and the idea of going out for your daily walk is just too daunting.

When your glucose control worsens, remember two things:

✔ If you're feeling reasonably well, even if your blood glucose levels climb up into the high teens (or even somewhat higher), there's no immediate danger to you. (The exception to this is if you have type 1 diabetes and are developing ketones. See Chapter 5 for a discussion of ketoacidosis.) A few days of blood glucose readings of 20 mmol/L will not damage your organs.

✔ Look at the higher glucose levels as a message that something is wrong and take corrective action. This may be as simple as adjusting your diet or restarting your exercise plan. Perhaps you've simply forgotten to refill a prescription for your diabetes medicines, in which case a trip to the pharmacy is in order. Or if you're unsure what has triggered the problem and what to do about it, then call your doctor or diabetes educator.

If your blood glucose readings have risen to the high teens or higher and you're feeling unwell (or if you have type 1 diabetes and you have developed ketones — see Chapter 5), then you need to seek immediate medical assistance. If you're very ill, proceed to the nearest emergency department. If you're not feeling all that badly, you may first contact your physician or diabetes educator. (As we discuss in Chapter 8, some diabetes educators are trained and empowered to assist you with these situations.)

Diabetes in Canada

Diabetes is a serious health problem, both for the individual with diabetes and for society as a whole. In Canada, more than 2 million people have diabetes (often not diagnosed). The older you get the more likely you are to have diabetes — some estimates suggest that as many as one out of every five people over the age of 60 in Canada has diabetes.

Canada is not unique in this realm. Indeed, virtually every country is experiencing alarming increases in the number of people being diagnosed with diabetes. The International Diabetes Federation (www.idf.org) estimates that 246 million adults currently have diabetes worldwide and that by the year 2025 this number will be over 380 million. The growth in the number of people with diabetes is mirrored by the growth in our collective waistlines, related to people having generally become more sedentary and not eating sufficiently healthfully. Another reason the number of diabetes cases has continued to increase throughout the world is that the lifespan of the population is increasing. What's the connection? Well, as a person ages, his or her chances of developing diabetes increases greatly. Along with obesity, age is a major risk factor for diabetes (though, as we age we also tend to gain weight, so it can be difficult to tease out which is the more important factor).

The yearly economic costs of diabetes in Canada are estimated to be a staggering $13 billion. That's not a misprint. That works out to about $6,000 for every man, woman, and child with diabetes, and may even be an underestimate.

Thankfully, governments in Canada are coming to grips with the need to improve diabetes services as well as working toward initiating preventive strategies. It's taken a long time, but Ministries of Health see the flow of red ink that diabetes causes and recognize that something must be done. Indeed, even since the first edition of this book was written just a few short years ago, Ian has observed new, concerted efforts from governments (and non-governmental organizations) across the country to improve how diabetes is managed (and prevented). And this is, simply put, a true thrill.

Chapter 3

Discovering the Cause of Your Diabetes

*Y*ou may not think that having a personal relationship with one of your body organs is possible or even desirable. Then again, maybe it's just that you haven't had a chance to meet some of them up close and personal. In which case, this chapter is just for you.

Ask most people what organ is involved with diabetes and a typical response would be "the pancreas." Indeed, the pancreas *is* a key player in diabetes, but it isn't the only one.

In this chapter, we take a look at the role each of the key participants plays in diabetes. (Incidentally, given the important role of genetics — as we discuss in Chapter 4 — two key participants are your parents. Which of course adds to the importance of picking your parents carefully, though that remains a little bit impractical, even with modern technology.)

How Your Organs Make Music

You may not think of your organs as being music makers (singing and other, ruder noises notwithstanding), but when it comes to controlling your blood glucose, your body is engaged in a wonderfully intricate symphony with each organ playing its part.

Glucose regulation starts the moment you begin to eat. When you ingest certain types of food, it gets broken down inside your gut into glucose, which is then absorbed across the lining of the small intestine into your blood. When inside your blood, the glucose travels around your body looking for a nice place to go. Some of the glucose gets used by your brain and some gets taken up and stored in your liver and muscles (in a form called glycogen). Your muscles use some of the glucose straightaway as they do their work. And fat cells store some of it as, well, fat (technically called triglycerides).

As you can see, several organs are involved in glucose metabolism. So, with apologies to Raquel Welch and Hollywood, now we can take a Fantastic Voyage inside our insides.

Presenting your pancreas

Unless you have diabetes, you probably don't ever think about that funny-looking organ tucked behind your stomach. Well, even if you do have diabetes, it's not likely that your dinnertime conversation centres on this tadpole-shaped (yuck!), 25.5-centimetre (10-inch) long, 80-gram (3-oz) organ. Figure 3-1 shows its location in your body.

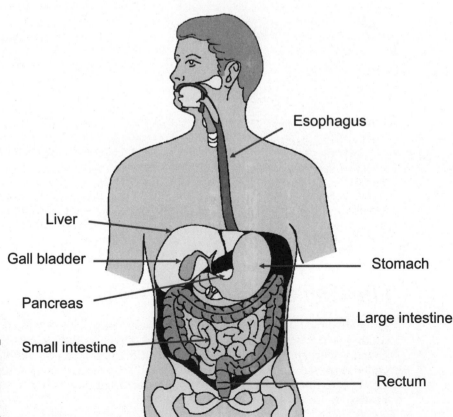

Figure 3-1: The abdominal organs.

The pancreas has two main functions. One is to produce enzymes, which are then released into your small intestine to assist with the breakdown of food. That is called the pancreas's *exocrine* function. The cells responsible for this take up 95 percent of the pancreas. People with diabetes seldom have a problem with this pancreas function.

Your pancreas's second task is called its *endocrine* function, and that has everything to do with your diabetes. Within the pancreas are clusters of hormone-producing cells called islet cells. The most important of these islet cells when it comes to diabetes is the beta cell. It is the beta cell that produces and releases into the blood stream a hormone called insulin. A normal pancreas has about 1.5 million islet cells. (If extracted and lumped together, these cells could fit inside a thimble. *Note:* Please do not try this at home!)

The pancreas also produces other hormones. One of these is glucagon. *Glucagon* can be thought of as an anti-insulin hormone because it acts in ways that oppose what insulin does. *Amylin,* another pancreatic hormone, works as a partner with insulin in keeping blood glucose under control. We discuss these hormones in more detail later in this section. Other pancreatic hormones (somatostatin and others) are either not involved with diabetes or are less important for blood glucose control and we don't discuss these further.

Looking at your liver

Perhaps we're admitting our bias here, but we feel bad for the liver. Apart from when people cook liver (and most people don't even like it), the only time it seems to get attention is when someone is suffering from hepatitis.

Your liver has many, many tasks to fulfill, including helping to rid your body of certain toxins and producing crucial proteins, such as clotting factors that prevent you from bleeding. The liver's role in glucose metabolism is to serve as a storage depot for excess glucose, removing it from or delivering it to the blood, depending on your body's needs at any given time.

Chewing the fat

You may know that if you're overweight, you're more prone to getting type 2 diabetes. But not all fat tissue is the same. There is fat inside the abdomen (called visceral fat) and there is fat in the abdominal wall and legs and arms (called non-visceral fat; how creative is that?). Depending on how much of each of these types of fat you have, your risk for getting diabetes will vary. We discuss this further in the next section.

The fat cells' role in glucose metabolism is to store extra glucose (as fat). For this reason, even if you were to entirely avoid fats in your diet, you could still easily gain excess weight if you were eating excess calories (such as ingesting too many carbohydrates). Imagine eating 2 dozen apples and half a kilo (1 pound) of icing a day. You wouldn't have seen an ounce of fat — not right away, that is. The fat would appear soon enough, though, but about a foot and a half lower than your lips!

Mentioning your muscles

When you walked into the bookstore or library to pick up this book, you were using your muscles and, without even thinking about it, your muscles were actively using glucose to do their work. Some of this glucose comes from stores within muscle and some comes from actively extracting glucose from your blood. When we think of muscles, we tend to think of power or strength. We should also think of fuel, because glucose is a key energy source that your muscles need to work properly.

Playing a beautiful melody

When things are going right, as soon as your blood glucose level rises after eating, your pancreas

- ✔ **Releases insulin into the bloodstream.** The insulin attaches to the lining of certain cells (such as muscle cells) and, as if a key has opened a door, the cells then allow the glucose to enter.

- ✔ **Releases amylin into the bloodstream.** Scientists haven't fully sorted out how amylin helps control blood glucose, but a main action appears to be slowing down how quickly food is absorbed into your body from the intestine.

- ✔ **Reduces how much glucagon it releases into the bloodstream.** The less glucagon in your bloodstream, the less glucose your liver will release. Your glucose goes up after eating, so having a lower amount of glucagon in your body as you eat is helpful because you don't need your liver to make additional glucose at that time.

At the same time that your pancreas is doing all those clever things, your intestines are releasing their own hormones, including GLP-1 and GIP. These hormones help prevent your blood glucose from going too high through several mechanisms, including increasing how much insulin your pancreas makes, slowing down how quickly food is absorbed into your body from your intestine, and reducing your appetite.

As soon as your glucose level falls back to normal, the pancreas shuts off production of insulin (good thing, too; otherwise we would always have low blood glucose — a condition called "hypoglycemia") and your glucose level immediately stabilizes.

If you haven't recently eaten, your body has to look elsewhere for glucose. Your insulin level will be low and your glucagon level high, and this allows your liver to release some of its stored glucose into the bloodstream and to make glucose out of protein, which it then releases into the blood. Your organs then use the glucose.

Your body even has a backup plan. Say you've been feeling unwell for a few days and haven't been eating properly. You may not have been eating enough to keep up with your body's demands for glucose, and your liver's stores of glucose (glycogen) and its ability to produce glucose may already have been exhausted. So where will your body turn for its source of fuel? Well, your clever body will, like a hybrid car, look for alternative fuels and start to break down fat tissue, which releases fatty acids into the blood. These fatty acids serve as an alternative source of energy to keep you and your organs going.

What Happens When Your Organs Hit the Wrong Notes?

The intricate system we describe in the previous section is the way things are supposed to work. And if they did, you wouldn't have diabetes. But you do have diabetes, so something has gone wrong. That's not your fault. You didn't want things to go wrong and you sure as heck didn't intentionally make things go wrong. So don't feel guilty.

If you have type 2 diabetes (far and away the most common form, as we discuss further in Chapter 4), then you typically have two different problems with insulin: You don't make enough insulin, and the insulin you do make does not work sufficiently well. We look at these issues in this section.

Insulin resistance

Almost all people with type 2 diabetes have *insulin resistance*. Insulin resistance means that certain tissues (such as fat and muscle) in your body resist the action of insulin. As a result, when you eat, even though your pancreas makes insulin, it doesn't work sufficiently well. Using the earlier analogy (see "Playing a beautiful melody" in the preceding section), your insulin can't unlock the key on the cell lining, so the glucose has a hard time entering your cells.

ANECDOTE

Slimming down your glucose readings

A colleague of Ian's recalls the time that a young woman with type 2 diabetes came to the office, two of her friends reluctantly in tow. "Doctor," she said, her voice ringing with frustration, "I know that I'm overweight, and that is part of the reason I have diabetes, but I wanted you to see my two friends here. They're the same weight and height I am, but they don't have diabetes. Why is that?"

Ian's colleague looked at the three ladies and then once again focused his attention on his patient. "Beth, I see your point. There can be many reasons why one person gets diabetes and somebody else does not. But at least in terms of body weight, not all pounds are created equal. Take a close look at your friends and you will find that even though they may have the same weight and height, their bodies look different. Your friends have their fat tissue evenly distributed on their bodies, but in your case you have it mostly on your belly. That makes you more insulin resistant. Lose that abdominal fat and I bet you will find that your glucose levels will improve."

Beth heeded the words and within a few months she was quite a bit trimmer — as were her glucose readings.

The degree to which you have insulin resistance is significantly related not just to how much fat tissue you have, but also to where it's located. Visceral fat (the fat within the abdomen) is the type of fat most likely to cause insulin resistance, followed by fat within the abdominal wall and fat elsewhere on your body. Insulin resistance (and type 2 diabetes) is, therefore, more common in people with an apple-shaped physique rather than a pear-shaped physique.

(Although we do not know for certain why someone has insulin resistance, there is rapidly emerging evidence that fat cells are responsible by causing inflammation in the body; indeed, some theories suggest that diabetes, heart disease, and other health problems share this common denominator.)

If you have a healthy pancreas, it can overcome a problem with insulin resistance simply by making more insulin. But if you have diabetes, your pancreas is unable to produce sufficient insulin. We look at this next.

Insulin deficiency

Although the initial problem if you have type 2 diabetes is insulin resistance, with time your pancreas's ability to produce insulin wanes so you now have two problems: insulin resistance and insulin deficiency. This one-two punch leaves you unable (without treatment) to move sufficient glucose from your blood into your cells. Instead, the glucose hangs around in your bloodstream and eventually it gets so high that it spills out into the urine, making both you and your urine the sweet things that you are.

Unfortunately, no proven way to prevent insulin deficiency from worsening exists and, as a result, almost all people with type 2 diabetes require more and more medication (including insulin therapy) as time goes by. ***Remember:*** This is not your fault!

If you have type 1 diabetes (which we discuss further in Chapter 4), your main problem is that your pancreas is unable to make insulin in the first place. As you eat, your blood glucose level goes up, and, try as it might, your pancreas is unable to respond. For this reason, all people with type 1 diabetes require insulin therapy. If you have type 1 diabetes and you're also overweight, you may also have insulin resistance; this is sometimes referred to as *double diabetes.*

The problems that we discuss above are often relative. In other words, if you have type 2 diabetes, your organs can partially respond to the insulin you have. And if you have only recently acquired type 1 diabetes, your body may still have *some* ability to produce insulin, but far less than you need.

Regardless of which type of diabetes you have, if you're not able to use glucose properly for fuel, your body starts to use other tissues for this purpose. You break down fat and, eventually, you break down muscles. The excess glucose that accumulates in your blood spills into the urine. And that is why, if you have uncontrolled hyperglycemia (high blood glucose), you may have noticed that you're losing weight and muscle bulk. But, of course, that either already is — or soon will be — behind you, because from this point on you're going to make sure that you control your blood glucose levels and stay healthy.

Insufficient, or ineffective (as seen with insulin resistance), insulin has the following effects:

— ∅ Source of energy

- ✔ Prevents your muscle cells from extracting glucose from your blood, therefore depriving your muscles of a source of energy and leading to high blood glucose levels.

- ✔ Prevents your fat cells from extracting glucose from your blood, therefore leading to high blood glucose levels.

- ✔ Allows your liver to release excessive glucose into your blood, therefore leading to high blood glucose levels.

- ✔ Leads to loss of fat and muscle tissue.

The discovery of insulin

When you were told you had diabetes, most likely you were anything but happy about it. But as badly as you may have felt, imagine if you were told you had this diagnosis back, say, in 1771, when *The Encyclopedia Britannica* described diabetes this way: "In the beginning, the mouth is dry . . . a heat begins to be perceived . . . the patient falls away, and the mind is anxious and unstable. In time the thirst greatly increases, the urine is plentiful and the body wastes. . . . There is a swelling of the loins . . . and . . . death is at hand."

And as for treatment, how about these commonly prescribed therapies: the oat cure (you ate pretty well nothing but oatmeal); overfeeding (sometimes with diets rich in sugar!); and, on the other side of the fence, starvation diets that were sometimes so awful that patients were kept locked in their rooms so they would not have access to food.

Until not too long ago, type 2 diabetes was uncommon. To have diabetes was to have type 1 diabetes. And to have type 1 diabetes before the discovery of insulin was to have a terminal illness. Imagine, therefore, the euphoria that greeted the discovery of insulin. It must surely have been equal to what the discovery of a universal cure for cancer would be nowadays. And it happened right here in Canada.

In 1889, a scientist discovered that if a dog's pancreas was removed, the dog became diabetic. This was the first strong clue that the pancreas and diabetes were intimately related. But how they were related remained a mystery.

In 1920, Dr. Frederick Banting, a Canadian surgeon from Alliston, Ontario, was working as a very junior lecturer at the University of Western Ontario in London. While preparing for a class, he read an article on diabetes and the pancreas, and that sparked an interest — soon to be an obsession — in finding out what secretion the pancreas might be making that prevents diabetes.

Dr. Banting, all of 29 years of age at the time, approached Dr. John Macleod, a professor at the University of Toronto, and asked permission to use a laboratory. Dr. Macleod agreed and assigned Charles H. Best, a science student, to assist. How was Best chosen for a role that was soon to make him world-famous? Through a rigorous selection process, you might think. Well, it wasn't quite like that. In fact, Best was picked by virtue of winning a coin toss!

Dr. Banting and Mr. Best (he wasn't a doctor yet) began their work in May 1921, and in December they were joined by J. B. Collip, a biochemist from the University of Alberta. After some initial setbacks (What would science be without setbacks?), they eventually purified a pancreatic extract that they felt could be given to people with diabetes.

On January 11, 1922, their extract was administered to Leonard Thompson, a 14-year-old boy in the Toronto General Hospital. The treatment was a dismal failure. Thankfully, the young scientists and Leonard were not deterred and, after some further work in the laboratory, they tried again on January 23. We do not know if they shouted "Eureka!" but they must have wanted to when they saw Leonard's glucose level fall and his well-being suddenly improve. The boy had been rescued from death. Insulin was born.

That is the end of one story and the beginning of another, for the subsequent personal rivalries between Banting and Best on the one side and Collip and Macleod on the other is the stuff of legend. The Nobel Prize in physiology or medicine was awarded to Banting and Macleod in 1923. Banting shared his portion with Best, and Macleod did likewise with Collip. Michael Bliss, a Canadian historian, has written an absolutely wonderful book, *The Discovery of Insulin,* which chronicles the story and is as entertaining and fascinating to read as any detective novel you're likely to come across.

Chapter 4

Looking at the Different Types of Diabetes

*Y*ou might think that diabetes is diabetes is diabetes. And, true enough, in many ways the various forms of diabetes have much in common. Everyone with diabetes is combating a tendency to have high blood glucose levels, and everyone with diabetes has to make appropriate dietary changes to enhance their health. And whether you're age 5 or 95, you must have proper eye care, proper foot care, and all the other things that go along with achieving and maintaining good health. Having said that, certain things are unique to the different forms of diabetes and require special attention.

Jim Tucker, a 50-year-old, assembly-line worker at a car plant, had always been healthy. Indeed, he never saw doctors. He was a hard-working man who enjoyed spending time playing ball in the summer and hockey in the winter. Over the past few months he had noticed that he was going to the bathroom night and day. And he was constantly thirsty. Thinking that he needed better nutrition, he had started to drink glass after glass of orange juice. But that didn't make him feel better. One day he got on the scale and realized that, although he was still overweight, during the past six months he had lost 7 kilos (15 pounds) without even trying. Jim was hesitant to see a doctor, but his wife finally convinced him that he had to get checked out. He went to see his family physician, a blood test was done, and a day later Jim got a call at work that he had to come in to see the doctor right away. His blood glucose level was 25. Jim's doctor told him the result and what it meant. Jim had type 2 diabetes.

Mary was a 5-year-old girl. She was a beautiful, healthy, and happy child, but had suddenly become irritable and in just a matter of days had started to look increasingly unwell. She was quickly losing weight and had started to wet her bed. Mary's parents became alarmed and took her to the local emergency department, where doctors found that she had a blood glucose level of 15 and that her urine contained a substance called ketones. Mary was diagnosed as having type 1 diabetes.

Fatima was pregnant with her third child. She had had no problems during the first two pregnancies, and with this one she also felt fine. As a matter of routine procedure, when Fatima reached her 24th week of pregnancy, her doctor sent her for a glucose tolerance test in which she drank a sugar-rich liquid and her blood glucose level was checked a couple of hours later. Her result was 11.2. Fatima's doctor diagnosed her as having gestational diabetes.

What do Jim, Mary, and Fatima have in common? That's easy to answer and takes but one word: diabetes. But if we were to write about how they differ, that would take a whole chapter. This chapter! In this chapter we look at the different forms of diabetes, determining what they have in common and how they differ.

Type 1 Diabetes and You

Type 1 diabetes is caused by destruction of the insulin-producing beta cells in the pancreas. This results in insulin deficiency which, without treatment, leads to a dangerous build-up of acid in the body called *ketoacidosis* (which we discuss in Chapter 5). Children, teenagers, and young adults are the most likely to develop type 1 diabetes, but it can occur at virtually any age. If you have type 1 diabetes, you need to inject insulin into your body if you are to stay healthy (or even alive!).

Type 1 diabetes used to be called *juvenile-onset diabetes* or *insulin dependent diabetes*. The problem with these old terms is that many people don't fit the descriptive titles. For example, many children who get diabetes actually have type 2 diabetes. And many adults who get diabetes actually have type 1 diabetes. Unfortunately, you're still likely to come across the outdated names because many people — including some health care providers — haven't caught up yet with the new terminology.

Identifying the symptoms of type 1 diabetes

Symptoms of undiagnosed or insufficiently treated type 1 diabetes are directly related to high blood glucose caused by lack of insulin. Symptoms of type 1 diabetes tend to come on quite quickly, usually over a matter of days or weeks. These symptoms include

- ✔ **Blurred vision:** When the glucose levels in your body undergo a big change, the fluid content of the lens of your eyes also changes. That, in turn, alters the way that light bends as it passes through your eyes and leads to blurring. Maybe you have noticed the way that a knife in a glass of water looks bent. It's much the same phenomenon. Your blurred vision will correct soon after you start insulin.

- ✔ **Fatigue:** When type 1 diabetes first strikes, you suddenly start to lose body fluids, muscle mass, and fat tissue, and you quickly become malnourished and are on the verge of being (or actually are) dehydrated. In the face of this onslaught, it's no wonder you feel fatigued. If you have type 1 diabetes, you probably recall how quickly your energy improved once you started insulin therapy.

- ✔ **Frequent urination:** As we explain in Chapter 3, passing lots of urine is a typical symptom of diabetes. You experience frequent urination because once your blood glucose level rises to above 10 or so (people without diabetes seldom have values above 8), glucose passes through the kidneys and spills into the urine, drawing extra fluids along the way.

- ✔ **Fruity breath:** When your body can't use glucose as a fuel, it looks for alternative sources of energy, one of which is fat tissue. As fat tissue breaks down, it releases acids called ketones and these typically make the breath smell fruity, very much like a candy mint. If lots of ketones are present, this can be a sign of a dangerous condition called ketoacidosis, which we discuss further in Chapter 5.

- ✔ **Increase in thirst:** Because you're losing excess fluids in the urine, you're at risk of getting dehydrated. Your clever body tries to prevent this by making you feel thirstier, which, of course, encourages you to drink more.

- ✔ **Weight loss and increased hunger:** If you have uncontrolled type 1 diabetes, you're passing urine that's rich in glucose and, thus, rich in calories. This wasted nutrition is going down the drain, in a manner of speaking. The body then starts to break down muscle and fat tissue. As your body wastes away, you become hungry as your brain encourages you to eat to make up for these losses.

Investigating the causes of type 1 diabetes

If you or someone you love has type 1 diabetes, after you get over the shock of hearing the news, the next thing you'll probably ask is, "How could this have happened?" And that's an excellent question. In fact, that is the same question scientists have been asking for many, many years, and it still goes unanswered.

Type 1 diabetes isn't contagious, and you can rest assured that you didn't get it from someone with diabetes sneezing on you or coughing on you. And you didn't get type 1 diabetes from eating the wrong foods, not exercising enough, or being under stress. In fact, you did nothing wrong at all. Type 1 diabetes is not something that you brought on; it is something that happened *to* you.

Type 1 diabetes is almost always an autoimmune disease, meaning that your body has been unkind enough to react against itself. (We say *almost* always because occasionally the insulin-producing beta cells are destroyed by unknown mechanisms.) Many different types of autoimmune disease exist, including certain types of thyroid disease and arthritis conditions such as lupus and rheumatoid arthritis.

Everyone makes antibodies to fight off infections, but in the case of type 1 diabetes, your body creates antibodies that have decided that your own insulin-producing islet cells of your pancreas are the enemy and have attacked these cells. This can be demonstrated by checking for certain antibodies in the blood stream, including islet cell antibodies, insulin antibodies, and glutamic acid decarboxylase (GAD) antibodies. It's seldom necessary to test for these antibodies outside of research settings (and in Canada, the cost for these tests is usually not covered by health insurance plans).

It's unknown why your immune system would turn against your pancreas, but a number of theories exist:

- At various times in our lives we develop viral infections and our bodies fight these off by producing antibodies. It could be that one of these viruses shared something in its appearance with an islet cell and the body's antibodies couldn't separate out the good guys (your islet cells) from the bad guys (the virus) and attacked both.

- Non-breastfed babies have a higher risk of developing type 1 diabetes. It could be that a protein in cow's milk causes the same sort of response as a virus and, just as we discuss in the preceding paragraph, leads to an antibody attack on your own pancreas. Bear in mind, however, that an association is not the same as cause and effect (for example, if you have blonde hair and blue eyes, your blonde hair did not cause your blue eyes, they simply occurred together).

✔ A virus may damage the pancreas by directly attacking it. Indeed, some small outbreaks of type 1 diabetes have supported this idea.

✔ As a result of normal chemical reactions in our bodies, we produce highly reactive molecules called oxygen free radicals. Despite the name, we can assure you that they bear no similarity to hippies from 1960s Berkeley, California. Oxygen free radicals can be produced in excess numbers by exposure to air pollution and smoking. It is possible that oxygen free radicals accumulate in and damage the pancreas.

✔ Certain chemicals are known to cause type 1 diabetes. One such example is a rat poison called Vacor, which, if ingested, can damage the pancreas.

Other theories exist as well (including the recently proposed, provocative idea that insufficient vitamin D due to lack of sun exposure in northern climates leads to type 1 diabetes), but the simple truth of the matter is that it's unknown what has caused your type 1 diabetes. One thing, however, that *is* known is that certain underlying genetic characteristics may make you more susceptible to getting type 1 diabetes. Individually they would not cause you to develop diabetes, but when taken together with some other trigger, they might.

The best possible illustration of how getting type 1 diabetes must be a combination of a genetic susceptibility *and* an environmental trigger is found in one extraordinarily simple fact. If you have type 1 diabetes and you have an identical twin (who would, therefore, have the same genes as you do), the likelihood of your twin getting type 1 diabetes is somewhere between 25 to 50 percent. If the cause were purely genetic, the odds would be 100 percent. Something else clearly must be at play here. But what? At this time, the answer is simply a mystery.

The great British prime minister Benjamin Disraeli may have been right when he said there are "lies, damn lies, and statistics," but when it comes to the inheritance of type 1 diabetes, certain statistics do seem to be true. In particular, if you have a parent or a (non-identical) sibling with type 1 diabetes, you have approximately a 5 percent risk of developing type 1 diabetes. This risk rises to about 30 percent if both your parents have type 1 diabetes.

Preventing type 1 diabetes

Although medical science currently has no proven way of preventing type 1 diabetes, very exciting research studies are currently underway looking at this very thing. Researchers are evaluating two types of preventative strategies:

✔ **Primary prevention:** This type of prevention aims to prevent diabetes before it starts. Possible candidates for primary prevention are people who are at particularly high risk of developing type 1 diabetes as reflected by having a family member (or members) with the condition, having certain antibodies in the blood (we discuss these in the previous section), and/or having genes that put them at increased risk.

An example of primary prevention is the administration of a vaccine (such as an experimental one, Diamyd, which is currently being studied). Another example is not giving infants cow's milk in case certain proteins in it may trigger diabetes. (This possibility is being evaluated by the TRIGR study: www.trigr.org.)

✔ **Secondary prevention:** This type of prevention aims to administer treatment to a person with diabetes as soon as possible after the disease is diagnosed, with a view to getting it to go away immediately. (And, if it then stayed away — without requiring further treatment — this would, in effect, be a cure.) An example of secondary prevention is taking a medicine that targets the immune system to try to get it to stop making antibodies that destroy the insulin-producing beta cells of the pancreas. (Although people with type 1 diabetes lack insulin, early on in the course of the disease they often still retain the ability to make *some* insulin: the goal of secondary prevention would be to maintain and enhance this ability.) As we say, this is experimental; at present there is neither a proven means of preventing type 1diabetes nor a cure for type 1 diabetes.

Unlike years ago, when scientists often worked in relative isolation, researchers now routinely pool their resources to improve their odds of success. TrialNet (www.diabetestrialnet.org) — of which the Hospital for Sick Children in Toronto is a member — is an organization that has a specific mandate to "perform intervention studies to preserve insulin-producing cells in individuals at risk for type 1 diabetes and in those with new onset type 1 diabetes." This type of intensive, integrated approach by researchers is wonderful news.

Type 2 Diabetes and You

Type 2 diabetes is caused by a combination of insulin resistance and insufficient insulin. (We discuss this in detail in Chapter 3.) Type 2 diabetes is much, much more common than type 1 diabetes (ten times more common, in fact). Whereas type 1 diabetes tends to develop in children and young adults, type 2 diabetes typically affects middle-aged or older people. Your likelihood of developing type 2 diabetes increases as you get older. Also, being overweight and sedentary puts you at particularly high risk of developing type 2 diabetes.

Although adults are most likely to be affected by type 2 diabetes, increasing numbers of children are also developing the condition. This appears to be directly related to affected children not being sufficiently physically active and being overweight. If you have type 2 diabetes and want to help protect your young child or grandchild from also getting type 2 diabetes, perhaps for their next birthday gift consider giving a YMCA/YWCA membership rather than a video game. Even better, while you're at it, get a membership for yourself, too, and go together!

Type 2 diabetes used to be called *adult-onset diabetes* or *non-insulin dependent diabetes,* but because children can develop type 2 diabetes, the former term didn't make sense, and because many people with type 2 diabetes require insulin therapy, the latter term didn't make sense either. For these reasons, these older terms have been abandoned. Nonetheless, not everyone has yet caught on to the new name, so you may still come across the older ones.

If you have type 2 diabetes and require insulin, you *still have type 2 diabetes,* not type 1 diabetes.

In Chapter 3 we talk about the cause of type 2 diabetes and how, with this condition, the pancreas is able to make insulin but the body's tissues aren't able to use it properly. This is called *insulin resistance,* and we look at it in more detail later in this chapter.

Type 2 diabetes gets a foot in the door

Nicholas had always been a very healthy man. Indeed, the last time he had seen a doctor was when he had his appendix taken out 10 years ago, when he was 40 years of age. The only reason he was now in the family doctor's office was at his wife's insistence. Starting a year ago, he had noticed some mild numbness in his right big toe. A month or two later, the same thing developed in his left big toe.

Nicholas wasn't a complainer and he figured it was just because of some new, overly tight-fitting shoes he had yet to break in. Nonetheless, as the months passed, things got worse and worse and now the numbness involved all his toes and had started to feel increasingly painful.

When his doctor examined Nicholas's feet, they looked healthy enough, but when the doctor pressed on the toes with a thin nylon rod, Nicholas hardly noticed. A few tests later and the doctor had made her diagnosis. Nicholas had diabetes. It was a shock for Nicholas. He had no recollection of having been overly thirsty or passing excessive quantities of urine. Indeed, he had felt perfectly fine otherwise. Not in a million years had he imagined that diabetes could show itself in such an unusual way.

If you have type 2 diabetes, you don't have a less severe or less important form of diabetes than if you had type 1 diabetes. You don't have a "touch of diabetes"; you have the real thing, meaning you require intensive therapy and equally intensive monitoring to keep yourself healthy. Don't let anyone try to convince you that if you're being treated with nutrition (diet) and exercise therapy alone, your diabetes is less serious than if you were on insulin. On the other hand, don't let anyone try to convince you that if you're on insulin, your condition must be worse than someone with diabetes who doesn't require insulin. All forms of diabetes are serious. And all people with diabetes are at risk of complications. But — and this is a big but — equally important, working with their health care team, all people with diabetes have the means to reduce that risk.

Type 2 diabetes is written as, well, type 2 diabetes, not type II diabetes. The little in-joke among diabetes specialists is that this nomenclature was chosen so that doctors wouldn't think it was to be called type eleven diabetes!

Identifying the symptoms of type 2 diabetes

Unlike type 1 diabetes, the symptoms of type 2 diabetes tend to come on gradually; often, so gradually that people who later discover they have the condition have discounted the symptoms, blaming them on something else. Perhaps before you were diagnosed as having type 2 diabetes, you attributed your weight loss to a new diet you had put yourself on. Or maybe you remember blaming your thirst on a particularly hot summer. Indeed, the symptoms of type 2 diabetes can come on so gradually and so imperceptibly that by the time it is discovered, your blood glucose may be extraordinarily high and, moreover, may have been high for so long that damage has already occurred to your body.

In fact, up to 50 percent of people with newly diagnosed type 2 diabetes already have some degree of damage to their bodies. It is for this reason that the Canadian Diabetes Association recommends people be routinely screened for diabetes; the goal is to try to make the diagnosis as early as possible so that treatment can be given before damage to the body occurs. The Cheat Sheet at the front of this book describes when screening should be done.

Many of the symptoms of (uncontrolled) type 2 diabetes are common to type 1 diabetes, including the following:

✔ Blurred vision

✔ Fatigue

✔ Frequent urination

✔ Increase in thirst

✔ Weight loss

Weight loss is more common with newly diagnosed type 1 diabetes, but also occurs fairly frequently with type 2 diabetes. Some other differences in symptoms exist, and the following ones are much more likely to be present with type 2 diabetes:

✔ **Heart disease, stroke, and peripheral vascular disease:** Heart disease, stroke, and peripheral vascular disease (blockage of arteries in the legs; also referred to as peripheral arterial disease) aren't symptoms per se, but are conditions that are commonly present in people with type 2 diabetes, often before type 2 diabetes is even diagnosed. If you have one of these conditions, we recommend you ask your doctor to test you to see if you have diabetes. (You will likely find your doctor has already done so.)

✔ **Numbness of the feet:** This isn't so much a symptom of high blood glucose as it is a symptom of nerve damage. If you have had high blood glucose levels for a number of years, you may develop an uncomfortable burning or numbness in your feet. This can be the first clue alerting you to the fact that you not only have diabetes, but that it has been there for quite some time. We discuss nerve damage further in Chapter 6.

✔ **Slow wound healing:** If you have high blood glucose levels, your body's ability to heal itself becomes impaired and you may find that seemingly minor cuts don't heal as quickly as they used to.

✔ **Yeast infections of the vagina and penis:** High glucose levels make the genital areas of your body prone to yeast infections. In a woman, this may manifest as vaginal discharge, and in a man, as a reddish rash at the end of the penis (balanitis).

Investigating the causes of type 2 diabetes

Although finding the initial trigger leading to type 1 diabetes has proved very elusive, medical science knows a lot more about why people develop type 2 diabetes.

Thrifty genes

In countries where people don't get enough food, people whose genetic makeup enables their bodies to use carbohydrates very efficiently have an advantage over the rest of the population because they can survive on the low food and calorie supplies. When these people finally receive ample supplies of food, their bodies are overwhelmed and they are more likely to become fat and develop diabetes. This may explain why people in developing countries are the most at risk to develop type 2 diabetes. The same theory may explain why First Nations have a higher risk of developing diabetes. This proposal is called the *thrifty gene hypothesis.*

When you were told you had type 2 diabetes, you may have thought of relatives of yours who shared the same problem. Indeed, you may have thought of many relatives who had diabetes. What you and your extended family have in common is, of course, more than being at risk for diabetes. You share many genes in common, including those that make you prone to getting diabetes. Note that the fact that your father or mother or sister or brother may have diabetes does not guarantee that you, too, will get it, but it does increase your risk.

If you have a parent with type 2 diabetes, you have approximately a 15 percent risk of developing type 2 diabetes. This risk rises to about 50 percent if both your parents have type 2 diabetes. If you have a sibling with type 2 diabetes, your risk is only 10 percent, but — and this is startling — if your sibling is your identical twin, your risk of developing type 2 diabetes rises to 90 percent. But before you throw your hands up in despair, please note there is a very, very large "but" here.

The "but" is that getting type 2 diabetes has more to it than family background alone. In addition to having relatives with diabetes, most people who acquire type 2 diabetes are overweight and sedentary. And recent scientific studies show overwhelming evidence that your risk of developing type 2 diabetes can be drastically reduced by making appropriate lifestyle changes. (As with many things diabetes — including getting type 2 diabetes — we refer you to Ian's diabetes mantra, "Problems are not inevitable, problems are not inevitable, problems. . . ." In other words, in many respects you can influence your diabetes health destiny.)

In the early stages of type 2 diabetes, you have plenty of insulin in your body (unlike people with type 1 diabetes), but the insulin isn't working effectively. As we discuss in more detail in Chapter 3, insulin is like a key that opens up the cells (especially your fat and muscle cells) to allow glucose to enter. In type 2 diabetes, this key is malfunctioning. This is called insulin resistance.

Although the initial problem with type 2 diabetes is that your insulin isn't working properly, as time passes, the pancreas also runs into difficulties and eventually can't make enough insulin. That's one of the main reasons that so many people with type 2 diabetes end up requiring insulin as time goes by. If you have type 2 diabetes and you require insulin to keep your blood glucose levels under control, this doesn't mean *you* have failed; it simply means that *your pancreas* has failed. And that is not your fault!

People often think that consuming sugar and experiencing stress cause type 2 diabetes, but in fact, they don't. Ingesting excessive amounts of sugar may bring out the disease to the extent that it makes you overweight, but that's quite different from saying sugar *causes* diabetes. Indeed, eating too much protein or fat will do the same thing. As for excess stress, it can make your glucose control worse if you already have diabetes, but it doesn't cause diabetes.

Preventing type 2 diabetes

Unlike type 1 diabetes, type 2 diabetes can be prevented, or at the very least delayed, according to a number of medical studies.

Type 2 diabetes typically occurs in people who are overweight and sedentary. (Like anything in life, exceptions exist, but over 90 percent of the time this is the case.) However, by losing weight and exercising regularly, you can reduce your risk of developing type 2 diabetes by over 50 percent. If you already have type 2 diabetes, then do your loved ones a favour and share this information with them so they can start making the necessary lifestyle changes to help them avoid getting (or at least delaying the onset of) type 2 diabetes.

To achieve this huge reduction in risk, all you need to do is lose 5 percent of your body weight and exercise for 150 minutes per week (which is only about 21 minutes a day)! Regarding weight loss, if you weigh 100 kg (220 lbs) and you lose 5 kg (11 lbs), you will drastically reduce your risk of diabetes. And this weight loss doesn't have to occur overnight; it can be over months and even years.

Research reveals that prevention is most likely to succeed with lifestyle therapy (that is, weight loss and exercise), but we must say that lifestyle change is often the most difficult prescription of all. Studies also show that you can achieve nearly similar benefits by using certain medications (particularly metformin or rosiglitazone). We discuss these medicines in Chapter 12. We believe that lifestyle therapy is a much, much, *much* better option for diabetes prevention than is medication. However, if you've repeatedly tried yet not succeeded with lifestyle change, talking to your physician about using medication to prevent diabetes is worth undertaking.

The aforementioned medical studies looked at people who already had problems with elevated blood glucose levels. They had prediabetes, meaning their readings were higher than normal but not high enough to classify them as having diabetes. We talk more about this condition later in this chapter.

You can determine whether or not you are overweight in several ways, including

- **Body Mass Index (BMI):** Calculating your BMI is the most commonly used technique to determine whether you're overweight. Basically, BMI is an indicator of whether you're the right weight for your height. It can be calculated — though nobody ever does it this way — by dividing your weight in kilograms by the square of your height in metres. Uh-huh. Realistically, you can just look it up on a graph (see Figure 4-1) or do what we do and use an online calculator (many are available, including www.nhlbisupport.com/bmi/bminojs.htm). A normal BMI is 18.5 to 24.9. Note that the normal range for BMI does *not* apply to pregnant or breastfeeding woman, nor does it apply to infants, children, or adolescents (nor to particularly muscular individuals).

- **Waist circumference:** Another way to establish whether you're overweight is to measure your waist circumference. Your health risk goes up if your waist circumference is equal to or greater than 88 centimetres (35 inches) for women, 102 centimetres (40 inches) for men.

When it comes to having too much fat in your body, not all fat is equal. If you have extra fat around your belly but not over other areas of your body, it puts you at much higher risk of getting type 2 diabetes than if you had extra weight distributed over all parts of your body. This is because fat over your midsection is more likely to cause insulin resistance (which we discuss earlier).

Knowledge is power. And now that you know the main risk factors leading to type 2 diabetes, you have the ability to lessen the likelihood of getting it. And if you already have it, reducing your BMI and your extra fat tissue can markedly improve your health anyhow. The point of finding out your BMI is not that you should get angry or frustrated with yourself. Rather, you know what the problem is and can now take steps (both figurative and literal) to improve it.

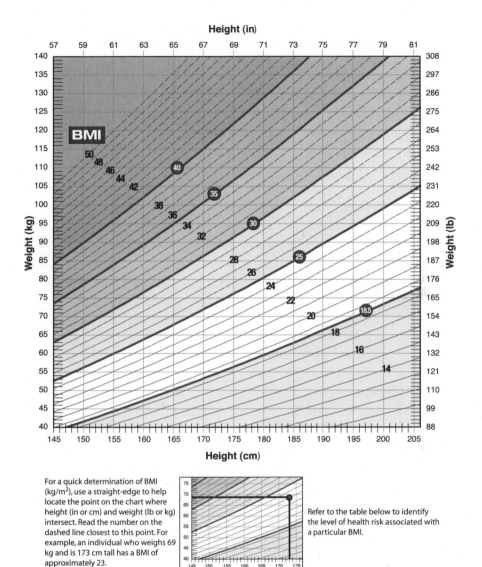

For a quick determination of BMI (kg/m²), use a straight-edge to help locate the point on the chart where height (in or cm) and weight (lb or kg) intersect. Read the number on the dashed line closest to this point. For example, an individual who weighs 69 kg and is 173 cm tall has a BMI of approximately 23.

Refer to the table below to identify the level of health risk associated with a particular BMI.

BMI	Risk of developing health problems
< 18.5	Increased
18.5 – 24.9	Least
25.0 – 29.9	Increased
30.0 – 34.9	High
35.0 – 39.9	Very high
≥ 40.0	Extremely high

Figure 4-1:
The Body
Mass Index.

Adapted from: WHO (2000) Obesity: Preventing and Managing the Global Epidemic: Report of a WHO Consultation on Obesity.

Key Differences between Type 1 and Type 2 Diabetes

Type 1 and type 2 diabetes are similar in many ways; however, they also have some important differences. Table 4-1 highlights some of these differences. (This table lists the *usual* characteristics seen with type 1 and type 2 diabetes — but frequent exceptions exist. For example, although type 1 diabetes typically develops in young people, middle-aged or even older people can also develop it.)

Table 4-1 Differences between Type 1 and Type 2 Diabetes		
	Type 1 Diabetes	*Type 2 Diabetes*
Age at time of diagnosis	Under 20	Over 40
Length of time present before diagnosis	Months	Years
Weight status at time of diagnosis	Normal or underweight	Overweight
Most common symptoms at time of diagnosis	Thirst, frequent urination, weight loss	Thirst, frequent urination, visual blurring
Insulin defect	Insufficient insulin (beta cell failure)	Ineffective insulin (insulin resistance) and, with time, insufficient insulin
Antibodies present to insulin and/or islet cells	Yes	No
Family history of diabetes	Sometimes	Almost always
Initial therapy	Lifestyle and insulin	Lifestyle (with or without medication)

You may come across the term LADA or Latent Auto-immune Diabetes of Adults. LADA refers to a slowly onsetting form of type 1 diabetes in adults. The most important thing to know about LADA is that because it slowly develops, doctors often mistake it for type 2 diabetes and treat it (unsuccessfully) with oral medications when, in fact, insulin is required. If you have been diagnosed with diabetes and you are not overweight yet your doctor recommends oral medicines rather than insulin, ask your doctor if you might have LADA and if you would be better served by insulin therapy. If he or she is uncertain, you should be referred to a diabetes specialist.

Gestational and Pregestational Diabetes and You

If you're pregnant (yes, that excludes you men, but read on, gentlemen — you do have something to do with your partner's pregnancy) and you didn't have diabetes prior to your pregnancy, during the course of your pregnancy you could acquire a form of diabetes called gestational diabetes. If you already have diabetes when you become pregnant, that is called pregestational diabetes.

Gestational diabetes is usually simply treated, and typically the pregnancy goes quite uneventfully. Pregestational diabetes is a more complex condition requiring more complicated monitoring and therapy.

If you have previously had gestational diabetes or if you already have diabetes, and you're considering snuggling up to your significant other tonight with the most amorous of intentions, be absolutely, positively sure that you combine your amoré with satisfactory contraception unless you've first read Chapter 7 (where we discuss pregnancy and diabetes in detail) and have determined that it's safe for you to get pregnant.

The Metabolic Syndrome and You

People who have insulin resistance (we discuss insulin resistance in Chapter 3) often also have other indicators which, taken together, put them at high risk of developing not only type 2 diabetes but heart disease also. When several of these indicators are present, you are said to have *metabolic syndrome*.

The definition of the metabolic syndrome varies depending on whose criteria one uses, but in Canada the most commonly used criteria are three or more of the following:

- Fasting blood glucose of 5.6 mmol/L or higher
- Blood pressure of 130/85 or higher

> ✔ Triglycerides of 1.7 mmol/L or higher (triglycerides are one of the fats in the blood)
>
> ✔ HDL cholesterol (the good type of cholesterol) less than 1.0 mmol/L (for men) or less than 1.3 mmol/L (for women)
>
> ✔ Abdominal obesity (a waist circumference of more than 102 centimetres — about 40 inches — for men; more than 88 centimetres — about 35 inches — for women)

The importance of having the metabolic syndrome diagnosed is controversial. Some people say it is very important because if you have the syndrome it means you are at greatly increased risk of having a heart attack, and knowing about it means you can take appropriate preventive actions (such as modifying your diet, getting your cholesterol level in order, and so on). Naysayers would tell you that the metabolic syndrome is simply a label and, what the heck, if you have high blood pressure or poor cholesterol, you *already* know that you have a problem that needs to be addressed.

The treatment of metabolic syndrome is, essentially, the treatment of its individual components. So if you have elevated blood glucose, high blood pressure, or abnormal triglyceride or HDL levels, you treat them with lifestyle measures and, if necessary, medication. Similarly, you treat abdominal obesity with lifestyle change (though we do discuss other treatment options in Chapter 10).

The bottom line: If you have metabolic syndrome, take that to be a wakeup call telling you that you need to make crucial lifestyle changes (and, when necessary, take helpful medications) in order to reduce the risk that the condition will deteriorate into diabetes, heart attacks, and other serious health issues. Your destiny is largely in your hands.

Prediabetes and You

Type 2 diabetes rarely appears suddenly. More commonly it's preceded by a period of time, which may last years, when your blood glucose levels are not high enough to say you have diabetes, but not low enough to say your levels are perfectly normal either. This blood glucose netherworld is called *prediabetes*. Note that having prediabetes is not the same as saying you have *borderline diabetes;* one can no more have borderline diabetes than one can be borderline pregnant.

Prediabetes is diagnosed if you have either *impaired fasting glucose* and/or *impaired glucose tolerance.* Impaired fasting glucose means your blood glucose level before breakfast is higher than normal (but not as high as someone with diabetes); that is, 6.1 up to and including 6.9 mmol/L. Impaired glucose tolerance means that your blood glucose level two hours after a meal is higher than normal (but not as high as someone with diabetes); that is, 7.8 up to and including 11.0 mmol/L.

If you've been diagnosed with prediabetes based on a fasting blood glucose test result (of 6.1-6.9 mmol/L), it is important that your doctor send you for a glucose tolerance test to exclude the possibility that you actually have type 2 diabetes.

Prediabetes is important to know about for two main reasons:

- **High risk of developing type 2 diabetes:** Think of prediabetes as an early warning system. It's an alert that you're at high risk of getting type 2 diabetes. Indeed, the risk of prediabetes developing into type 2 diabetes is as much as 10 percent in any year and about 90 percent over ten years (hence the reason for calling this condition prediabetes). Not good odds, eh? But there is a "but": Despite the name, prediabetes doesn't *have* to progress to type 2 diabetes. Following the measures we outline in the section "Preventing type 2 diabetes," earlier in this chapter, will substantially improve your odds of avoiding (or, at the very least, delaying) diabetes.

- **High risk of heart attack and stroke:** Having prediabetes means you are at very high risk of developing hardening of the arteries (atherosclerosis), which can ultimately lead to heart attacks and strokes. However, this does not have to happen. Aggressive treatment of prediabetes and other risk factors for vascular disease can keep you healthy. This treatment involves paying attention to your diet, being physically active, achieving a healthy weight, making sure your blood pressure and lipids (cholesterol and triglycerides) are good, and, of course, not smoking.

Although the term *prediabetes* is very apt in that it hammers home the message that impaired fasting glucose (IFG) and impaired glucose tolerance (IGT) are huge risk factors for getting type 2 diabetes, it implies an inevitability about something that we know is not necessarily inevitable. IFG and IGT don't have to lead to diabetes.

Recognizing Other Types of Diabetes

The great majority of diabetes cases fall within the categories we discuss in this chapter (that is, type 1, type 2, and gestational diabetes), but other types (dozens in fact) of diabetes exist, including the following:

- **Destruction of pancreatic tissue due to pancreatitis:** Severe inflammation of the pancreas *(pancreatitis)* may so badly damage the insulin-producing beta cells of the pancreas that you lose the ability to produce insulin.

- **Damage to the pancreas due to excess iron:** Another disease that damages the pancreas (and can potentially damage the liver, heart, and joints also) is *hemochromatosis.* This genetic condition results from excessive absorption of iron into the blood. When the blood deposits too much iron into these organs, damage can occur. Because hemochromatosis leads to increased skin pigmentation, it is sometimes called *bronze diabetes.*

- **Maturity Onset Diabetes of the Young (MODY):** MODY is the former name for a group of rare genetic diseases in which young, non-overweight people develop a condition similar to type 2 diabetes. We discuss this further in Chapter 15.

- **Drug-induced diabetes:** Some medicines can cause diabetes. Prednisone (and similar drugs) is a type of steroid that is wonderful at treating some very serious diseases (such as asthma), but unfortunately has the potential to cause diabetes, especially if used in high doses for long periods of time. Some blood pressure medicines (for example, hydrochlorothiazide), some newer psychiatric medicines (for example, risperidone and clozapine), and niacin (a medication used to lower triglyceride levels) can occasionally do this also. That does not mean you should never take these medicines. What it does mean, however, is that if you are taking one of these medicines and you have symptoms of diabetes (which we discuss earlier in this chapter), you should see your doctor to have your blood glucose level checked.

- **Hormonal disease-induced diabetes:** The following is a partial list of hormonal disorders that can lead to diabetes by causing insulin resistance:

  - **Acromegaly:** This is a pituitary gland disorder involving excess levels of growth hormone.

  - **Cushing's Syndrome:** This is a disease in which the body produces excess amounts of steroid hormones similar to prednisone.

  - **Glucagonoma:** This is a rare tumour of the pancreas that leads to over-secretion of glucagon hormone.

  - **Hyperthyroidism:** This is a condition in which the thyroid gland produces excess quantities of thyroid hormone.

  - **Pheochromocytoma:** This is an adrenal gland disorder in which too much adrenaline (or similar hormones) is made.

ANECDOTE

Breathing easy but experiencing drug-induced diabetes

Mohammed was a 55-year-old man with a long history of severe bronchitis. He came to the emergency department because he was having increasing difficulty catching his breath despite taking a number of different "puffers." The emergency room physician prescribed prednisone and advised Mohammed to follow up with his family doctor in three weeks.

Within a couple of days, Mohammed's breathing had started to improve and he was feeling very encouraged. A week later, however, he found himself having to get up during the night to go to the bathroom. Initially he blamed this on his prostate, but it kept getting worse and worse, and by the time he saw his doctor a week later, he had already lost 4.5 kilos (10 pounds) and was feeling miserable.

Hearing Mohammed's story, his doctor immediately sent him to the laboratory, and the subsequent result confirmed his suspicion: Mohammed's blood glucose level was high — 25 mmol/L. Fortunately, by that time his breathing had improved and he was able to quickly come off the prednisone. Within two weeks his glucose level had returned to normal and his diabetes symptoms resolved. Mohammed's story is an example of drug-induced diabetes; in this case, due to prednisone.

Part II
How Diabetes Can Affect Your Body

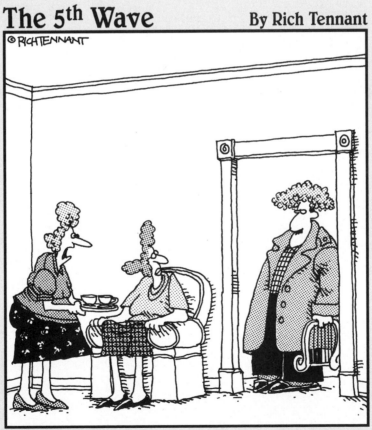

The 5th Wave   By Rich Tennant

"Oh dear, it's Troy's Harpo-glycemia. I can always tell — fatigue, confusion, the compulsion to play the harp in a trench coat and fright-wig...."

In this part . . .

Diabetes can have profound effects on your body. This part explains these effects, how they occur, the kinds of symptoms they produce, and what you and your health care team can do to treat them and, even better, to prevent them.

This part also looks at the special issues surrounding diabetes and pregnancy and discusses measures that will help you to have a healthy pregnancy and a healthy baby.

Chapter 5

Handling Low and High Blood Glucose Emergencies

*B*lood glucose control in diabetes involves two separate issues. On the one hand, you have your long-term goal of maintaining good glucose levels to feel well and to avoid damaging your body as time goes by. On the other hand, you sometimes face situations when glucose control suddenly deteriorates and requires urgent attention. We address the long-term issues in Chapter 6. In this chapter we discuss those circumstances that require immediate action.

With the exception of mild hypoglycemia (low blood glucose that you can manage yourself), you should treat all the issues we look at in this chapter as medical emergencies. Don't try to treat these complications by yourself. Contact your health care team or, if necessary, call 911. In this chapter we discuss when and whom to call.

Understanding Hypoglycemia (Low Blood Glucose)

Hypoglycemia is a blood glucose level below normal. That much is straightforward. The problem is defining precisely how low a normal blood glucose can be. This is a subject of some controversy in the medical community, with widely varying numbers used. However, the Canadian Diabetes Association 2008 Clinical Practice Guidelines (upon which this book is based) consider hypoglycemia to be a blood glucose level of less than 4.0 mmol/L (*if* you are taking certain medications like insulin injections).

Your body doesn't function well when you have too little glucose in your blood. Your brain needs glucose to allow you to think properly, and your muscles need the energy that glucose provides in much the same way that your car needs gasoline to run. As we discover in this chapter, diabetes in and of itself does not cause hypoglycemia; rather, certain *treatments* for diabetes can cause hypoglycemia.

Having diabetes isn't fair. It's unfair to get it. It's unfair to develop complications. And it's especially unfair that those people with diabetes who try the hardest to stay healthy are the most prone to getting hypoglycemia. If you have poorly controlled glucose levels with values running between 15 and 20, you may not feel great, but you are highly unlikely ever to run into significant problems with hypoglycemia. But if you look after yourself meticulously and keep your blood glucose levels in the 4 to 8 range, you are at much greater risk of having hypoglycemia. Fortunately, it is possible to have excellent control and, at the same time, to minimize the risk of getting hypoglycemia. It ain't easy, but it is doable. We discuss how to do it later in this section.

Not every person develops symptoms of hypoglycemia at the same level of blood glucose. Some people notice it at blood glucose levels of 3.8, others only when their blood glucose level is between 2 and 3. Moreover, a person might notice it on one occasion when his or her blood glucose level is below 3.6 and that *same* person might not notice it on another occasion until it's below 3.2. You also need to remember that glucose meters aren't perfect. You may have already discovered that you can check your reading seconds apart and find discrepancies of up to 15 percent. That doesn't mean your blood glucose level changed that much in that brief interval. It simply means the machines aren't precision instruments. (But if your machine gives readings — checked moments apart — that differ by *more than* 15 percent, have your device checked to make sure it isn't malfunctioning.)

Looking at the symptoms of hypoglycemia

Doctors traditionally divide the symptoms of hypoglycemia into two major categories:

- **Autonomic symptoms** are symptoms (such as tremors and palpitations, as we discuss below) that are due to the effects of the hormones (especially epinephrine, also called adrenaline) that your body sends out to counter low blood glucose. They are called autonomic symptoms because they arise from the *autonomic* (automatic in a sense) part of your nervous system.

> ✔ **Neuroglycopenic symptoms** are symptoms (such as <u>confusion</u> and <u>disorientation</u>, as we discuss later in this section) that are due to your brain not receiving enough glucose. *Neuroglycopenic* is derived from *neuro* (referring to the nervous system), *glyco* (glucose), and *penic* (insufficient).

The severity of hypoglycemia can be classified as

> ✔ **Mild:** Autonomic symptoms are present and you're able to treat yourself.
>
> ✔ **Moderate:** Autonomic and neuroglycopenic symptoms are present and you're able to treat yourself.
>
> ✔ **Severe:** Hypoglycemia is bad enough that you require someone else to assist you. Unconsciousness may occur. (With severe hypoglycemia, the blood glucose is typically less than 2.8 mmol/L.)

(handwritten note in left margin:) Severe = BS< 2.8

The main reason to know this classification is so that you and your health care providers are sure to be on the same page. Otherwise, there could be miscommunication and inappropriate advice given to you. For example, if you are on insulin and you tell your doctor you had a "severe low," your doctor may interpret this as per the above definition and give you advice — like substantially reducing your insulin dose — based on that. But if by "severe low" you *actually* meant you felt really, really crummy, but in fact your blood glucose was only slightly decreased (say, 3.6 mmol/L) and you were able to easily treat yourself by drinking a glass of pop, then you would likely receive very different advice from your doctor.

If you take medicines (such as insulin) that can cause hypoglycemia, for your own safety it would be very wise to wear a medical alert bracelet or necklace. At the very least (though certainly not as good), carry some form of identification in your purse or wallet noting that you have diabetes. You may never need them, but it's a good idea to be prepared just in case. We've had more than one patient who has received necessary emergency care (for hypoglycemia) that might not have been given if a passerby had not seen the person's medical alert and instead mistakenly assumed he was drunk. (We've also had patients who were hypoglycemic and, as a result, driving erratically, but who might have been arrested for suspected drunk driving if the police officer hadn't noticed the person's medical alert stating that they had diabetes. And speaking of driving, we discuss this topic in detail in Chapter 18.)

Most people with diabetes go their entire lives without ever experiencing even a single episode of *severe* hypoglycemia. The vast majority of the time, if you are experiencing hypoglycemia, the early-warning autonomic symptoms kick in and allow you to quickly rectify the problem.

A sweet first date

Alan (one of the authors of this book) heard a story about a young man who had gone on a blind date. He and his date went to a bar where they had a drink before dinner. As he sat there, he began to say, "Sugar, baby, sugar, baby, sugar, baby."

At first his date was offended (perhaps she thought he was performing a poor Austin Powers routine), but she then realized that he had a glazed look in his eyes and noticed that he was wearing a bracelet identifying him as having diabetes. He was suffering from hypoglycemia and needed glucose. She helped him out (we discuss how to do this in the section "Treating hypoglycemia"), and he felt better soon thereafter. Alan isn't sure whether the rest of their date was similarly sweet.

Autonomic symptoms

Autonomic symptoms are your best friends. They're your warning system alerting you to a problem of low blood glucose and demanding that you attend to it before it progresses to the more dangerous neuroglycopenic stage (which we discuss shortly).

Autonomic symptoms are

- Anxiety
- Hunger
- Nausea
- Palpitations (noticing a rapid or excessively forceful heartbeat)
- Sweating
- Tingling (numbness)
- Trembling (shaking of your body, especially the hands)

[handwritten margin note: epinephrine = fight or flight]

As you look through the above list, you may realize you've had some or all of these symptoms at various times in your life, even if you've never been on medicine that could cause low blood glucose. The reason: These symptoms can occur in *any* situation where epinephrine levels are high, and that includes so-called fight-or-flight situations where you're under extreme stress. (Examples are if you're about to write a difficult exam, about to have a job interview, or are writing a book on diabetes and your editor calls you to let you know your manuscript is due . . . yesterday. Eeek.)

Because symptoms such as sweating or palpitations, which can indicate hypoglycemia, can also occur in situations such as stress, where your blood glucose level may actually be perfectly normal, you should conclude that you have hypoglycemia only if you have demonstrated a low blood glucose level on your glucose meter.

Shortly after you begin therapy for high blood glucose, you may find that you're experiencing autonomic symptoms, suggesting you have hypoglycemia even though your blood glucose levels may not be low. This is perfectly normal — it will take a few days for your body to become accustomed to having normal blood glucose levels, at which point your symptoms will resolve (that is, they'll go away).

If you are on medications such as insulin or a sulfonylurea (sulfonylureas are medicines that help reduce blood glucose, as we discuss in Chapter 12), it's quite possible that you recall having had at least one episode where your hands started to shake, you became sweaty and hungry, and you recognized that something wasn't quite right. You probably reached for your glucose meter, checked your blood glucose level, and found it to be somewhere in the low 3s. You likely took some sugar candies or a glass of juice or pop and felt better within a few minutes. Congratulations: You successfully diagnosed, treated, and cured your first patient. Feel free to write the rest of this chapter. Oh, never mind, we'll do it.

Neuroglycopenic symptoms

Neuroglycopenic symptoms are much more of a problem. These symptoms are most definitely not your friends — quite the opposite. Whereas autonomic symptoms alert you to a problem, neuroglycopenic symptoms often interfere with your ability to recognize and deal with hypoglycemia. By the time these symptoms develop, your blood glucose level is usually profoundly low and has become a true emergency. These symptoms include

Profound low Emergency

- ✔ Confusion
- ✔ Difficulty concentrating
- ✔ Difficulty speaking
- ✔ Dizziness
- ✔ Drowsiness
- ✔ Headache
- ✔ Loss of consciousness (coma)
- ✔ Seizures

- ✔ Tiredness
- ✔ Vision changes (such as double vision or loss of vision)
- ✔ Weakness

People lose their ability to think clearly when they become hypoglycemic. They make simple errors, and other people often assume that they're drunk. Suffice it to say, if Albert Einstein were having an episode of hypoglycemia, he may have ended up mistakenly deciding E = mc. And if similarly affected, Wayne Gretzky would have been the not-quite-as-Great One. Fortunately, adult brains have an amazing capacity to put up with insults like hypoglycemia, and long-term damage to the brain from low blood glucose almost never occurs. Because the brains of infants and young children are more sensitive to injury, however, it's especially important to avoid severe hypoglycemia in this age group (we define severe hypoglycemia earlier in this section).

Considering the causes of hypoglycemia

Hypoglycemia doesn't cause diabetes. Now, in another attempt to dispel popular misconceptions, we wish to hereby announce that diabetes doesn't cause hypoglycemia. Remember, you read it here first. Certain medicines used to *treat* diabetes can cause hypoglycemia, but hypoglycemia is not caused by diabetes in and of itself. Indeed, if you have diabetes and are being treated purely with lifestyle measures (nutrition and exercise therapy), you will *never* experience hypoglycemia.

Hypoglycemia is always unintended. Ideally, your blood glucose levels would always be normal — never high, never low. Unfortunately, we seldom have that degree of success with our imperfect therapies. A number of the medicines we use to prevent blood glucose levels from being too high have the potential to drop them too low. These medicines are

- ✔ **Insulin:** Unlike insulin made by your pancreas, insulin you inject does not have the ability to turn itself off the instant you no longer need it. An injection of insulin will help to reduce your blood glucose level, but it also has the potential to drop your level excessively. This drop is called an *insulin reaction.* (You may have heard the term *insulin shock* used in reference to particularly bad insulin reactions. Insulin shock is not a scientific term, however, and can be misleading. Indeed, we would prefer the term never be used. Accordingly, we won't be using it beyond this brief explanation.) We discuss insulin therapy in detail in Chapter 13.

- ✔ **Sulfonylurea medicine:** As we discuss further in Chapter 12, medicines from this family have the potential to cause low blood glucose. This is particularly true of glyburide.

✔ **Meglitinides (and d-phenylalanine derivatives):** Never do we, as diabetes specialists, consider ourselves luckier than when we attend conferences where these medicines are discussed. Oh no, not just because they're important drugs to know about. No. We consider ourselves fortunate because at these conferences we learn how to pronounce them! Don't worry; no one uses these names anyhow. Doctors pretty well just use the trade names (GlucoNorm, Starlix) for drugs currently available within this group. These drugs, like sulfonylureas, make the pancreas release extra insulin and have the potential to cause hypoglycemia.

Although these medicines can cause hypoglycemia, you can improve the odds that they won't by taking certain precautions. We discuss these precautions later in this chapter.

Treating hypoglycemia

The vast majority of episodes of hypoglycemia are mild (or moderate; see the definitions of these terms earlier in this section) and you will be able to deal with them easily. Nonetheless — particularly if you have type 1 diabetes — severe episodes can and do occur, so it is best for you and your loved ones (and friends, workmates, and so on) to know what to do in the event that this happens to you. In this section we look at these important issues.

Treating mild and moderate hypoglycemia

If you find that your blood glucose level is low, then you must ingest some sugar to restore your level to normal. The Canadian Diabetes Association (CDA) recommends that if you have mild to moderate hypoglycemia (that is, you are still awake and aware enough to take things by mouth), you should take the following steps:

✔ **Step One:** Eat or drink 15 grams of a fast-acting carbohydrate such as

- Three 5-gram glucose tablets (for example, BD glucose tablets)

- Five 3-gram glucose tablets (for example, Dextrosol tablets)

- 175 mL (³/₄ cup) of juice or regular (not diet or sugar-free) pop (but see the tip following this list)

- 15 mL (3 tsp) honey

- 15 mL (3 tsp) table sugar dissolved in water

✔ **Step Two:** Wait 15 minutes, and then retest your blood. If your blood glucose level is still less than 4 mmol/L, ingest another 15 grams of carbohydrate.

✔ **Step Three:** If your next meal is more than one hour away, or you are going to be physically active, eat a snack, such as half a sandwich or cheese and crackers. The snack should contain 15 grams of carbohydrate and a source of protein.

Despite what most people think (and do), orange juice (or milk or, especially, glucose gel) is not as effective as products like Dextrosol because it raises glucose levels and relieves you of symptoms more slowly. Nonetheless, if you have some O.J. and it's handier than an alternative, it will work.

Because acarbose (Glucobay) — see Chapter 12 — slows down absorption of sucrose, if you are taking this medicine and you develop hypoglycemia, you should be treated with glucose (such as Dextrosol), not sucrose (such as fruit juice).

If you are hypoglycemic and you're about to eat a meal, you should *first* treat your hypoglycemia with a fast-acting carbohydrate as described above. This will ensure that your blood glucose is brought up rapidly.

Because the symptoms of hypoglycemia are so unpleasant and because hypoglycemia is understandably scary, you may find yourself taking candy after candy until you feel better without actually giving time for the first treatment to take effect. Then, when all that sugar you have just ingested gets absorbed into your system, you may find that your glucose level is up into the teens. It is best, therefore, to give the first treatment time (as described above) to work before you take another.

Dealing with severe hypoglycemia

Because your mental state may be impaired when you have hypoglycemia, you need to make sure that your friends or relatives know in advance what hypoglycemia is and what to do about it. Having people around you who are aware is especially important if your hypoglycemia is so bad that you are unconscious or nearly so, in which case you will be unable to swallow properly. In this circumstance, people should *not* try to feed you, because you could choke. Instead, your helper should administer glucagon (see the "Using glucagon" section) to you, and also should call 911 to summon an ambulance. If you experience milder hypoglycemia, where you are alert but somewhat confused and unable to obtain an appropriate sugar source, then your helper simply needs to find one for you and help you to ingest it.

Inform people about your diabetes and about how to recognize hypoglycemia. Let them know where you store your emergency supplies (such as the glucose tablets you use to treat hypoglycemia). Don't keep your diabetes a secret. The people close to you will be glad to know how to help you.

Using glucagon

Glucagon is available by prescription in a package called a glucagon kit. This kit includes a syringe and 1 mg of glucagon, one of the major hormones that raises glucose, which your helper should inject into your leg muscle (the buttock and arm can also be used). (Half that dose — that is, 0.5 mg — should be used if you are treating a child 5 years of age or less.) The injection of glucagon raises the blood glucose, and within 15 to 20 minutes you will likely become fully alert.

If you have just experienced a severe episode of hypoglycemia and you required an injection of glucagon, then once you have fully come around and are again able to swallow properly, you should consume some quick-acting hypoglycemia treatment (see the list earlier in this section) followed by food to help prevent your redeveloping hypoglycemia as the glucagon wears off.

Some people are, understandably, just too nervous or too intimidated to take it upon themselves to administer glucagon. In that case, they should just call an ambulance.

Remember that when you pick up the glucagon kit from the pharmacy, the person who is most likely to be giving it should go with you. The pharmacist *must* sit down and explain to both of you how it is given.

Like most medicines, glucagon has an expiration date after which it may not work sufficiently well. For this reason, as soon as you pick up your glucagon kit, find out when it will expire and mark on your calendar a few weeks in advance of the expiration date a reminder for you to pick up a new kit.

If you live, work, or play in an area where emergency health care services are more than just minutes away, it's especially important for you to have a glucagon kit. Do you snowmobile? Hunt? Hike? Boat? Do you live in a remote area? Does your job take you into the bush? All of these situations would warrant having a supply of glucagon readily available. Keep in mind the Boy Scouts' motto: Be prepared.

If you are the parent of a young child, you likely know all too well the phrases "I'm not hungry" or "I don't want to eat." These typically relatively harmless situations, however, take on a potentially much more serious meaning if your child has diabetes and is receiving insulin therapy. In this case, without food, your child will be at risk of hypoglycemia. If your child is receiving insulin, refuses food, and then develops mild hypoglycemia (or is about to), you can give her mini-doses of glucagon. The glucagon will help ward off or reverse hypoglycemia. We recommend you speak to your child's diabetes specialist or diabetes educator to find out more information on when you would use glucagon and the doses to administer.

Notifying your health team

If you have experienced severe hypoglycemia — even if you quickly recovered — it's crucial that you notify your family physician, your diabetes specialist, or your diabetes educator(s) so that they can make appropriate adjustments to your therapy to lessen the likelihood of your having another severe attack. If you're feeling well and have fully recovered from the episode, you don't have to call your health care team right away, but it would be wise to get in touch with them within a day or two.

Preventing hypoglycemia

Not everyone with diabetes experiences hypoglycemia. As we discuss earlier in this chapter, if your treatment is lifestyle therapy alone, you won't have low blood glucose. However, most people with diabetes at some point will require use of medicines (such as insulin or a sulfonylurea) that will put them at risk of hypoglycemia.

Although no foolproof way to avoid hypoglycemia exists, you can follow the following techniques:

- **Don't miss or delay meals:** Because pills and insulin that are used to reduce blood glucose do not have the good sense to know exactly when to stop working, like the famous battery-operated bunny, they sometimes tend to keep going and going. (Precisely how long depends on the particular type of pill or insulin that you are using; we discuss this in Chapters 12 and 13.) That would be fine if your glucose level is still high, but not so fine if your level has come back to normal, as it most likely will have by the time your next meal rolls around. If your meal is unduly delayed, the medicine may pull your glucose level down too low.

- **Plan your exercise:** Exercise is an essential component of your diabetes therapy (particularly if you have type 2 diabetes), as we discuss in Chapter 11. But it's important for you to be aware that exercise accelerates the rate at which glucose moves from the blood into muscle (where it's used as fuel) and, thus, can cause you to have hypoglycemia. By all means *do* exercise; however, if you know from experience that when you perform a certain type or amount of exercise you develop hypoglycemia, speak to your diabetes educator or physician about how to adjust your medicines or diet to reduce the risk of developing low blood glucose. Often the solution is something as simple as having a small snack before (or even while) you work out. The worst thing is to have hypoglycemia every time you exercise; we can't imagine a stronger disincentive to exercising than that!

✔ **Have a bedtime snack:** Eating a bedtime snack is not necessary for most people with diabetes unless you're taking evening doses of insulin and your bedtime blood glucose level is less than 7 mmol/L, in which case a bedtime snack containing at least 15 grams of carbohydrate and 15 grams of protein will help you avoid having a low reading overnight. If you find that going to bed with a higher glucose level does not prevent overnight lows, then you should take a snack even if your bedtime reading is higher than 7 mmol/L. (As we discuss in Chapter 13, if you are on insulin it's a good idea to periodically test your blood glucose level at about 3 a.m. to make sure it is not going low overnight without your having recognized it.)

[handwritten note: only if BS < 7mmol]

✔ **Change your oral hypoglycemic agent or insulin therapy if necessary:** If your current treatments are resulting in hypoglycemia, speak to your physician about whether you would benefit from a change to your diabetes medicines. This may be something as simple as a small dose change or as major as changing to a different medicine altogether.

✔ **Pay close attention to your symptoms of hypoglycemia:** By knowing what symptoms you typically get when you have hypoglycemia, you will be able to recognize hypoglycemia faster and treat it earlier.

✔ **Avoid (or minimize) the use of other drugs that can cause hypoglycemia:** Several drugs (not specifically being used to treat your diabetes) that you may take from time to time have the potential to lower your blood glucose levels. These drugs include alcohol and *high* doses of aspirin (ASA). We further discuss important issues about alcohol in Chapter 10. If you are experiencing hypoglycemia, make sure you review *all* your medicines (and any alternative and complementary therapies; we discuss these in Chapter 14) with your doctor to see if you should make some changes.

✔ **Set higher blood glucose targets:** For some people, despite their (and their diabetes team's) best efforts, recurring hypoglycemia is still a problem. (This is rarely the case unless you have type 1 diabetes.) In this situation, the only way to avoid repeated episodes of hypoglycemia may be to set blood glucose goals somewhat higher than the CDA target (see Chapter 9). We recommend you discuss with your doctor and your diabetes educator what your specific targets should be.

✔ **Wear a continuous glucose monitoring system (CGMS):** These recently developed devices continuously measure your (interstitial fluid) glucose level and alarm you if your level is heading too low. They are particularly suited to people with type 1 diabetes on insulin pump therapy. We discuss CGMS in detail in Chapter 9.

If you are on intensified insulin therapy (see Chapter 13), episodes of hypoglycemia are inevitable. Ian has found that, as a very rough rule of thumb, to achieve excellent overall blood glucose control, you can expect to have *mild*

hypoglycemia about two to three times per week. More frequent hypoglycemia may put you at undue risk of severe hypoglycemia. On the other hand, if you are on intensified insulin therapy and you are *never* experiencing episodes of hypoglycemia, your average blood glucose level is probably too high.

We discuss additional tips for people on insulin therapy in Chapter 13. We discuss issues surrounding driving and hypoglycemia in Chapter 18.

Coping with hypoglycemia unawareness

Hypoglycemia unawareness is a condition in which you lose your ability to recognize when your blood glucose level has fallen below normal. Samantha, one of Ian's patients, had this condition.

Samantha was 28 years old. She had developed diabetes when she was only 5 years of age. Samantha was a highly motivated patient and was monitoring her blood glucose levels many times per day. With aggressive use of insulin, nutrition therapy, and exercise, she was able to keep her glucose readings generally between 3.8 and 7.6. Recently, while she was at work, her boss had found her staring vacantly into space. He was able to get her to drink some juice and she quickly came around, but the next day the same thing happened again. Two days later, her husband awakened to find Samantha soaking wet in bed beside him. He couldn't awaken her. He tested her blood and found her glucose level to be 1.8. He gave her an injection of glucagon (see above for a discussion about glucagon) and over the next 15 minutes she gradually awakened. Later that day, she went to see Ian in the office, her therapy was adjusted, and soon thereafter she was able to once again recognize when her blood glucose levels were too low.

A condition like Samantha's can occur for several reasons:

- **Repeated hypoglycemia:** If you have been experiencing frequent hypoglycemia — even if mild — your autonomic warning system (such as sweating and palpitations; see the "Autonomic symptoms" section, earlier in this chapter) may start to fail and the first clue that you have low blood glucose can be when you are confused and unable to look after yourself. The best way to correct this is, *under your diabetes specialist's guidance,* to somewhat reduce your insulin doses to avoid any and all hypoglycemia for a few weeks at which point your doses can typically be again increased with restoration of hypoglycemia awareness.

- **Longstanding diabetes:** Occasionally, if you have had diabetes for a very long time (generally speaking, we are talking decades), your autonomic warning system may fail and, as Samantha's situation above, the first clue there is a problem may be when you become confused. Setting higher blood glucose targets may be required. Also, using a CGMS (see the "Preventing hypoglycemia" section and Chapter 9) may be helpful.

✔ **Other drugs impairing your ability to recognize hypoglycemia:** Several drugs can interfere with your body's ability to produce autonomic symptoms. Such drugs include beta blockers (such as propranolol), which are often used to treat heart disease and high blood pressure. If a medication is responsible, your physician (in consultation with you) will need to determine if another medication may be substituted. Another drug that some of you may have passing acquaintance with is alcohol, which, if used in sufficient quantities that impair your alertness, can blunt your ability to recognize when you're hypoglycemic. We discuss alcohol and diabetes in detail in Chapter 10.

Dealing with Ketoacidosis

If you have type 1 diabetes, you're at risk for developing a dangerous, temporary condition called *diabetic ketoacidosis* (typically just called ketoacidosis or by its abbreviated form, DKA) in which your blood glucose level is high (typically above 14) *and* you have excess quantities of a type of acid called *ketones* in the blood. High blood glucose *without* the presence of ketones does not indicate DKA. (Though, of course it might indicate your glucose control is pretty crummy, but that is a different story.)

Ketoacidosis requires urgent attention because, if severe, it can be life-threatening. Occasionally, the first clue that you have type 1 diabetes is when you become ill with ketoacidosis. More commonly, DKA occurs after you already know that you have the disease.

Exploring how ketoacidosis develops

As we discuss in Chapter 2, the main source of energy for your muscles is glucose. And for glucose to be used properly you must have sufficient insulin in your body. If you have type 1 diabetes, you lack the ability to produce insulin and, thus, you need to give it to yourself by injection.

But what happens if your body requires more insulin than you are giving? Several things can happen:

✔ Your blood glucose levels will climb (because the glucose can't get into your cells without sufficient insulin to help it).

- Your body will start to break down fat (and muscle) because it can't use glucose as a fuel.

- As fat tissue breaks down, it releases acids (ketones) into the bloodstream.

The result is that you develop ketoacidosis.

Investigating the symptoms of ketoacidosis

These are the symptoms of ketoacidosis:

 - **Extreme tiredness and drowsiness:** If your DKA is mild, your tiredness may also be mild, but as your DKA worsens you will feel increasingly drowsy, and if your DKA becomes severe you can lose consciousness.

 - **Fruity breath:** The presence of ketones in your system gives your breath a fruity, not unpleasant, odour. Most people with DKA do not notice it even though it might be apparent to bystanders.

 - **Nausea, vomiting, and abdominal pain:** It is noteworthy that many people with diabetes — and many doctors also, by the way — mistakenly attribute these symptoms to stomach flu (*gastroenteritis*) even when they are due to DKA. (Of course you *may* simply have the flu, but a doctor should come to this conclusion only after DKA has been excluded.)

 - **Rapid breathing:** You experience rapid breathing when your blood is so acidic that your body tries to compensate by ridding itself of acids through the lungs.

The Canadian Diabetes Association recommends that people with type 1 diabetes test for ketones

- During periods of acute illness when elevated blood glucose readings are present

- When before-meal blood glucose readings are above 14 mmol/L

- When symptoms of DKA (see above) are present

 Ketoacidosis occurs rarely in type 2 diabetes. Nonetheless, if you have type 2 diabetes and you develop typical symptoms of DKA, it would be a good idea to check for ketones.

Although ketones can be tested in the urine (by urinating on test strips; several companies make these strips), it is preferable to test for them in the blood (with use of the Precision Xtra ketone testing meter; this is the only blood ketone tester available in Canada).

If you notice that you have symptoms of ketoacidosis and you test your blood ketone level and find it to be elevated (0.6 mmol/L or higher), in most cases the safest and best thing to do is to go to the closest emergency department. However, if your symptoms are mild and you are fortunate enough to be working with a diabetes educator who is both trained — and empowered — to deal with DKA (and is immediately available), you can first contact her or him for detailed advice.

Understanding the causes of ketoacidosis

Ketoacidosis is caused by a *relative* lack of insulin. And no, this does not mean that it is caused by your first cousin Sally not having enough insulin. (Though perhaps she doesn't. We wouldn't know.) When we say *relative* lack of insulin, we mean that the amount of insulin in your body — no matter how much there is — is not enough for your body's needs. It follows, then, that DKA will develop in one of two general circumstances:

- ✔ **You are missing insulin doses:** If you have type 1 diabetes, your pancreas is unable to manufacture insulin, so you must give yourself insulin. If you miss doses, your body quickly detects this and your metabolism will promptly suffer. (See Chapter 13 for a detailed discussion of insulin.) The occasional missed dose of rapid-acting or regular insulin isn't likely to harm you, but if you miss several consecutive doses, you'll be at substantial risk for developing DKA.

- ✔ **You aren't taking high enough doses of insulin:** It's quite possible that day to day you give yourself a fairly similar quantity of insulin and get along quite nicely, thank you very much. That's great. But if you're experiencing some additional stress (emotional or, more commonly, physical) on your body, you will likely require higher doses of insulin to meet your body's increased needs. Examples would be if you develop, say, pneumonia or a kidney infection.

If you have type 1 diabetes, you depend on insulin injections not only to preserve your health, but to preserve your life. Even if you're feeling rotten and aren't eating anything, you *cannot* forgo taking your insulin. In fact, you may need to give yourself *more* insulin than usual. The sickest patients that diabetes specialists ever see are those people with diabetes who, unfortunately, either weren't given this advice or knew it but didn't follow it. If you have type 1 diabetes, please follow this advice. It may save your life.

Not just cabin fever

Beth was a 13-year-old girl who had had type 1 diabetes for three years. After visiting a friend at a cottage, she came down with terrible diarrhea. She spent the better part of the day on the toilet, but with her mom's encouragement, she was able to drink lots of fluids. Beth usually required three injections of insulin per day and her total daily dose of insulin was generally about 20 units. When she became ill, her blood glucose level rose to 22 mmol/L and her blood started to test slightly positive for ketones.

Beth contacted her diabetes educator, who advised her to test her blood glucose every 2 hours and told her to take extra rapid-acting insulin every 2 hours if her blood glucose level was elevated. Over the next 12 hours she ended up taking an *extra* 30 units. By the next day, Beth was feeling back to normal, her glucose levels were normal, she had no ketones in the blood, her insulin doses were back to usual, and she was out playing with her friends.

Beth was thrilled. Her mom was thrilled. Her educator and her doctors were thrilled. Everyone was thrilled, in fact, except for Beth's friend, who felt terribly guilty when they found out their lake water was contaminated with giardiasis and as a result Beth had developed "beaver fever."

Treating ketoacidosis

Ketoacidosis is a serious condition that requires very careful treatment. If you have *very mild* DKA, and you are fortunate enough to have a diabetes educator who is empowered to do this, you will possibly be treated as an outpatient under their very, very close supervision. The following will probably be part of your treatment:

- ✔ **Ensuring proper hydration:** Achieved by making sure you're drinking sufficient quantities of fluids.

- ✔ **Giving yourself frequent insulin injections:** You may be asked to give yourself injections of rapid-acting insulin as often as every two hours.

- ✔ **Testing your blood:** You will need to check your blood glucose and blood ketone levels often.

If you have anything more than very mild DKA, you should be treated in a hospital. The treatment will consist of the following:

- ✔ **Administering insulin:** This is usually done intravenously.

- ✔ **Ensuring proper hydration:** Achieved by intravenous administration of fluids.

✓ **Restoring proper potassium and mineral balance:** This is achieved by intravenous or oral administration of potassium and, at times, calcium, phosphate, magnesium, and bicarbonate.

✓ **Testing your blood:** Oh yes, where would we be without blood testing? You will likely be poked and prodded quite a bit, but fortunately that can usually be done by inserting a small tube into a blood vessel that can, in a sense, be turned on and off at will (sort of like a tap), so you may not have to be jabbed afresh each time.

✓ **Looking for the cause:** If the reason for your having developed DKA is not apparent (like missing insulin doses, for example), you may require additional blood and urine tests, X-rays, and so on to try to determine what may have triggered the episode (pneumonia, for example).

Preventing ketoacidosis

How truly wonderful it is that what was once both unavoidable (and fatal!) is now almost always avoidable. It does, however, take a fair bit of effort to accomplish this. The key measures to prevent DKA are

✓ **Monitor, monitor, monitor:** Often the earliest signs of developing DKA are rising blood glucose readings. If you're testing your blood frequently, you may well detect a problem before it gets out of hand.

✓ **Take your insulin:** Whatever you do, don't fall into the trap of figuring that if you're feeling unwell and aren't eating or drinking properly, you don't need insulin. Trust us; you *do* require insulin (possibly more than usual).

Hyperosmolar Hyperglycemic State

The name *hyperosmolar hyperglycemic state* refers to a situation where tremendously excessive levels of glucose are in the blood. *Hyper* means "larger than normal," *osmolar* has to do with concentrations of substances in the blood, and *glycemic* has to do with blood glucose. In other words, the blood is simply too concentrated with glucose.

Hyperosmolar hyperglycemic state (fortunately, abbreviated HHS) occurs in people with type 2 diabetes. Like ketoacidosis, HHS is a medical emergency; unlike ketoacidosis, HHS *always* requires treatment in a hospital. (As we discuss later in this section, HHS is virtually always triggered by a serious illness — such as pneumonia, for example. Because both HHS and the illness triggering it are serious conditions, people so affected are typically very, very ill; hence the need for hospitalization.)

Hyperosmolar hyperglycemic state goes by a variety of other names, including hyperosmolar hyperglycemic nonketotic coma, hyperglycemic hyperosmolar nonketotic coma, and hyperglycemic hyperosmolar nonketotic state. What all these terms share in common is that they are a mouthful to say and impossible to remember!

Identifying the symptoms of the hyperosmolar hyperglycemic state

The symptoms of HHS arise in part from the effects on the body of very high glucose levels and in part from whatever condition (for example, a heart attack) triggered it. In terms of the high glucose levels — values as high as 100 are not unheard of — symptoms may include the following:

- ✔ Frequent urination
- ✔ Excessive thirst
- ✔ Dry mouth
- ✔ Leg cramps
- ✔ Weakness and lethargy
- ✔ Unconsciousness

The diagnosis of HHS is actually quite straightforward. If a person with known type 2 diabetes develops extraordinarily elevated blood glucose levels with evidence of dehydration and without the typical blood chemistry picture of ketoacidosis, the diagnosis is readily made.

If you measure your blood glucose regularly — and more frequently if you are feeling unwell — you will probably never develop HHS because you'll notice if your blood glucose is getting high and you'll take corrective action before it reaches a critical level.

HHS requires immediate and skilled treatment at a hospital. If you think you may have it, go to the nearest emergency department. The great majority of the time, however, it is not the affected person who recognizes the problem; it is a loved one (or, in the case of nursing home residents, a nurse) who detects something is wrong. The affected person is usually too sick to even know that they are unwell.

Not all elevations of blood glucose indicate HHS. If you're feeling well, you don't have the symptoms described above, and your blood glucose level is only mildly to moderately elevated (10 to 25 mmol/L or so), you probably don't have HHS. It may mean, however, that you need to speak to your health care team about improving your overall glucose control.

Examining the causes of the hyperosmolar hyperglycemic state

HHS is most common among elderly people with diabetes, though it can occur in younger individuals. Whereas ketoacidosis (see the preceding section) most often occurs when people haven't been taking sufficient insulin, HHS is most likely to occur if you have some additional serious illness that has triggered it. This illness may be, for example, a stroke, a heart attack, or a severe infection such as pneumonia.

Typically, HHS develops in an infirm person whose diabetes is reasonably well controlled until some additional factor (like those just mentioned) develops. Whereas an otherwise healthy person with type 2 diabetes would recognize the presence of the additional problem and seek medical attention, an infirm individual may not know something is amiss or may not be able to deal with it. The person then becomes increasingly unwell from the additional illness, the worsening blood glucose levels, and dehydration. Indeed, HHS leads to profound dehydration.

Treating the hyperosmolar hyperglycemic state

Similar to the treatment of ketoacidosis, HHS treatment includes the following:

- **Administering insulin:** This is usually done intravenously. (Incidentally, insulin is less important than restoring proper hydration, and often insulin can be stopped altogether within a few days.)

- **Ensuring proper hydration:** Achieved by intravenous administration of fluids. This is absolutely essential. Dehydration in HHS is usually very, very severe.

- **Restoring proper potassium and mineral balance:** This is achieved by intravenous or oral administration of potassium and, at times, calcium, phosphate, magnesium, and bicarbonate.

- **Testing your blood:** Monitoring of blood glucose levels as well as electrolytes, calcium, magnesium, phosphate, and other key blood constituents is crucial.

- **Looking for the cause:** HHS is almost always caused by something in addition to diabetes. A physician must make a meticulous search for this other cause; this search will likely include blood and urine tests, X-rays, and heart tests, among other things.

Even with the best possible therapy, the death rate for HHS is high because most people who suffer from it are elderly and have other serious illnesses that both trigger it and complicate treatment.

Preventing the hyperosmolar hyperglycemic state

Hyperosmolar hyperglycemic state can be prevented in two broad ways, depending on where you or your loved one lives:

- **In the community:** If you or a loved one has type 2 diabetes and lives in the community, follow the treatment plan detailed in this book. With proper therapy (including nutrition, exercise, medicines, and so forth), you will likely never develop HHS. And, importantly, if despite following proper therapy, your blood glucose levels keep climbing, contact your health care team to see if your treatment program needs to be adjusted or if a new health issue has come up that has made things worse.

- **In nursing homes:** If you or your loved one has diabetes and resides in a nursing home, speak to the staff (or the physician) to ensure that blood glucose levels are being checked regularly and even more often when you or your loved one is not feeling well. That way, if the blood glucose level is progressively climbing, it can be picked up rapidly and dealt with before it spirals out of control.

Chapter 6

As Time Goes By: Handling Long-Term Complications

*Y*ou may think that diabetes has made your life more complicated. And, of course, it has. What with having to alter your diet and your exercise pattern, having to monitor your blood glucose levels, needing to take medicines, and so on, you may feel that it is all one big hassle. And who could blame you? But the thing is, our long-term objective is not to make your life more difficult but to make it easier. And because looking after your diabetes *before* you run into complications is immeasurably easier than dealing with complications *after* they develop, you have to know how to protect yourself from diabetes damage or, if damage is already present, how to minimize its impact.

This chapter discusses the long-term complications that diabetes can cause, the best ways to avoid them, how to recognize them, and how to deal with them if they are already present. (We deal with acute glucose problems in Chapter 5.)

For a detailed discussion of many of the conditions mentioned in this chapter and, particularly, the medicines used to treat them, we unabashedly refer you to *Understanding Prescription Drugs For Canadians For Dummies,* a book Ian co-wrote with his rheumatologist wife, Dr. Heather McDonald-Blumer.

Complications Aren't Inevitable

As you read through this chapter you will come across complications that you will deem, correctly, to be minor, and others that will scare the pants (if that is your chosen attire) off you. Please, please do yourself and us a favour and if you see something that frightens you, keep repeating to yourself the following mantra: Complications aren't inevitable, complications aren't inevitable. . . .

Not only are most long-term complications avoidable, but if they do occur they can take years to fully develop. For this reason, if complications are creeping up on you, you must ensure they're detected early and treated promptly so that you minimize the risk of their worsening.

Ian was invited to speak to parents of teens with diabetes. As Ian spoke to the parents, a social worker colleague spoke to their children. Ian remarked to the parents how, with the excellent therapies now available, we could do so much to keep their children healthy. Afterwards, Ian's colleague mentioned to him that the children had, to a soul, told him that they figured it was just a matter of time until they went blind, or had amputations, or needed dialysis. Ian was aghast: These poor kids must have felt awful, and all based on misinformation. Complications are *not* inevitable. So, if like these youngsters, you've also had this misapprehension, we are ever so thankful you're now reading this chapter so that you'll be fully informed.

Preventing and minimizing complications require you to invest lots of energy, but hey, you're worth it. By the way, if anyone who doesn't have diabetes has the temerity to tell you it's easy, ask them to try it, and see how many takers you get!

Also, if you do develop complications from your diabetes, *never* feel guilty and don't ever let anyone point an accusing finger at you. As anyone who has ever been in a fender-bender knows, life happens and sometimes one's best efforts are confounded.

Categorizing Long-Term Complications

Many of the problems we discuss in this chapter can be lumped into two broad categories:

✔ **Organ damage due to narrowing or blockage of the small blood vessels** (called *microvascular disease* or *microvascular complications*): Microvascular complications include damage to the eyes (retinopathy), kidneys (nephropathy), and nerve endings (neuropathy). Microvascular disease is primarily the result of inadequate blood glucose control. (We look at this problem further later in this section.)

✔ **Organ damage due to narrowing or blockage of the large blood vessels** (called *macrovascular disease* or *macrovascular complications*): Macrovascular complications include damage to the brain (for example, stroke), heart (for example, heart attack), and legs (for example, amputations). Macrovascular disease is particularly likely to occur if you smoke or inadequately control your blood pressure and cholesterol. The relationship of high blood glucose to macrovascular disease is controversial. (We discuss this in the sidebar "Does reducing high blood glucose prevent macrovascular complications?")

The bad news: Macrovascular disease is the cause of death of 80 percent of people with diabetes. The good news: Macrovascular disease is often preventable and always treatable.

TECHNICAL STUFF

How high blood glucose leads to small blood vessel damage

Although doctors aren't certain precisely how high blood glucose levels cause microvascular complications of diabetes (or how other factors exert their impact), here are a couple of current theories.

Advanced glycated end products (AGEs) are one of the substances that damage tissues. AGEs can damage the eyes, the kidneys, the nervous system, and other organs in your body. You always have glucose in your blood, and some of that glucose attaches to substances in your bloodstream to form *glycated* (glucose-attached) products. In this way, when glucose attaches to *hemoglobin* (the molecule that carries oxygen in your blood and delivers it to the body's tissues), hemoglobin A1C is formed. (We discuss hemoglobin A1C in Chapter 9.) When glucose attaches to *albumin,* a protein in the blood, glycated albumin is formed. Glucose can similarly attach to red blood cells and

white blood cells, as well as to other cells and molecules in the bloodstream. When glucose attaches to these body substances, their functioning may be impaired.

Your body handles a certain level of glycated substances. But when your blood glucose is elevated for prolonged periods of time, the level of glycated cells and substances becomes excessive, and this may damage your body's tissues.

The *polyol pathway* — a pathway that glucose can take as it is *metabolized* (broken down) — is another potential source of diabetes damage to your body. Through the polyol pathway, glucose is metabolized to become a product called *sorbitol,* a member of a class of substances called *polyols.* Elevated blood glucose levels lead to excess sorbitol levels in many tissues, where it can damage them.

Does reducing high blood glucose prevent macrovascular complications?

Studies have convincingly proven that reducing high blood glucose hugely lowers the risk of *microvascular* complications such as retinopathy, nephropathy, and neuropathy. Whether reducing high blood glucose similarly reduces the risk of *macrovascular* complications like heart attack and stroke has been a subject of controversy.

Two very large and compelling studies found that people with *recently diagnosed* type 1 or type 2 diabetes had their risk of heart attack and stroke substantially reduced by good blood glucose control, but other studies looking at people with more longstanding diabetes (many of whom already had macrovascular complications) did not find similar results. These studies, taken together, strongly suggest that good blood glucose control is, indeed, important in preventing heart attack and stroke, but it needs to be strived for (and achieved) early on. Also, while you're striving for good blood glucose control, follow other proven protective measures such as keeping your blood pressure and cholesterol in check, not smoking, following a healthy diet, exercising regularly, and so on. We discuss these key measures in this chapter and throughout this book.

If you have been diagnosed recently as having type 2 diabetes, you may have already had it for a number of years without knowing it and, as such, you potentially already may have developed complications that you had no idea were present. For that reason, your physician must carefully check to determine if you have any evidence of damage to your body — even if you were diagnosed yesterday. This chapter as well as the Cheat Sheet in the front of this book detail what you and your doctor should look for.

Eye Disease

A variety of different types of eye problems can occur in people with diabetes. Some eye diseases, such as *glaucoma* (raised pressure within the fluid of the eye) and *cataracts* (cloudiness of the lens of the eye), also occur in people without diabetes, though you're more likely to get them if you have diabetes.

The eye disease of greatest concern to people with diabetes is *retinopathy* — damage to the back (retinal) surface of the eye — including *macular edema* (a form of retinopathy in which fluid leaks into the macula from adjacent blood vessels). Retinopathy is the leading cause of blindness in Canada.

Retinopathy

Diabetic retinopathy refers to several different types of injury to the back surface of the eye. This surface allows you to see the world around you. The earliest feature of retinopathy is a tiny ballooning of small blood vessels, called *microaneurysms.* One stage later in severity is the development of small areas of bleeding called *dot hemorrhages* or slightly bigger ones called *blot hemorrhages.* These changes, collectively referred to as *non-proliferative retinopathy,* do not cause loss of vision.

Sometimes retinopathy progresses to a more serious stage *(proliferative retinopathy),* which, if untreated, can threaten your eyesight. Abnormal blood vessels can form *(neovascularization).* These vessels are fragile and have the potential to bleed, which, in turn, can both obscure vision and lead to a potentially catastrophic *retinal detachment.*

Macular edema, swelling of the macula (the area of the retina where light focuses and vision is sharpest), occurs when the blood vessels lining the retina become sufficiently damaged that fluid leaks from these vessels into this part of the eye.

If by this point you are not frightened out of your mind — or, for that matter, even if you are — you might wish to see pictures of these different features. Go to Google (www.google.ca) and type in any of the terms above, then click Images. For the greatest number of results, use *"diabetic retinopathy"* as your search term and you will come up with thousands of images.

Pregnancy can cause retinopathy to worsen rapidly. If you have pre-existing diabetes and you are considering getting pregnant (see Chapter 7), you must see an eye doctor *before* you try to get pregnant, then regularly during your pregnancy. (This does not apply to gestational diabetes since retinopathy does not develop in this condition.)

If you look in the mirror one day and see that you have pinkeye or that you have a small area of bleeding in the whites of one of your eyes, you can rest assured that these are not features of diabetes eye damage. Diabetes damages the *inside* of the eyes, not the *outside.*

How you can prevent retinopathy

You must keep reminding yourself of what we said at the outset of this chapter: Damage to your body from diabetes — including serious eye disease — is not inevitable. By paying careful attention to your diabetes and having appropriate monitoring by health care professionals, you can minimize the likelihood of running into eye damage.

Here are the most important ways to protect your vision:

✔ Maintain excellent blood glucose control (see Chapter 9).

✔ Maintain excellent blood pressure (see the section "Heart and Circulatory Disease," later in this chapter).

✔ Maintain excellent lipids (see the section "Abnormal Cholesterol and Triglyceride Levels (Dyslipidemia)," later in this chapter).

✔ Don't smoke (reason number 4,362, last time we checked).

✔ Obtain regular, expert eye care from a highly skilled optometrist or oph-thalmologist.

As we discuss in Chapter 2, if your blood glucose levels are going through a major change (high to normal, or normal to high), you may develop temporary visual blurring. This is *not* a sign of retinopathy.

If you have had chronically poor blood glucose readings and are then placed on aggressive (as it should be!) treatment to improve things, retinopathy may initially worsen *if* you already have it. Ultimately, better blood glucose control will help protect your eyes, but because of the initial potential for worsening, you must see an eye doctor shortly after starting aggressive blood-glucose-lowering treatment. Most doctors don't know this, so you may have to tell them. Feel free to show them this page. Don't worry about offending your doctor. No doctor in the world knows everything. (Just ask their kids.)

No drugs are of proven value in treating retinopathy (although many studies are currently underway), but laser surgery is an excellent treatment option. Sometimes, for particularly severe cases, an operation — called a *vitrectomy* — is done in which fluid (and any blood that is present) is removed from the back portion of the eyeball and replaced with a sterile solution.

Contrary to what is commonly thought, ASA (for example, Aspirin) does *not* increase the risk of serious bleeding within the eye. If you need to take ASA (see the next section), having diabetic retinopathy should not prevent you from taking it unless your eye doctor has very specific concerns for your par-ticular situation.

Screening for retinopathy

These are the Canadian Diabetes Association (CDA) recommendations for *initial* retinopathy screening:

✔ If you have type 1 diabetes, you should first be assessed by an expert eye specialist five years after the onset of diabetes if you are age 15 or over.

✔ If you have type 2 diabetes, you should first be assessed by an expert eye specialist at the time of diagnosis.

Which eye doctor should you see: An optometrist or an ophthalmologist?

As you read this chapter you may be thinking to yourself, "Boy, I'd better make sure I see my eye doctor." You bet. But which one? Should you see an optometrist or an ophthalmologist? An optometrist is trained to detect eye disease and can prescribe glasses, but he or she is not a medical doctor and cannot perform eye surgery. An ophthalmologist is a medical doctor who is trained to detect and treat eye diseases — with medicines and, if necessary, surgery. An optician, by the way, is someone who is trained to fit you with glasses but not to detect or treat eye disease.

If you do not have diabetes eye disease and simply need to have routine screening to ensure your eyes are in good health, it doesn't matter whether you see an optometrist or an ophthalmologist. If, however, you have diabetes eye damage — especially if it's severe — you should be referred to an ophthalmologist. The key thing is to see a highly skilled eye specialist.

These are the CDA recommendations for *follow-up* visits with your eye specialist:

- ✔ If you *have* retinopathy detected at the time of initial screening, then, depending on the severity of your eye damage, you should see your eye specialist every year or, if necessary, even more often.

- ✔ If you do *not* have retinopathy detected at the time of initial screening, you should see your eye specialist

  - Every year if you have type 1 diabetes

  - Every one to two years if you have type 2 diabetes (Ian, however, admittedly perhaps being overly cautious, advises *all* his patients without retinopathy to be re-screened annually.)

Nowadays, in addition to an eye exam, retinal photographs are often taken. These photographs are an excellent way of detecting and recording eye damage and providing a permanent record for future comparison. The charge for these pictures is typically between $30 and $50.

When an eye doctor examines your eyes (with an ophthalmoscope), he will need to first put eye drops in your eyes to dilate (widen) your pupils so he can see your retina. This will typically make your eyesight distorted (and very sensitive to light) for a few hours until the drops wear off. For this reason, take someone with you to your eye appointment so that he or she can drive you home.

Scanning for sore eyes

One of Ian's patients is a man who uses a bar code reader to scan his grocery store purchases. The device has a speech synthesizer, so that whenever he is looking for, say, a can of chicken soup, he will scan the cans on his shelf and, *presto,* he knows it's not *pesto* (rather, his bar code reader announces the can's contents as indccd, being chicken soup).

Some provincial health insurance plans will pay for only one optometry visit (but an unlimited number of ophthalmology visits) per year. We don't like this policy, but hey, we don't make the rules. (Sure wish we did, though.)

Cataracts

A *cataract* is an opaque (cloudy) area of the lens of the eye that, if large enough, can lead to blurred vision. Cataracts tend to be more common in people with diabetes, even at a young age. Cataracts can be surgically removed by a fairly routine operation. The entire lens is removed, and an artificial lens is put in its place. With removal, you have an excellent chance for the restoration of your vision.

Glaucoma

Glaucoma is high pressure inside the eye. If untreated it can lead to damage to the optic nerve and, ultimately, blindness. Glaucoma is found more often in people with diabetes than in people without diabetes (but is common in both). Fortunately, medical treatment (typically with eye drops) can lower the eye pressure and save your eyesight. Eye doctors check for glaucoma on a routine basis.

Resources to help you if you are blind or visually impaired

In the event you need them, many devices are available to assist you, including the following:

✔ Glucose meters that have speech capability (well, they will talk to you, but don't bother trying to speak to them; not yet anyhow). We discuss glucose meters in Chapter 9.

✔ Insulin pen devices that click as you dial them. This makes it easier to keep track of how much insulin you are about to give. We discuss insulin pen devices in Chapter 13.

Many Internet resources are also available to assist you. We list particularly helpful Web sites in Appendix C.

Heart and Circulatory Disease

Although we (physicians and patients) talk about heart *disease,* in fact what we should be doing is talking about heart *diseases.* Most commonly, the term *heart disease* refers to *coronary artery disease* (CAD), which is also known as *coronary heart disease,* but people with diabetes can also run into other heart ailments, as we discuss later in this section.

Other circulatory problems that people with diabetes are at special risk for include the following:

✔ *Peripheral vascular disease* (abbreviated as PVD; also known as *peripheral arterial disease,* which is abbreviated as PAD): This is a problem with blockage of the arteries that carry oxygen to your legs and feet. PAD can lead to amputations.

✔ *Cerebrovascular disease (CVD)*: This is a problem with blockage of the arteries that carry oxygen to the brain. CVD can lead to strokes.

Circulatory diseases account for the death of 80 percent of people with diabetes (by causing heart attacks and strokes). This is a terrifying statistic. And it's why in this section we discuss in detail the various ways you can help avoid these diseases and, if you have them already, how you can keep them under control.

Coronary artery disease and heart attacks

The heart is, essentially, a pump. An amazing, complex, wonderful pump (when was the last time you went to the hardware store and bought a pump that was likely to last for 80-plus years?), but a pump nonetheless.

Coronary artery disease (CAD) is the term for blockage (plaque) within the arteries that supply blood to the heart muscle (the *coronary* arteries). Plaque is composed of a mixture of cholesterol, fat, and calcium. The presence of plaque within blood vessels is called *atherosclerosis.* Because the blood vessels become very stiff from all this scarring, atherosclerosis is commonly referred to as *hardening of the arteries.*

The most common symptoms of coronary artery disease are chest discomfort (angina) and shortness of breath. Other symptoms can include dizziness or fatigue. Symptoms of coronary artery disease are especially likely to occur if you are exerting yourself, such as walking up a hill or climbing a flight of stairs.

If ever you develop symptoms like those just described, you must arrange to see your doctor promptly. If, however, you experience chest discomfort or shortness of breath that lasts more than a few minutes, you must call 911 and be taken by ambulance to hospital. You should *never, ever* drive yourself to hospital if you think you are experiencing a heart attack. (And don't get your loved one or next-door neighbour to drive you, either, unless of course they happen to be a paramedic and have an ambulance parked in the driveway!)

Determining if you are at high risk of a heart attack

Although, in general terms, having diabetes increases the risk of heart attack, this risk is not the same for all people with diabetes. For example, a 22-year-old who has had type 1 diabetes for only one year is at very low risk of having a heart attack, and a 65-year-old who has had diabetes for 30 years and is a smoker with high blood pressure and high LDL cholesterol is at very, very high risk. This is important to know because, although everyone with diabetes should do their best to be healthy, extra precautions need to be undertaken if you are at high risk of having a heart attack.

High risk is defined as having a 20 percent or greater ten-year risk of dying from heart disease or having a nonfatal heart attack.

If you have diabetes and *any* of the following are true, then you are at high risk:

- You are a man 45 years of age or older.

- You are a woman 50 years of age or older.

- You are over the age of 30 and you've had diabetes for more than 15 years.

- You have macrovascular disease (coronary artery disease, peripheral arterial disease, or cerebrovascular disease; we discuss these conditions in this chapter).

- You have microvascular disease (retinopathy, nephropathy, or neuropathy; we discuss these conditions in this chapter).

- ✔ You have very high blood pressure (systolic blood pressure of more than 180).

- ✔ You have very high cholesterol (LDL of more than 5.0).

- ✔ You have two or more of the following: Smoking, high blood pressure, high (LDL) cholesterol, a close family member (father, mother, sister, brother) who developed heart disease or a stroke at a young age.

Preventing a heart attack

The Canadian Diabetes Association recommends the following heart attack–prevention strategies for *all* people with diabetes:

- ✔ Follow a healthy lifestyle by eating healthfully, exercising regularly, and striving to achieve a healthy weight. We discuss these issues in detail in Chapters 10 and 11.

- ✔ If you smoke, quit. If you don't, don't start. We discuss this further right after this list.

- ✔ Keep your blood pressure within target (less than 130/80). We discuss this in more detail later.

- ✔ Keep your A1C no higher than 7. Your A1C is an indicator of your overall blood glucose control. We discuss A1C in Chapter 9.

The Canadian Diabetes Association recommends the following *additional* heart attack–prevention strategies for people with diabetes who are at *high risk* (we look at how you can determine this in the preceding section):

- ✔ Take ACE inhibitor or ARB medication. (ACE inhibitors work by blocking (inhibiting) the action of the *a*ngiotensin *c*onverting *e*nzyme. ARBs work by blocking the action of a protein (angiotensin) from acting on its receptor; that is they are *a*ngiotensin *r*eceptor *b*lockers.) Medicines from these families reduce the risk of heart attack. The best known of these medicines is ramipril (Altace), which is an ACE inhibitor.

- ✔ Take ASA "based on (your physician's) individual clinical judgment." We look at this challengingly worded and controversial subject later in this section.

- ✔ Take cholesterol-lowering medication targeting your LDL to be 2 mmol/L or less and targeting your total cholesterol divided by HDL to be less than 4. The preferred medication is a statin drug. (We discuss this in more detail in the "Abnormal Cholesterol and Triglyceride Levels (Dyslipidemia)" section, later in this chapter.)

Quitting smoking

More than one patient has told us that quitting cigarettes is easy; they've done it hundreds of times! Okay, so quitting *is* easy; but to remain a quitter is difficult. Still, it can be done, *if* you're ready.

Quitting cold turkey is the best option for some people. For others, using a nicotine patch (available over-the-counter) or a prescription medication like Zyban (bupropion) or Champix (varenicline) is helpful. If you've tried quitting but have gone back to smoking, then try again the next day. And if that doesn't work, try again the next day. The key to success is not giving up. Ignore your failures and start your efforts afresh each day. Ultimately you can and will succeed.

Taking ASA

ASA (Aspirin being one commonly used variety), acting as a mild blood thinner (a so-called anti-platelet drug), is of proven value in preventing heart attacks in people who do *not* have diabetes. It is of less proven value for people who *have* diabetes. The Canadian Diabetes Association Clinical Practice Guidelines indicate

- ✔ If you have diabetes *and* have (stable) cardiovascular disease, "low dose ASA therapy (81–325 mg) may be considered." Clopidogrel (Plavix) — another type of mild blood thinner — can be used instead if you have side effects from ASA.

- ✔ If you have diabetes and do *not* have cardiovascular disease, the role of ASA is unclear. The Canadian Diabetes Association Guidelines, referring to this situation, note that "the decision to prescribe ASA . . . should be based on individual clinical judgment. . . ."

Because ASA is so safe for the vast majority of people, Ian's philosophy is to routinely recommend its use for his patients *with known* cardiovascular disease. And because most people with diabetes ultimately develop (and die from) cardiovascular disease, and because it can be hard to know when it has developed, Ian typically recommends ASA for his patients who are *at high risk* for this condition. We look at how you can determine if you're at high risk in a preceding section.

Do not use ASA if you are less than 21 years of age because its use in this age group increases the risk of developing a serious neurological condition called Reye syndrome. Also avoid using it if you have a bleeding disorder or have had recent internal bleeding. Before you start taking ASA therapy, we recommend you first discuss with your doctor the pros and cons of taking this medicine.

Cerebrovascular disease and strokes

The same processes that affect the *coronary arteries* (the arteries that feed the heart with oxygen) can affect the arteries to the brain. This is called cerebrovascular disease (CVD). CVD can lead to strokes.

Having read the preceding paragraph, you may already have concluded that if cerebrovascular disease and coronary artery disease have a similar underlying process, then the risk factors leading to CVD are probably the same. You're right.

If you want to know what therapies you can use to prevent having a stroke, read the previous section, where we talk about ways to prevent heart disease. The same information applies.

Peripheral vascular disease (problems with circulation to the legs and feet)

Diabetes can do many scary things. For most people, high up on this intimidating list are perfectly justified fears about poor circulation leading to amputations. Poor circulation to the legs is called *peripheral vascular disease* (PVD) or *peripheral arterial disease* (PAD) and is due to atherosclerosis obstructing the flow of blood. It is caused by the same factors that lead to coronary artery disease and cerebrovascular disease. Similarly, you can avoid it by following the measures that we describe earlier in this chapter.

A diabetes educator that Ian works with recalls the time, many years ago, when she was sitting in a room with a 45-year-old man whose diabetes had been recently diagnosed. After they had chatted for a while, the doctor entered the room and nonchalantly said to his patient, "You may as well start preparing for your amputations now. It's just a matter of time, after all." The poor man's face sank. The doctor was clearly heartless and tactless, but even worse, he may have had some reason for saying this. The knowledge and therapy we had back then were vastly inferior to what we have nowadays, and this particular doctor had likely had all too much experience in seeing the devastation that could occur.

But — drum roll please — we've got news for him (and you). It's most definitely *not* just a matter of time. Amputations are almost always avoidable. But the time to start your program of healthy foot maintenance is *now*. Think of it the way you would car maintenance: Much better to keep your car in a top state of repair than to run into engine problems halfway between Quebec City and Montreal on a –30°C Christmas Day (Ian speaks from experience, as you may have suspected).

Far and away the most common symptom of PVD is an aching discomfort in your calves as you walk. This is called *intermittent claudication* (usually abbreviated to *claudication*). Generally speaking, the sooner the discomfort occurs when you walk, the worse are the blockages in the arteries.

If PVD is very severe, it can lead to changes in the feet, including the following:

- Pale appearance
- Loss of hair
- Constant pain in the toes
- Small, usually red or black spots on the tips of the toes
- Open sores or ulcers on the bottom or sides of the feet

If you have developed any of the above symptoms, let your family physician or diabetes specialist know; however, if you have developed an open sore or ulcer on your foot, you may have an infection and you need to seek *immediate* medical attention.

Peripheral vascular disease is difficult to treat, but helpful therapies are available, including medications and, in some cases, surgery to open or bypass a blocked artery. You must not smoke and must control your cholesterol and blood pressure. Your physician can also discuss certain helpful types of exercises that you can perform, or, alternatively, can refer you to a specialist in this field.

Numerous reasons not to smoke exist, but we want to make special mention of the influence of smoking on PVD. Smoking will make you much more prone to PVD. Even more important, if you continue to smoke when you *already have* PVD, it is a certainty you will develop worsening circulation problems and you will put yourself at enormous risk of developing foot ulcerations and gangrene. Trust us; you will not be a happy camper if this happens.

We talk more about foot care later in this chapter (see "Foot Disease in Diabetes").

The lowdown on high blood pressure

High blood pressure is a common health problem regardless of whether or not you have diabetes. It is, however, especially common among people with diabetes. Not that diabetes *causes* high blood pressure; it's just *associated* with it. Yet another unfair thing about having diabetes (as if there weren't enough already).

The medical term for high blood pressure is *hypertension*. You may have noticed that your doctor refers to your blood pressure as being *something* over *something* (140 over 90, for example). The first number represents the *systolic* value and the second number the *diastolic* value. The systolic value is the amount of force exerted by the heart when it contracts to push blood around the body. The diastolic value is the pressure in the large arteries in-between heart contractions.

Keeping your blood pressure *normal* is essential. High blood pressure can lead to all sorts of problems — particularly if you have diabetes — including the following:

- Blindness (hypertension aggravates retinopathy)
- Heart attacks
- Kidney failure
- Strokes

Now, we didn't design that list to depress you. We want to alert you to the importance of the issue, because with proper therapy you can help avoid these problems. Indeed, modern medicine has very, very effective therapy for high blood pressure.

What exactly is normal blood pressure? This should be such a simple question to answer, but in fact it isn't. It seems that each year some new study comes out showing that we should be aiming lower. Ian recalls being at a lecture where a highly respected blood pressure specialist facetiously said, "If your patient can still stand up, then their blood pressure is still too high!" Suffice it to say, if you have diabetes, your target blood pressure is less than 130 over 80 (usually written as 130/80 — which, by the way, is not to say you should divide 130 by 80 and walk out of your doctor's office thinking your blood pressure is 1.625. A blood pressure of 1.625 would likely make an earthworm dizzy!).

Never let your doctor (including us!) or any other health care provider simply report to you that your blood pressure is good or fine or okay, or some other equally vague and ultimately meaningless term. If he doesn't volunteer what your measurement was, ask him to write the number down in your blood glucose logbook (we talk more about logbooks in Chapter 9) or, even better, on the Cheat Sheet at the front of this book. Furthermore, if your blood pressure is above target (remember, target is less than 130/80), ask your doctor how you and he or she are going to improve it. Do not settle for second-rate blood pressure control. We're talking your health here!

The CDA recommends that you have your blood pressure measured every time you see your doctor for a diabetes-related visit (since diabetes can affect pretty well all your body, that would mean almost every visit).

The following are treatments for high blood pressure:

- Diet (limiting salt and alcohol)
- Exercise
- Weight control
- Medicines (an ACE inhibitor or ARB — see earlier in this section — is a particularly good choice; however, often a combination of two, three, or even four different medicines is required)

Some medicines used to treat hypertension can have an effect on your blood glucose control. For example, hydrochlorothiazide (HCT) has the potential to make blood glucose levels go up, and beta blockers can reduce your awareness of low blood glucose. This doesn't mean these drugs are bad or shouldn't be used, but pay especially close attention to your blood glucose levels if you are prescribed these drugs. (If HCT is going to make your readings rise, it will most likely happen shortly after you first start taking the medicine.)

Abnormal Cholesterol and Triglyceride Levels (Dyslipidemia)

In this section we look at the importance of keeping your lipids (cholesterol and triglyceride levels) in check and how to achieve this. Unlike when Ian first started medical school (some time, according to Ian's children, between the Jurassic and Cretaceous periods), nowadays we have excellent therapy that allows almost everyone to reach their lipid targets.

Many types of lipids exist, but you should be aware of these five important ones:

- **HDL:** This stands for *high density lipoprotein*. You want your HDL to be high because it helps protect your blood vessels; it removes cholesterol from the walls of your arteries. HDL is thought of as the *good* cholesterol. You can remember this by the phrase "A **h**igh **H**DL keeps you **h**ealthy."

- **LDL:** This stands for *low density lipoprotein*. You want your LDL to be low. LDL is thought of as the *bad* cholesterol. You can remember all of this by the phrase: "**L**DL is **l**ousy and should be **l**ow."

- **Triglycerides:** These are the main fats in the blood. Their role in the development of atherosclerosis is not quite as proven as LDL and HDL; however, it's wise to keep your triglycerides in the normal range (see below).

- **Total cholesterol:** This is a measure of a combination of various forms of cholesterol.

- **Total cholesterol/HDL ratio:** Just as it sounds, this is a ratio of total cholesterol to HDL cholesterol and is used in helping to decide if you require treatment. The lower the ratio, the better.

The CDA recommends that you have your lipid levels checked at the time of diagnosis of your diabetes and then every one to three years (more frequently if treatment has been initiated or changed).

You should be fasting when your blood sample is taken to measure your lipids, because this allows for a more precise determination of your levels. When your doctor fills out the requisition for your lipid measurement, make sure he or she writes on the requisition precisely how long you should fast. If your doctor doesn't do this, the lab may tell you that you must be fasting for 14 hours before they will do the test. That can be dangerous if you are taking certain oral hypoglycemic drugs (we discuss these in Chapter 12) or, especially, insulin (Chapter 13). If you are on these medicines, *never* fast for anywhere near 14 hours unless you have first checked with your doctor. In most cases an 8-hour fast is sufficient.

Looking at healthy cholesterol levels

Although pretty well everything you read about cholesterol discusses how bad it is, in fact, cholesterol is an essential substance required for maintaining healthy cells and manufacturing certain vitamins and hormones. Problems arise when we have too much cholesterol or too much of the wrong type.

If your lipid levels are abnormal — particularly if you have additional risk factors for heart disease — you are at increased risk for developing hardening of the arteries *(atherosclerosis),* which can, in turn, lead to strokes, heart attacks, and amputations. These are the Canadian Diabetes Association (CDA) recommended targets for people *at high risk* of a heart attack (to determine if you are at high risk see "Determining if you are at high risk of a heart attack" earlier in this chapter):

- ✔ **LDL:** Less than or equal to 2.0 mmol/L. Achieving this is the most important priority in lipid management.
- ✔ **Total cholesterol/HDL:** Less than 4.0.

The CDA does not set a specific lipid target for people who are *not* at high risk of a heart attack. (However, most people with diabetes are at high risk and should, therefore, strive for the above-mentioned goals.)

Although the CDA does not have a specific treatment target for triglycerides, they note that a triglyceride level of less than 1.5 mmol/L is considered optimal.

For people with diabetes, the most common problem is high LDL, low HDL, and high triglycerides.

Keeping your lipids under control

You can improve your lipids in these ways:

- ✔ Achieve (and maintain) a healthy weight (for more, see Chapters 10 and 11)
- ✔ Eat healthfully (see Chapter 10)
- ✔ Exercise regularly (see Chapter 11)
- ✔ Take medication (we discuss this next)

Most of the cholesterol in your body is actually manufactured *by* your body (your liver, to be precise). Although you may be able to limit your cholesterol intake, getting your liver to stop making cholesterol is quite different. The liver's tendency to make too much cholesterol is often genetically determined. Thus, lifestyle therapy (diet, exercise, weight control) is often not sufficient to bring your lipids into line — and medication becomes necessary. A common mistake is for people to stop taking their medicine after they have completed their first prescription, mistakenly thinking that they no longer need it. Unless you change livers (which we imagine is not very likely), you'll need to continue to take the medicine.

The preferred medicine to get and keep your LDL cholesterol level in target is a *statin,* of which several exist, including the particularly widely prescribed Lipitor (atorvastatin). Statins are very, very safe (indeed, so much so that in the U.K., one type of statin is even available without a prescription). The most common side effect is muscle aching, which goes away promptly after discontinuing the medicine.

If a statin isn't working sufficiently well, Ezetrol (ezetimibe) or a fibrate is often *added.* Other, less frequently used medicines to treat dyslipidemia are cholestyramine, and, if your main problem is very high triglycerides, nicotinic acid (also known as niacin). (Nicotinic acid is not often used as it can have significant adverse effects, including increasing blood glucose, skin flushing, and itching.)

Because statins lower your risk of a heart attack even if your lipids are within target in the first place, the Canadian Diabetes Association advises that statins should be used "for all people with diabetes considered at high risk" of a heart attack *regardless* of what your lipid levels are without such treatment.

Some medicines, like simvastatin (Zocor), that are used to improve cholesterol levels work better if taken in the evening, whereas others, like atorvastatin (Lipitor), work equally well regardless of what time of day you take them. If you are prescribed cholesterol-lowering pills, be sure to ask your doctor or pharmacist when to take them.

Kidney Disease

Think of your kidneys as filters. And what amazing filters they are. Not only can they rid your body of toxins that are produced as a normal by-product of metabolism, but also they can maintain your salt and water balance, keep the level of acids in your body under control, and release hormones that regulate your body's production of blood. Sometimes it seems the only thing these amazing filters can't do is help make coffee (though they do help you get rid of it!).

Unfortunately, diabetes can damage the kidneys. In fact, diabetes is the most common cause of kidney failure in Canada. Fortunately, this damage is largely preventable.

Diagnosing diabetes kidney damage

It takes years and years for diabetes to cause kidney damage. That means you have lots of opportunity to prevent damage from occurring. A doctor's earliest clue that a problem exists is the discovery of excess levels of *albumin* (a type of protein) in your urine. This is called *microalbuminuria* and can be screened for with a very simple urine test (a urine *albumin/creatinine ratio;* abbreviated as *ACR*), which can be performed any time of day. A normal ACR is less than 2 if you are a man, less than 2.8 if you are a woman. Your doctor should be testing your ACR routinely (see the Cheat Sheet at the front of this book to find out how often), because it won't cause symptoms to alert you that there's a problem. If damage progresses, it leads to larger quantities of protein in the urine and can cause your feet and legs to swell (edema). If things continue to worsen, your kidneys can become unable to purify your blood of toxins. This last stage is called *kidney failure* and typically makes people feel unwell in many ways, including causing fatigue, weight loss, and, if severe, confused thinking. (Incidentally — and contrary to popular wisdom — kidney damage from diabetes does *not* cause back pain.)

Because the ACR can be temporarily elevated due to conditions *not* related to diabetes kidney damage (such as menstruating, having recently done heavy exercise, having very high blood glucose levels, having heart failure, or having a kidney or bladder infection), your ACR should not be tested until these other conditions have passed. Additionally, if you have an elevated ACR, unless it is extraordinarily high your urine will need to be retested to verify the problem is persisting before it is concluded that you have kidney malfunction.

If you have evidence, on blood or urine testing, of having more advanced kidney damage, your doctor may ask you to do a urine collection, which is basically what it sounds like: collecting your urine (for 24 hours) in a jug, with which the lab will provide you. This is done to more precisely measure your kidney function. It's a hassle to do ("Hmm, I wonder if I properly labelled that yellow jug I put in the office fridge?"), so fortunately it's not necessary to do it routinely.

The CDA guidelines recommend that an additional kidney test called the blood creatinine level be performed from time to time (see the Cheat Sheet for the exact frequency). Your creatinine level is used to estimate your GFR (glomerular filtration rate), which is a measure of how efficiently your kidneys are able to purify your blood. This test is done to monitor your kidney function. A particularly important reason to do this test is that recent studies tell us that quite a few people will develop kidney damage without first having microalbuminuria; in other words, an abnormal creatinine (and GFR) may be the first clue that a problem exists. (In many of these cases, the kidney damage may be due to a condition — such as high blood pressure — not directly related to your diabetes.)

Treating diabetes kidney damage

The most important factors leading to diabetes kidney disease are inadequate blood glucose control and elevated blood pressure. Other, unknown (perhaps genetic) factors must be present, too, because most people with diabetes never develop kidney malfunction. Because it's impossible to predict whether you'll always have healthy kidneys, taking all possible precautions to protect these important organs is crucial.

With appropriate therapy, not only can you substantially reduce your risk of developing kidney damage, but if you already have it, you can help prevent it from worsening or, in some cases, undo some of the damage. We've sure come a long way from the time, not so very long ago, when once you had diabetes kidney damage, it inevitably got worse and worse.

These are the ways to protect your kidneys from diabetes damage:

- ✔ Excellent blood glucose control
- ✔ Excellent blood pressure control
- ✔ Medication (either a member of the ACE inhibitor family or a member of the ARB family) if you have microalbuminuria. (We define microalbuminuria earlier in this section.)

ACE inhibitors and ARBs will occasionally lead to potentially dangerous accumulation of potassium in the body and can, rarely, make kidney function worse, not better. For these reasons, one to two weeks after you start taking one of these types of drugs (or have the dose increased), your doctor should send you to the laboratory for a blood test to check your potassium and creatinine levels. Although the creatinine typically goes up shortly after starting ACE inhibitor or ARB therapy, it shouldn't rise by more than 30 percent. If it does, that may signify worsening kidney function caused by the drug, and your doctor may tell you to stop taking the medicine.

Getting a second chance

Sandra was 13 years old when she found out she had diabetes. Over the next 10 years she didn't look after herself all that well. In fact, she seldom checked her glucose readings, hardly ever saw her doctor, and never met with her diabetes educators. Now, however, she was "getting her act together," as she herself said when she came for her appointment with Ian.

She was engaged to be married and had new interest in her health. Ian ran some basic investigations and determined that Sandra had excess albumin in her urine. Sandra was devastated.

Now that she was keen to be healthy, she felt guilty about her "past sins" (as she called them).

But Sandra was a determined woman and put her full effort into looking after herself and her diabetes. She got her glucose under control, quit smoking, and started ACE inhibitor medicine. Over the next year her urine albumin level returned to normal. Ian has rarely seen a happier face than Sandra's the day he told her the good news.

If you have diabetes kidney damage, you're at high risk of cardiovascular damage and you'll need to take protective action. We discuss these precautions in detail earlier in this chapter.

If, despite every effort, your kidneys have progressed to the point where they have almost completely stopped working, you'll require dialysis (a method of purifying the blood) or a kidney transplant.

Neuropathy (Nerve Damage)

Nerve damage from diabetes is a very common but *very* preventable problem. Many different types of nerve damage exist, and this topic alone could fill an entire book. Most forms are uncommon or downright obscure, however, so in this section we concentrate on the more frequent types of nerve damage that you should be aware of.

You can think of the nervous system as a complex network of electrical circuitry with signals going in every direction as messages are relayed from one part of your body to another. Suffice it to say that no computer system yet designed has even 1 percent of the complexity of the human nervous system. Shakespeare sure knew of what he spoke when he said, "What a piece of work is man."

The most important factor leading to neuropathy in people with diabetes is elevated blood glucose levels. Nonetheless, because other causes exist (such as certain types of vitamin deficiency, overuse of alcohol, and so on), your doctor will need to exclude these.

Peripheral neuropathy

The peripheral nervous system is made up of the nerves that travel from the spinal cord to the *periphery* of your body, including your arms and legs. Peripheral neuropathy is damage to the nerves that make up the peripheral nervous system.

Looking at the symptoms of peripheral neuropathy

The most common symptoms of peripheral neuropathy are abnormal sensations (usually collectively — though not always technically accurately — referred to as *dysesthesiae*) such as a burning or numb feeling in the toes (and, if more advanced, other areas of the feet also). Other sensations that can be experienced include throbbing; aching; prickling; sharp, shooting pains; or even a tickling. Sometimes, people say they feel like they are walking on marbles. If neuropathy progresses, it can lead to lack of ability to perceive pain. Although lack of pain is wonderful when you are having an operation, it is not a good thing when it comes to your feet, because in the absence of pain you may not recognize when a sore or injury has developed.

Diagnosing peripheral neuropathy

Peripheral neuropathy is usually diagnosed on *clinical grounds,* which is a fancy way of saying that doctors generally make the diagnosis based on what symptoms you are having and what they find upon examining you. One very helpful and very easily performed test is to see if you can recognize the feel of a thin nylon rod *(a 10-gram monofilament)* when it is pressed against your foot (in particular, the big toe). We discuss additional issues in foot care later in this chapter.

The 10-gram monofilament test tells us crucial information. If your test is abnormal, it means that you're at much greater risk of developing a foot ulcer, and, as you may recall, foot ulcers can lead to gangrene (and, ultimately, put you at risk for amputation). You can see an online demonstration of how this test is done and you can order your own (free) monofilament at the LEAP (Lower Extremity Amputation Prevention) Web site (www.hrsa.gov/leap/fivestep.htm).

Treating peripheral neuropathy

Although no cure is known for peripheral neuropathy due to diabetes, very helpful therapies are available, including the following:

- ✓ **Meticulous foot care:** Because peripheral neuropathy is a key factor in putting people at risk of amputation, you require meticulous foot care to protect yourself from this complication. We discuss this in detail later in this chapter.

- ✓ **Excellent blood glucose control:** Bringing your blood glucose levels down is a key measure both to help prevent further nerve damage and, if your neuropathy is very mild, to reverse existing damage. Yet another reason (we must be up to a hundred by now) for making sure your blood glucose control is as good as possible.

- ✓ **Medications that act on nerves:** The most commonly used of these medicines are amitriptyline, gabapentin (Neurontin), and pregabalin (Lyrica). If the area of discomfort is very small, you can try applying a topical medicine called capsaicin. (Because capsaicin is derived from chili peppers, you might think that it could really sting if it got in your eyes. And you would be right. After you apply the capsaicin to your feet, make sure you wash your hands really well before you touch *anything* else.)

- ✓ **Analgesics (pain relievers):** For mild symptoms, acetaminophen (Tylenol and many other brands) is helpful. If your symptoms are more severe or not sufficiently responding to the other therapies we mention here, using narcotic-containing analgesics such as codeine (often in combination with acetaminophen) can be very helpful.

  You may come across very, very heavily promoted (by the manufacturer) non-prescription drug therapies to ease the pain of diabetic peripheral neuropathy. Unfortunately, at least as of the time of this writing, minimal scientific data supports their use. We look forward to properly done studies of these drugs and cross our fingers they will show benefit. Until these are available, we advocate skepticism regarding their use.

 If your symptoms aren't well controlled despite trying the various measures listed above, you might consider contacting the neurology department of a university-affiliated hospital to see if you are eligible to participate in any ongoing research studies.

Autonomic neuropathy

The autonomic (automatic) nervous system works behind the scenes, controlling many body functions that you don't directly control, including bowel and bladder function. Autonomic neuropathy is nerve damage to the autonomic nervous system. This occurs quite commonly if you have had diabetes for a long time, but often the symptoms are (incorrectly) assumed to be caused by something else. Some of the most common problems encountered include the following:

- ✔ **Sexual dysfunction:** We discuss this further in Chapter 7.

- ✔ **Disorders of the stomach and large intestine:** We discuss these in the next section.

- ✔ **Bladder difficulties:** You may lose your ability to recognize an urge to empty your bladder even when it is full (*neurogenic* bladder). This leads to retention of urine within the bladder, which in turn can make you more prone to urinary tract infections and, in the most severe cases, kidney malfunction. The most common symptom that may alert you to the development of bladder malfunction is the repeated passage of only tiny quantities of urine (basically a problem with overflow akin to water dripping down the sides of an over-filled glass).

- ✔ **Abnormal heart rate:** Your heart normally has the ability to slow down and speed up to match your body's needs. If you develop damage to the part of the autonomic nervous system that helps regulate your heart, your heart may end up beating too fast.

- ✔ **Sweating problems:** Excess sweating can occur. One very unusual and intriguing problem is the development of sweating over the forehead as you start to eat your food. This is called *gustatory* sweating.

These are some other, important forms of neuropathy to be aware of:

- ✔ Numb fingers due to compression of a nerve in the wrist *(carpal tunnel syndrome):* We discuss this condition later in this chapter, in the section, "Musculoskeletal Problems (Muscles, Joints, and Such)."

- ✔ Weakness of a muscle controlling eye movement *(extra-ocular muscle palsy):* In this condition, one of the muscles that controls eye movement becomes damaged, which typically leads to double vision. Fortunately, this problem spontaneously corrects, but that can take a number of weeks or even months to come around.

- ✔ Numbness on the side of the thigh *(lateral femoral cutaneous nerve syndrome):* In this condition, also known as *lateral femoral cutaneous nerve entrapment* or, more colourfully, *meralgia paresthetica,* the lateral femoral cutaneous nerve, which is located on the side of the thigh, is damaged, causing numbness in this region. This problem typically spontaneously resolves with time.

Recently, a number of researchers have noted a high prevalence of hearing loss among people with diabetes. The reasons for this aren't yet fully clear, but it could be that nerve damage within the ear is a main factor. We expect this issue to be further sorted out over the next few years. If you think you have hearing loss — whether or not you have diabetes — be sure to report this to your doctor so that you can have it looked into and, if necessary, treated.

Having diabetes and reading about the various neuropathies that can occur may make you feel either discouraged or alarmed, or both. Although that makes perfect sense, remind yourself that most of these complications are avoidable by having the best possible blood glucose control. Ultimately, we hope the closest you'll ever get to a nerve problem will be when you try to get a date with that cute neighbour of yours.

Mental Health Problems

Over the past few years physicians have become increasingly aware of how common mental health problems affect people with diabetes. We discuss these here.

Depression

If you have diabetes, you're more likely to develop depression, and, conversely, if you have depression, you are more likely to develop (type 2) diabetes. The first of these seems, at first glance, to be readily explained given the hassles — both physical and mental — that diabetes poses. But that's only a partial explanation because many people with diabetes, despite handling these stresses just fine thank you very much, still develop depression. The reason for this is unclear. It is similarly unclear why people with depression are more likely to develop diabetes. (In yet another example of what's new is old, Thomas Willis, a famous British physician, observed in 1674 that "diabetes is caused by sadness or long sorrow.")

Researchers have looked at factors such as whether depression could lead to diabetes because people who are depressed may be more likely to not eat healthfully, may be less likely to exercise, and so on, but these factors also do not fully explain things. Suffice it to say, if you have diabetes and are feeling blue, don't ignore it. Dealing with depression is of paramount importance, both for its own sake and also because if you're depressed you are much less likely to pay attention to looking after your diabetes. We discuss depression further in Chapter 1.

Dementia

People with diabetes are more prone to dementia. Sometimes this is due to cerebrovascular disease (which we discuss earlier in this chapter, in the section "Heart and Circulatory Disease") and, for unclear reasons, sometimes this is due to Alzheimer's disease. Until more is known about the relationship between diabetes and dementia (and likely even when it is), we recommend following the key measures of good diabetes care we espouse throughout this book — particularly, striving for excellent blood glucose levels, blood pressure, and lipid control.

Digestive Disorders: Problems of the Stomach, Intestines, and Liver

Your gut can be thought of as a long, hollow tube extending from your mouth to your anus. Stretched end to end it would reach over 8 metres (25 feet); once again, please do *not* try this at home! Diabetes can affect the gut in a variety of ways:

- *Diarrhea* can occur for one of several reasons, including damage to the nerves that control intestinal function and excess numbers of bacteria (bacterial overgrowth) within the bowel. Depending on the specific nature of the problem, your doctor may prescribe either antibiotics or medicine to slow down bowel function.

- *Gastroparesis* is a condition in which your stomach becomes less efficient at propelling food into your small intestine. As a consequence, you may find that you get full very quickly as you eat. Additionally, because nutrients don't get absorbed as efficiently (nutrients get absorbed almost exclusively from the small bowel, not the stomach), your blood glucose control may become erratic.

  Doctors treat gastroparesis with medicines (such as metoclopramide and domperidone) that enhance stomach emptying. Also, if you are taking rapid-acting insulin with meals, your doctor may recommend you take this insulin *after* your meal rather than the conventional before-meal administration. (We discuss this further in Chapter 13.)

Diabetes can also affect the liver. If you have diabetes — particularly if your blood glucose control isn't very good — your liver may accumulate very excessive quantities of fat, a condition unimaginatively but straightforwardly called *fatty liver* (or, more fully, *nonalcoholic fatty liver disease*). It was long thought this was a pretty harmless condition, however, recent evidence suggests it may lead to the development of a much more serious condition: *cirrhosis of the liver*.

The first clue your doctor may have that you're developing liver damage is often the finding, on routine blood tests, of an elevated liver enzyme level (such as an *AST*). Key aspects of treating fatty liver are weight control, exercise, optimizing blood glucose and lipid levels, and avoiding alcohol. Evidence also suggests that metformin and TZD medication may help (we discuss these drugs in detail in Chapter 12).

Although not caused by diabetes, *celiac disease* is a quite common intestinal disease in people who have type 1 diabetes. Celiac disease is a condition in which the lining of the small intestine, in genetically susceptible individuals, becomes damaged by exposure to a substance called gluten (this is a protein found in wheat, rye, and barley). This damage leads to inconsistent absorption of nutrients from food into your body and, as a result, may lead to erratic blood glucose control. Fortunately, avoiding ingesting gluten-containing foods (and other gluten-containing products) allows the bowel to heal. This treatment, however, needs to be continued lifelong. Celiac disease is diagnosed by performing a blood test and having an *endoscopy* in which a flexible fibre-optic tube is swallowed and passed through the stomach into the small intestine where a biopsy is obtained.

Foot Disease in Diabetes

The most serious threat to your foot is an ulcer, because this can lead to infection, gangrene, and, ultimately, the need for amputation. (This sequence of events is often triggered by seemingly minor trauma.) For this reason, you need to keep your feet healthy and happy. You must develop an obsession with your feet. A veritable love affair with your feet. Indeed, you must develop a foot fetish!

In a sense, foot disease is really a combination of many of the different topics we cover in this chapter. Typically, a person with diabetes who runs into foot problems has a combination of peripheral neuropathy and peripheral vascular disease (PVD) and may have skin problems as well (which we discuss in the next section). Because neuropathy and PVD are most common if you're older and, especially, if you've had diabetes for many years, the following precautions — though applicable to all people with diabetes — are particularly important to follow if you've already got numbness or lack of sensation in your feet or if you're known to have impaired circulation in your legs.

Protecting your feet

Here are things you can do to protect your feet:

- ✔ **Look at your feet:** Inspect your feet carefully at least once a day. Usually this is most convenient after you complete your shower or bath. Check your toes (including between your toes) and check your soles and the sides of your feet. You are looking for cuts, cracks, calluses, flaking skin (which may indicate a fungal infection called *athlete's foot*), dry skin, sores, blisters, and foreign bodies. (No, this doesn't refer to Carla Bruni — or Nicolas Sarkozy for that matter. It refers to things like splinters or even tacks, which, if you have significant nerve damage, could be imbedded in your foot without your even knowing it.) Most important, you are looking for openings in the skin, such as ulcerations (which appear as small holes in the skin surface), and areas of redness with heat and pus (which likely indicate an infection). If you choose to discover on the Web what a diabetic foot ulcer looks like, be forewarned that Internet sites invariably show only the most grisly, worst-case scenarios. It's actually hard to find images on the Net of the early, mild type of foot ulcer that is much more common than these horrific cases.

  Your doctor should also inspect your feet regularly — at least annually and more often if you're known to have foot problems or are at high risk for them. Help your doctor help you: If your doctor hasn't checked your feet recently, while you sit in the examining room waiting for her to join you, take off your shoes and socks and, when the doctor joins you, ask her to have a look at your feet. (If she tells you it's not necessary, feel free to blame us and tell her we felt it was necessary.)

- ✔ **Determine if you have a lack of sensation:** As we discuss in the section on peripheral neuropathy, diabetes can make you less able to feel pain in your feet, and this puts you at much higher risk of developing foot ulcers. Touch different parts of your feet (with your finger or, even better, with a monofilament as we discuss earlier) to see if the sensation is impaired in any areas. If your sensation is impaired (and in fact even if it isn't), you should avoid using a heating pad on your feet.

- ✔ **Wear your shoes on your hands before you wear them on your feet:** Before you put on your shoes, look and feel inside them (with your fingers, not your toes) to make sure that they don't contain any errant pebbles, tacks, paper clips, or any other object that could damage your feet. And speaking of shoes . . .

- ✔ **Buy only very comfortable, well-fitting shoes.** (If you have new shoes, break them in by wearing them initially for no more than one to two hours at a time.) The heels on your shoes should be under 5 centimetres

(2 inches) high. And before you put on those comfortable, low-healed shoes (without over-the-counter insoles — they can cause blisters), make sure the socks you use are not overly tight. Because your feet may swell over the course of the day, be sure to buy your shoes in the late afternoon (that is when your feet will be at their largest).

Long-term diabetes complications — including foot complications — are more likely to develop the longer you've had diabetes. So if you are an 18-year-old woman who's had diabetes for one year and you're wondering if it's okay to wear high heels to your high school prom, it is. Well, from a diabetes standpoint anyhow.

✔ **Keep your feet well groomed:** Your toenails must be kept short (but not too short). Cut them straight across (use an emery board to smooth the edges). Better yet, have someone else cut them for you, especially if you have impaired feeling in your feet or impaired eyesight. Keep the *soles* of your feet from getting overly dry. (If dryness is a problem for you, apply a good skin lotion in the morning and at bedtime.) Keep the *spaces between your toes* from getting overly moist by applying liberal quantities of powder after you bathe. Remember, you want the spaces between your toes to be dry and the soles of your feet to be moist.

✔ **Check your feet for calluses.** These are often a trigger leading to foot ulceration. If you have calluses, corns, or warts, you should not treat them yourself; have a professional deal with them (generally, a podiatrist is the best person to see for these problems).

✔ **Test the waters:** You would never dive into unknown waters, right? Well, you should never *step* into unknown waters either, even in your own bathroom. Before you step into a bath, use your hand (or, even better, your elbow) to make sure the water is not too hot.

✔ **Remember that *Barefoot in the Park* was only a movie:** It may have been okay for Jane Fonda and Robert Redford to go barefoot in the park (assuming they do not have diabetes), but it is not okay for you. Also, it's not okay to go barefoot in the dark (even in your own home) because you never know what you are about to step on — or *in* for that matter. Your feet are just too valuable to risk injuring them.

✔ **Don't soak your feet:** You may be surprised to read this, but soaking your feet is seldom a good idea because it can make the skin overly soft and fragile (think waterlogged) and actually increase your risk for getting a foot infection. If you really want to soak your feet, ensure the water is not too hot *and* limit your soaks to no more than 10 to 20 minutes.

✔ **Don't smoke:** 'Nuff said, says Ian. Alan is even more blunt: If you smoke, you are asking for an amputation. Yeah, that's blunt.

Inspecting your feet

If you see an open sore on your foot — in particular if pus and/or surrounding redness is present — you *must* seek *immediate* medical attention because you likely have an infection. If you have a foot infection, time becomes of the essence. Every day that goes by without proper treatment increases your risk of the infection worsening, potentially leading to amputation. Tragically, Ian has seen dozens of people who had amputations that could have been avoided if only they had followed the simple advice contained in this section. (If, however, you have only a minor cut or scratch, clean it with soap and water and then cover it with a dry dressing. Be sure to change the dressing daily.)

If you're unable to lift your feet up close enough to your eyes to inspect them, you can try using a mirror propped up against a wall (like you see in shoe stores) or you can buy a mirror with an angled handle. We prefer a telescoping self-examination mirror. If you buy this, be sure to get one that comes with a light. These can be hard to find in retail outlets; one online Canadian source that sells such a device is Diabeters (www.diabeaters.com).

Here's one other simple, effective, and very inexpensive way to have your feet inspected: Ask a loved one to check your feet for you. Don't worry about asking. Remember, if they love you, they love *all* of you.

Skin Disease in Diabetes

You may already have discovered that to cope with diabetes it sometimes helps to have a thick skin, in a manner of speaking. Well, we'll save for another time our discussion about how to deal with well-meaning but irritating casual acquaintances who insist on acting like diabetes police by instructing you about what you can and cannot eat. In this section we focus on the less figurative thick skin that people with diabetes can get as well as other skin problems that are of special importance.

You don't have to be concerned about many serious skin problems, but you should watch out for the following:

- **Lipohypertrophy:** This is a build-up of fatty tissue under the skin in areas of repeated insulin injection (especially if you are reusing your needles — which, by the way, we don't advocate). It appears as bumps — sometimes as large as tennis balls (or even cantaloupes!). It isn't a danger in and of itself, but it's of major importance in another way. Insulin absorption from areas of lipohypertrophy is erratic and, not surprisingly, causes erratic blood glucose control.

Never inject insulin into areas of lipohypertrophy. By avoiding inject-ing insulin into these affected areas, the lipohypertrophy will gradually shrink, but it can take years to see much improvement. (Many people with diabetes treated with insulin develop a favourite spot to inject and repeatedly use this same area; this is a sure-fire way of promoting lipo-hypertrophy.)

✔ **Sores on the feet:** Take *any* wound, ulcer, sore, or other form of skin breakdown on the feet very seriously. See the section "Foot Disease in Diabetes" earlier in this chapter for more information.

Some skin problems may raise worries but in fact are fairly harmless. These include the following:

✔ **Acanthosis nigricans:** This is a dark, velvety increase in pigmentation on the back of the neck and the armpits in some people with type 2 dia-betes. (It can also occur without type 2 diabetes if you have insulin resis-tance.) It isn't dangerous and doesn't require treatment.

✔ **Bruising:** This may occur at insulin injection sites.

✔ **Nail infections:** The medical term for this is *onychomycoses*. People with diabetes commonly develop fungal infections of the toenails. The affected nails appear thickened and yellow-brown. The problem is not serious in and of itself, but if you have a fungal nail infection, you should pay special attention to the health of the skin around the nail to make sure that your nail is not irritating it (and making it red, abraded, or sore). Infected nails can be treated with anti-fungal medicine, but this is usually unnecessary. The nails can be quite difficult to cut, in which case we recommend that you have it done professionally (by a podiatrist or other professional foot professional).

✔ **Necrobiosis Lipoidica Diabeticorum:** Try saying that quickly three times (assuming you can pronounce it in the first place)! This mouthful of a disease (fortunately abbreviated as NLD) affects the legs and feet (rarely the upper limbs) and presents itself as reddish-brown, shiny patches. The skin is often thinner in these areas. Only rarely does it lead to significant problems apart from its cosmetic importance. No particu-larly effective treatment exists, but corticosteroid medication injected into the affected area or applied topically is sometimes used. Typically, NLD fades with time.

✔ **Thickened skin:** As mentioned in the introduction to this section, people with diabetes can have thickening of the skin. This is felt as, well, thick skin. It is not important and will not make you unwell.

✔ **Vitiligo:** People with this condition lose normal skin pigmentation and look very pale. Vitiligo is not unique to diabetes, but type 1 (not type 2) diabetes does put you at increased risk of developing it. Vitiligo has cos-metic importance (especially for African Canadians), but is not a threat to your health.

✔ **Xanthomata:** These are small, yellow marks that can occur in a variety of parts of the body, especially the eyelids (where they are called xanthelasma). Their importance is confined to the fact that they are often a clue that your lipids may be abnormal (see earlier in this chapter for a discussion about lipids).

Musculoskeletal Problems (Muscles, Joints, and Such)

The *musculoskeletal system* in your body is made up of your muscles, bones, joints, and connecting material (such as ligaments and tendons), all of which allow for movement and locomotion. When most people think diabetes, they usually don't think of musculoskeletal problems, but, for unknown reasons, these too (alas) can occur. The most important types are as follows:

✔ **Carpal tunnel syndrome:** In this condition the *median nerve* gets compressed as it travels through the wrist. It can cause a feeling of numbness in the hand (particularly the thumb, index, and middle fingers). Carpal tunnel syndrome can occur for many reasons, diabetes among them. Treatment is geared toward avoiding precipitating factors (such as *repetitive strain injury,* as can occur with prolonged typing) and, if necessary, splinting, medication, or even surgery can be used.

✔ **Diabetic hand syndrome:** In this condition the hands feel stiff and sore. As you might imagine, many people without diabetes can also develop similar symptoms. Treatment is with anti-inflammatory medication and physiotherapy.

✔ **Frozen shoulder:** Even during another muggy summer heat wave, you can run into problems with a frozen shoulder. *Frozen shoulder* is a condition where your shoulder joint becomes stiff (and sometimes a bit painful) as a result of inflammation in the capsule that surrounds the joint. Treatment options include physiotherapy, anti-inflammatory medication, steroid injections into the joint (this procedure is most often done by either a *rheumatologist* — that is, an arthritis doctor — or an orthopedic surgeon), and, in severe cases, surgery.

Gum Disease in Diabetes

If diabetes can affect you from head (hair loss) to toe (peripheral neuropathy), inside (atherosclerosis) and out (necrobiosis), is it any wonder that it can even affect your gums? Regrettably not. But like so much in the world of diabetes, this complication, too, is one you can avoid with proper attention to your health.

Elevated glucose levels within your mouth can promote the growth of bacteria. These germs can attack the gums, causing *gingivitis* (gum infection), which in turn can lead to problems with your teeth and, of greater concern, blood infections. Conversely, gingivitis, like other infections in your body, can make your blood glucose control worse.

The required treatment is one that your mother (or father, of course) likely prescribed for you when you were 5 years old. Brush your teeth twice a day, floss your teeth once a day, and see your dentist regularly. It's that simple.

Chapter 7

Diabetes, Sexual Function, and Pregnancy

*A*s diabetes specialists, for us nothing is quite so thrilling and rewarding as seeing "one of our moms" as she proudly holds her healthy newborn. We look at this beautiful scene and know that until the past few decades, women with diabetes seldom were fortunate enough to enjoy the miracle of creating a new life. Getting pregnant was difficult, miscarriages were common, and birth defects were all too frequent. But nowadays that has all changed. The great majority of women with diabetes can have successful pregnancies and healthy infants. Achieving such a wonderful outcome isn't easy — indeed, it's a ton of work for the mom-to-be — but it can be done. We see it all the time.

And, of course, sexual intercourse remains the starting point for most babies. People with diabetes — both male and female — can have problems with sexual function, but, once again, very effective therapies are now available for what used to be treated quite ineffectively or ignored (by both doctors and patients) altogether.

This chapter discusses how you can overcome problems with sexual dysfunction related to diabetes as well as the important things you should know about in order to have a healthy pregnancy.

Erectile Dysfunction Due to Diabetes

If carefully questioned, up to 50 percent of all males with diabetes will acknowledge having difficulty with sexual function. This difficulty usually takes the form of *erectile dysfunction,* the inability to have or sustain an erection sufficient for intercourse.

Another form of sexual dysfunction that can occur with longstanding diabetes is called *retrograde ejaculation,* wherein you are able to achieve a normal erection and experience a normal orgasm, but no semen emerges from the penis, having instead been sent the reverse direction into the bladder. This is not a serious problem and requires treatment only if you wish to father a child.

Why the spirit may be willing, but the penis isn't

Erectile dysfunction (ED) in a man with diabetes is usually due to poor blood supply and/or nerve damage to the penis. Nonetheless, you and your doctor must not fall into the all-too-common trap of assuming that if you have diabetes, every conceivable problem you might develop must be diabetes related. People with diabetes can encounter the same problems as everyone else. Or, as Henry Kissinger (or Golda Meir, some would argue) famously said, "Even paranoids have enemies." Some non-diabetes-related causes of erectile dysfunction include the following:

- **An adverse effect from medication:** This is particularly common with medicines such as beta blockers, thiazide diuretics, and some antidepressants.

- **Hormonal abnormalities:** Insufficient levels of the male hormone testosterone or excess levels of a pituitary hormone called prolactin can interfere with normal sexual function.

- **Psychological factors:** Problems such as stress and depression can interfere with normal sexual function.

- **Trauma and other physical abnormalities of the penis:** Peyronie's disease, for example, causes a curvature of the erect penis which, if severe, can make intercourse difficult. See the anecdote below.

Psychological factors — whether anxiety, stress, depression, or something else — leading to erectile dysfunction are, of course, no less important to address than any other cause, including diabetes. Your family physician can help determine whether a psychological factor is the cause of your sexual difficulties, and effective therapy is available to help you.

Ron, a 30-year-old man, came to see Ian in the office for a routine appointment. He said everything was going well and that he had no complaints. As he regularly does, Ian asked if Ron had had any problems with his erections. Ron denied any difficulties but didn't sound very convincing and, with a bit of prompting, acknowledged that something was amiss. He said he was getting erections but they "weren't straight." Ian arranged for Ron to meet with a urologist (a doctor who specializes in urinary tract and genital problems), who found that Ron had developed some scar tissue on his penis that was making his erections curved (Peyronie's disease). Ron was successfully treated and immeasurably happier at the time of his next office visit.

The moral of Ron's story is twofold: First, your doctor is there to help you — *all* of you! — so you should feel free to bring up *any* problems you are experiencing; and second, neither you nor your doctor should automatically assume that every symptom you have is necessarily related to your diabetes.

You can help protect yourself from developing erectile dysfunction by

- Maintaining good blood glucose, blood pressure, and lipid control
- Avoiding the consumption of excess quantities of alcohol
- Not smoking (Smoking leads to blockage of the arteries, including the arteries that supply blood to the penis.)

Many men are hesitant or downright embarrassed to bring up their ED problems with their doctor, often to the point of not mentioning it at all. That's understandable, but it's also a shame. Your doctor sees hundreds of men with the same problem you have, and his or her obvious comfort discussing this issue will immediately put you at ease.

How to improve erectile dysfunction

Fortunately, many different therapies are available to treat erectile dysfunction, with an overall success rate of over 90 percent. Some treatments are geared toward correcting specific reversible causes (such as stopping a medicine if it is causing your problem). Other treatments include the following:

- **Oral medications (Cialis, Levitra, Viagra):** These are members of the PDE5 (phosphodiesterase type 5) inhibitor family of medicines. You can't miss the plethora of advertising for these drugs. The benefits are well known. Each of these drugs has somewhat different properties but they are more similar than dissimilar. Some people respond better to one of these drugs than another, so, if one doesn't work, discuss trying another with your doctor.

PDE5 inhibitors are not free of the potential for side effects. Some men experience headaches, facial flushing, or indigestion. These drugs can also cause a temporary colour tinge to a man's vision as well as increased sensitivity to light and blurred vision. These side effects tend to decline with continued use of the medicines.

One important group of men must not take these medicines. Men who have chest pain due to coronary artery disease (see Chapter 6) often take nitrate drugs (such as nitroglycerine). The combination of a PDE5 inhibitor and nitrates may cause a significant and possibly fatal drop in blood pressure.

✔ **Injection into the penis:** Several types of medicine can be injected directly into the penis to create an erection. The most commonly used is a medicine going by the trade name Caverject. This may sound pretty nasty, but if you can overcome the understandable fear of giving yourself a needle in the penis, you'll find that the amount of discomfort is usually minimal and that this type of therapy is often very effective.

✔ **Suppository in the penis:** This form of therapy involves inserting a small amount of medicine (MUSE) directly into the urethral opening at the tip of the penis. The success rate is not as good as with the two previously mentioned options.

✔ **Vacuum device:** This is a tube that fits directly over the penis and, with the use of a connected pump, allows for blood to fill the penis, at which point an erection is achieved and a rubber band is placed around the base of the penis to prevent the blood from escaping. Some men find the device cumbersome to use, but in general it is quite effective, and we feel that this is an under-used therapy.

✔ **Implanted penile prosthesis:** If none of the other measures in this list is helping, another option is to have a prosthesis surgically implanted directly into the penis. A variety of types are available, some of which create a permanent erection while others have an implanted pump (placed in the scrotum) that allows for creation of an erection on an on-demand basis. As with a car, the fancier the equipment, the more expensive the device and the more things that can go wrong, but in general this is a very successful treatment.

Viagra — and other drugs from this family — are almost always the first treatment used. If you do not respond to this type of therapy, we recommend you be referred to a urologist — they are the experts when it comes to treating erectile dysfunction — to see if you might benefit from one of the other treatment options listed above.

Dealing with Female Sexual Problems Related to Diabetes

Sexual problems in women with diabetes have, regrettably, not received nearly the attention that male sexual difficulties have. Some types of female sexual dysfunction, though not unique to people with diabetes, are more common for them. Fortunately, treatment is available that will allow you to have an active and pleasurable sex life. Here are the most frequent issues you are likely to encounter:

- **Vaginal dryness:** The most common causes are poor glucose control, nerve damage, impaired blood flow, or estrogen deficiency. Vaginal dryness makes intercourse more difficult and less pleasurable (lubrication increases vaginal sensitivity) — sometimes even painful. It can be treated with lubricants that are water-based (such as K-Y Jelly) or oil-based (such as vegetable oil). Water-based lubricants are easier to clean up. Oral stimulation by your partner may also assist in lubricating the vagina. If you are menopausal, lack of estrogen could be the main cause of your vaginal dryness, in which case vaginal estrogen preparations (which are much safer than oral estrogen) may be an option for you. To know if vaginal estrogen therapy is a suitable option for you, ask your doctor to review your specific situation.

- **Vaginal yeast infections:** Diabetes and, in particular, poor blood glucose control can make you prone to recurrent vaginal infections. Improving your glucose control and taking an antifungal medicine would be in order.

- **Vaginal thinning:** Menopause leads to lower levels of estrogen and this, in turn, can cause not only vaginal dryness (see the first item in this list) but can also cause the lining of the vagina to become thin. In this case vaginal estrogen therapy may be an option for you.

- **Decreased genital sensation:** Nerve damage can lead to reduced sensitivity around the genital area and this, in turn, can reduce sexual enjoyment. Treatment options include gentle stimulation by touch or by use of a hand-held vibrator gently applied to the clitoris.

- **Bladder problems:** If you have difficulty controlling your bladder, you may experience leakage during intercourse. Try to empty your bladder before intercourse. Other treatments, depending on the cause of the problem, include medication or surgery (bladder suspension).

- **Adverse effects from medications:** Some medicines — particularly some types of antidepressants — can interfere with sexual function. If you have recently started a new medicine only to find your sexual function becomes impaired, speak to your doctor about possibly switching to a different medicine.

✔ **Psychological factors:** Many different psychological factors can influence your ability to enjoy sexual relations, including poor self-image if you are dissatisfied with your appearance or if you are concerned that your partner may be dissatisfied with your appearance. As you work with nutrition therapy, weight loss (if you are overweight), and exercise to improve your glucose control, you may find you're seeing yourself (and your partner is seeing you) as more attractive, and that, in turn, may be the best therapy of all for your sexual dysfunction. If you're feeling anxious, stressed, or depressed, it would be wise for you to speak to your doctor about this to see what kind of help he or she can offer. In some cases your doctor may wish to refer you to a specialist for therapy.

Pregnancy and Diabetes

If you have diabetes, pregnancy does complicate matters; often quite a bit. Nonetheless, it can and will still be a period of joy, excitement, and anticipation. You will not likely ever have another time when the efforts you apply to your diabetes are so crucial, and you can be assured you'll have many people working with you all the way.

When we talk about diabetes and pregnancy, we distinguish temporary, pregnancy-related diabetes *(gestational diabetes)* from diabetes that was present before you got pregnant *(pregestational diabetes)*. (Technically, gestational diabetes refers to *any* form of diabetes discovered during pregnancy. However, in the overwhelming majority of cases, when diabetes is found during pregnancy, it is temporary, pregnancy-induced diabetes, not pregestational diabetes.) The implications, risks, and treatment are very different for each of these types.

Gestational diabetes

Gestational diabetes (abbreviated as GDM which is short for *gestational diabetes mellitus*) occurs in women who had normal blood glucose levels before pregnancy, but who run into elevations of blood glucose *during* pregnancy. The degree of glucose elevation is so mild that symptoms of hyperglycemia (see Chapter 2), such as increased thirst and visual blurring, do not develop. (Of course you may develop a frequent urge to pass urine during your pregnancy, but that is not due to gestational diabetes; it is due to a growing future gymnast having decided to test out his or her skills by doing flips on your bladder or, as Ian's wife used to say, doing "bladder dancing.")

Gestational diabetes is very common, developing in about 4 percent of pregnancies. This percentage is much higher in certain populations; for example, it develops in up to 18 percent of pregnancies in Aboriginal peoples. Most women with GDM have otherwise uneventful pregnancies and perfectly healthy babies. The reason we look for and treat GDM is to take good odds for a successful pregnancy and make them even better.

Exploring the causes of gestational diabetes

As you might imagine, many hormonal changes take place during pregnancy, not the least of which is the release of hormones produced by the *placenta*. These placental hormones increase insulin resistance (see Chapter 3 for a discussion of insulin resistance). In a normal pregnancy, the pancreas can respond to this challenge by increasing the amount of insulin it makes so that your blood glucose control would remain normal. If you develop GDM, it means that your pancreas cannot respond sufficiently, so your blood glucose levels rise above normal.

Diagnosing gestational diabetes

The Canadian Diabetes Association recommends every pregnant woman be tested for GDM. The way you should be tested for GDM is as follows:

- **50-gram challenge:** When you reach 24 to 28 weeks into your pregnancy, your doctor should order this test. It requires you to drink a sweet drink containing 50 grams of carbohydrate. You don't have to be fasting for this test. One hour after you drink the fluid, the laboratory will draw a blood sample from your arm to check your glucose level.

  - If your test result is less than 7.8 (mmol/L), it is normal and you do not have GDM.

  - If your test result is 7.8 up to (and including) 10.2, your doctor should send you for a glucose tolerance test (which we discuss next).

  - If your test result is 10.3 or higher, you have GDM and no further testing is required to make the diagnosis.

- **75-gram glucose tolerance test (GTT):** An abnormal 50-gram challenge is not sufficient to indicate that you have GDM (unless your result is 10.3 mmol/L or higher). All the 50-gram challenge does is determine whether you have a strong enough likelihood of having GDM to proceed with the next stage of screening — that is, a GTT. For this test, after you fast for eight hours, a health care professional will draw blood from you *before*, and then one and two hours *after*, drinking a sweet drink containing 75 grams of carbohydrate. You have GDM if you have *two* or more abnormalities on the GTT; that is, two or more of the following results:

- Fasting blood glucose 5.3 mmol/L or higher
- One-hour blood glucose 10.6 mmol/L or higher
- Two-hour blood glucose 8.9 mmol/L or higher

If you have only one abnormal reading, you have *impaired glucose tolerance (IGT) of pregnancy*. This has a similar impact on pregnancy as GDM, and the Canadian Diabetes Association recommends it be treated the same way.

If you are at high risk for GDM (as is the case if, for example, you have previously had GDM, if you've previously delivered a large infant, if you're 35 years of age or older, if you have a BMI of 30 or greater — see Chapter 4 — or if you are a member of a high-risk population such as being of Aboriginal, Hispanic, South Asian, Asian, or African descent), then you should be tested during your first trimester (that is, the first one-third of your pregnancy). If your test result is normal, you should be re-tested periodically throughout your pregnancy.

Treating gestational diabetes

As with other forms of diabetes, the most important part of the treatment of gestational diabetes is what *you* do for you, not what others do for you, so it is essential that you be provided with the necessary tools. When these cornerstones of therapy are not sufficient, medications are added.

Non-medication therapy

These are the key non-medication therapies used to treat your GDM:

- ✔ **Education:** Your doctor should refer you to a diabetes education centre where you will meet with a dietitian and a nurse educator who will provide you with the knowledge you need to help control this condition. Your doctor should also refer you to a diabetes specialist. The diabetes specialist will typically coordinate your diabetes care, help teach you about your GDM, review your blood glucose readings, and manage any medication you require for your GDM treatment.

- ✔ **Proper nutrition:** Your dietitian will set you up with a healthy eating program. This program will be geared toward assisting with blood glucose control while allowing for appropriate weight gain and ensuring adequate nutrition. Your carbohydrate intake will be distributed over three meals and at least three snacks (one of which will be at bedtime). Think of this as a therapeutic indulgence! Your target weight gain will be based, at least in part, on your pre-pregnant weight.

- ✔ **Exercise:** Because GDM is associated with insulin resistance, and because insulin resistance is improved (though not eliminated) by exercise, daily exercise can help control your blood glucose readings. We're not talking marathon running here; even just taking a daily walk can help. Your doctor or diabetes educator can provide you with other exercise recommendations based on your specific circumstances and stage of pregnancy.

Medication therapy

If your blood glucose readings are too high (we discuss blood glucose targets in the next section) despite one to two weeks of lifestyle therapy (that is, nutrition and exercise) then medication is required. Because of its proven safety and effectiveness in treating GDM, insulin is almost always the preferred drug. (We discuss principles of insulin therapy in Chapter 13.) The idea of having to give yourself insulin may not sound particularly pleasant, but bear in mind two things:

✔ Unlike taxes and Canadian winters, insulin won't be forever. The moment you deliver your baby, you'll discontinue your insulin.

✔ Your efforts during your pregnancy will help you have a healthy baby. What could possibly be a better reward than that?

The Canadian Diabetes Association recommends oral medication (instead of insulin) be used only for women with GDM who either decline insulin therapy or are taking insulin but, basically, are missing so many doses that it's not doing much good. The only recommended oral medications are glyburide and metformin. (We discuss these drugs in Chapter 12.) In the future, should there be sufficient scientific evidence that oral medications are as safe and effective as insulin, it's likely that their use will become more recommended.

If you take insulin, you'll find that your insulin requirements progressively increase as your pregnancy goes along. This is perfectly normal. Your diabetes educators and diabetes specialist will help you adjust your insulin doses (and, indeed, will teach you how to adjust them on your own).

Monitoring gestational diabetes

In order for you and your health care team to know if your treatment program is successfully controlling your blood glucose levels, you will need to perform certain tests:

✔ **Blood glucose testing:** Most diabetes education centres (DECs) will be able to provide you, free of charge, with a glucose meter (though not necessarily the blood glucose test strips), and will show you how to use it and how often to test (this may be as much as four or more times per day; the frequency of testing will depend on what kind of therapy you are on). See Chapter 9 for more on glucose meters.

These are the Canadian Diabetes Association target blood glucose readings for GDM:

- Fasting and before meals: 3.8 to 5.2 mmol/L

- One hour after meals: 5.5 to 7.7 mmol/L

- Two hours after meals: 5.0 to 6.6 mmol/L

"One hour after meals" refers to one hour after you first *begin* your meal. Similarly, "two hours after meals" refers to two hours after you begin your meal.

Whether it's best to test one hour after a meal or two hours after a meal is a subject of controversy. Some doctors advocate choosing whichever of these times produced the highest value during your GTT (a test we explain in the section "Diagnosing gestational diabetes," earlier). Some doctors recommend you choose whichever of those two times is most convenient for you, and some doctors feel it doesn't matter. Your doctor will make his or her own recommendation for you.

✔ **Urine ketone testing:** Your diabetes educators will also teach you how to test your urine for ketones. *Ketones* are a type of acid that, when present in the urine, may indicate that you are not consuming an adequate diet (in which case it is wise to call the dietitian to review your diet). Urine ketone testing is typically done once daily, first thing in the morning. You should have hardly any ketones in your urine.

Understanding the potential complications for the mother

Most moms with gestational diabetes sail through their pregnancy with no complications and deliver perfectly healthy babies. Serious complications seldom occur. If you have gestational diabetes, you do face an increased likelihood that you'll end up delivering by Caesarian section because you will be at risk of having a big baby (see the next section), and your obstetrician may determine that it would be unsafe for you to deliver vaginally.

Considering the potential complications for the baby

Your baby will likely be completely fine. Your baby will *not* be born with diabetes and your baby will *not* be at greater risk of birth defects. Two important possible complications exist:

✔ **Macrosomia:** This is the medical term for a large baby. Elevated blood glucose levels put your infant at higher risk of being large (which can complicate delivery). Medical science typically assumes the baby to be at risk of being large because if the mom's glucose levels are high, that glucose travels through the placenta into the baby's circulation and it is akin to overfeeding the baby in the uterus. Things may indeed be that simple; but in medicine, whenever things seem really simple, one can't help but be reminded of a famous quote from H. L. Mencken: "For every complex question there's a simple answer . . . *and it's wrong.*" The reason for a baby having macrosomia is likely far more complex and related to other maternal metabolic factors, genetics, and other undetermined issues.

✔ **Hypoglycemia:** This is low blood glucose, and your baby may develop it shortly after being born. It is usually easily treated by giving your baby sugar water to drink.

Other complications (such as the baby having low calcium) occur far less frequently.

If you have GDM and you deliver a large baby, you may find the hospital staff (including, alas, some doctors) look at you reproachfully (egads!) and suggest or even directly say to you that your baby is large because you didn't adequately look after your diabetes and, in particular, that your blood glucose control was insufficient. However, if you're like the overwhelming majority of women with GDM that we see in our practices, you've delivered a large infant *despite* conscientiously looking after yourself and maintaining excellent blood glucose control. In other words, the fact that your baby was large had *nothing* at all to do with anything you did or did not do. Maybe you were simply destined to have a big baby, pure and simple. Or maybe your baby was big unrelated to anything to do with your blood glucose control. In either case, you have two choices: You can either correct the staff on their misapprehension or you can grin and bear it. Your call. Don't feel guilty; the reality of the situation is that you've done nothing wrong and, indeed, have done most everything right!

Knowing what to do after you've had your baby

Now that you've had your baby, you no longer have gestational diabetes, but there remain some very important things left to do (in addition to the million other responsibilities you now have!):

✔ **Breastfeeding:** Breastfeeding has many benefits for both mom and infant, with special additional benefits if you've had GDM — evidence suggests that breastfeeding may reduce your risk *and* your child's risk of subsequently developing type 2 diabetes. It may also help prevent your child from becoming overweight.

✔ **Following a healthy lifestyle:** If you have (or have previously had) GDM, you are at very, very high risk of developing type 2 diabetes. You can, however, substantially reduce this risk by following a very healthy lifestyle after you have your baby. Do your utmost to achieve and maintain a good weight. Eat healthfully. Exercise. After all, you've got a family to stay healthy for!

✔ **Being screened for type 2 diabetes:** Because having had GDM means you are at high risk of subsequently developing type 2 diabetes, you will need to be screened for this from time to time. The Canadian Diabetes Association recommends the following:

- Between six weeks and six months of delivery, you should have a 75-gram glucose tolerance test. See the following Tip for additional information.

- You should have ongoing periodic screening for type 2 diabetes (see the Cheat Sheet at the front of this book for the scoop on this).

- You should be screened for type 2 diabetes *prior to* any future pregnancies. This is very important because if you have developed type 2 diabetes and then get pregnant, the implications are far, far greater than was the case when you had GDM. We discuss this in detail later in this chapter (see "Pregestational diabetes").

Many women never end up having their glucose tolerance performed after they've delivered. (This happens for a variety of reasons, including the fact that, after you deliver, the doctor that monitored your GDM during the pregnancy may no longer be involved in your care. Also, you are likely going to be run off your feet looking after your newborn and, even if your doctor previously discussed the need for the test with you, in the hectic life that is new motherhood, it simply may not happen.) To avoid missing this important test, we recommend that you and the doctor (likely your diabetes specialist) who's been helping you with your GDM during the pregnancy organize the post-pregnancy GTT *before* you deliver. Doing so may be as simple as you being given the necessary lab requisition toward the end of your pregnancy and noting on your calendar when you are to have it done. (And don't forget to be in touch with your doctor a few days after the test to get the results and to find out what is to be done if it's abnormal.)

- ✔ **Keeping an eye out for the development of symptoms of hyperglycemia:** If you start having symptoms of high blood glucose (we talk about how high blood glucose makes you feel in Chapter 2), promptly see your doctor to have your blood glucose level checked.

Facing fears about gestational diabetes

When Dominique first found out that she had gestational diabetes, she was certain that meant that her baby was going to be huge. She had heard that "it's always like that." She had also heard from well-meaning but uninformed friends that her baby would probably have diabetes. When Ian met her for the first time, he spent almost the entire interview reassuring Dominique, not warning her.

By the time the appointment was over, newly aware that, with proper attention, her pregnancy would almost certainly be smooth and her baby would be the picture of health, she was smiling ear to ear. As she passed through the waiting room, Ian smiled equally broadly as he overheard Dominique say to a seated, anxious-appearing pregnant woman, "Hey, don't worry, everything's going to be just fine!"

Pregestational diabetes

Pregestational diabetes is diabetes that you had *before* you became pregnant (and will still have after you deliver), whereas *gestational* diabetes is diabetes that is acquired during pregnancy and that resolves once you have had your baby. If you have type 1 or type 2 diabetes and you get pregnant, then you have pregestational diabetes. If *only* the father has diabetes, none of this discussion applies to you. Only when the mother has diabetes do these issues apply.

If you have diabetes and get pregnant, you have an excellent chance that everything will go well for you and, nine months down the road, your dreams will be fulfilled and you'll hold a beautiful, bouncing, healthy baby. You are, perhaps, waiting for a "but." If so, then you're right. Everything *can* go well for you, *but* to achieve your dream you must follow many precautions. We hate to be dogmatic, but we feel so strongly about the issue of pregestational diabetes that in this section we are going to sound far more "black and white" about things than pretty well anywhere else in this book.

Although the odds are good that you won't run into serious problems during your pregnancy, the risk of complications is very real. We look at these next.

Knowing what can happen to the mom

Thankfully, most pregnant woman with pregestational diabetes don't run into problems, but there is an increased risk of the following:

- **High blood pressure and toxemia:** *Toxemia* is a condition of raised blood pressure and fluid retention leading to swelling and, at times, more serious complications. High blood pressure can be treated with medications. Toxemia generally requires hospitalization and early delivery.

- **Deterioration in eyesight:** This rarely occurs unless you have at least some retinal damage before you get pregnant. If severe, you may require retinal laser surgery. We discuss diabetes eye disease in more detail in Chapter 6.

- **Deterioration in kidney function:** This rarely occurs unless you have kidney malfunction *before* you get pregnant. We discuss diabetes and kidney function in Chapter 6.

- **Insulin reactions (including severe insulin reactions due to hypoglycemia unawareness):** Because you will be keeping your blood glucose levels under exceptionally tight control, you will likely experience more frequent hypoglycemia than ever before. You will also be more prone to hypoglycemia unawareness and, as a result, severe hypoglycemia (particularly toward the end of your first trimester). We discuss hypoglycemia unawareness and severe hypoglycemia in more detail in Chapter 5.

Knowing what can happen to the fetus and baby

Most of the time the fetus and baby are perfectly healthy, but there is an increased risk of the following:

- **Miscarriage:** Miscarriages are more common if your blood glucose control is poor in the early stages of pregnancy. If your control is excellent in early pregnancy, your risk of a miscarriage is much less.

- **Birth defects:** The medical term for birth defect is *congenital anomaly.* This is the most dreaded complication of all, but fortunately it's largely preventable. If your blood glucose control at the time you get pregnant and for the first 12 weeks or so thereafter (when your baby's organs are forming) is excellent, your risk of having a baby with a congenital anomaly is about the same as if you never had diabetes (about 2 to 3 percent). On the other hand, if your blood glucose control is poor during this critical period of time, your risk is as high as 30 percent. An astounding difference, indeed. And one that you can directly influence.

- **Other health problems:** These include difficulty breathing, prematurity, small or large size, and disorders of body chemistry such as low blood glucose or low calcium. Your baby will *not* be born with diabetes.

We hope that as you read through the two preceding intimidating lists you noticed the recurring theme that these complications are usually avoidable. Most women with pregestational diabetes do *not* experience these complications!

Reviewing things to do before you get pregnant

To maximize your likelihood of having a healthy pregnancy and a healthy baby, here's what you should do *before* you get pregnant:

- **Be in regular touch with your health care team.** We discuss the members of the health care team and their respective roles in Chapter 8. Reviewing with your diabetes specialist whether it's safe for you to proceed with trying to conceive is essential. Safety will be determined based largely on the other factors in this list.

- **Achieve excellent blood glucose control (A1C 7 or less).** Your A1C level (this is measured on a blood sample) reflects your overall blood glucose control for approximately the last three months. Having an excellent A1C at the time of conception and for the first few months of pregnancy will dramatically lower your risk of miscarrying or having a baby with a birth defect. Target pre-conception A1C is 7 or less, but reaching a value of under 6 is even better (though very difficult to achieve). We discuss A1C in detail in Chapter 9.

✔ **See your eye specialist.** Because retinopathy (we discuss retinopathy in Chapter 6) can rapidly progress during pregnancy, having your eye doctor assess the health of your eyes *before* you get pregnant is crucial.

✔ **Have your kidneys tested.** If your kidneys are healthy before you get pregnant, they'll almost certainly remain healthy during your pregnancy. But if your kidneys are damaged to begin with, your kidney function can significantly worsen during pregnancy. Your doctor can assess your kidneys through very simple blood and urine tests (as we discuss in Chapter 6).

✔ **Have your blood pressure tested.** Having high blood pressure before you get pregnant puts you at much higher risk of running into more severe blood pressure problems during your pregnancy.

✔ **Have your medicines reviewed.** Your doctor will need to review any medicines you are taking, and if they're unsafe to take during pregnancy (as is true, for example, of ACE inhibitors, ARBs, and cholesterol-lowering *statin* medicines), you will need to stop taking them. If you have type 2 diabetes treated with oral hypoglycemic agents (see Chapter 12), you will need to stop taking them and start on insulin well before you try to get pregnant. (The exception is if you have infertility related to a condition called polycystic ovary syndrome (PCOS), in which case your obstetrician may advise you to take metformin to help you get pregnant and, typically, to discontinue it after you do.)

✔ **Ask questions.** Nothing in your life will ever be as important as your quest to have a healthy baby. If you have questions about the impact of your diabetes on your pregnancy, *ask*. Ask your family doctor, ask your diabetes specialist, ask your diabetes educators, ask your obstetrician; ask *anyone* who is a part of your health care team. As well, don't forget to make sure your partner is fully involved. Your partner needs to know what you're going to be contending with.

✔ **Take folic acid supplements.** Taking folic acid supplements is important to help prevent certain types of birth defects (see the sidebar "Folic acid supplements during pregnancy"). Take 5 mg per day starting three months *before* you get pregnant and continuing until you are 12 weeks pregnant at which time the dose is reduced to 0.4 mg to 1 mg per day which is continued until you complete breastfeeding.

✔ **Take a multivitamin.** Take a multivitamin starting three months before you get pregnant and continuing until you have completed breastfeeding.

There are available multivitamin preparations that contain folic acid. This will save you taking an extra pill. Be sure, however, that your multivitamin contains the appropriate amount of folic acid (as described in the preceding bullet) for your stage prior to, during, and after pregnancy.

Folic acid supplements during pregnancy

Folic acid supplements taken during pregnancy will help reduce the risk of your baby developing *neural tube defects*. These are serious disorders where a part of the central nervous system fails to develop normally and can result in the fetus having a form of impaired brain growth (anencephaly) or a spinal disorder (spina bifida). Neural tube defects occur in the very earliest stages of pregnancy — usually before you would even be aware that you are pregnant. Women with diabetes are at higher risk of having a baby with neural tube defects.

Managing your health while you are pregnant

Congratulations. You have done everything you had to, and you are now a proud, though perhaps apprehensive, mother-to-be. So what next? These are the things that you will need to do during your pregnancy:

- **If you drive, get a rewards card for your favourite gas station.** You'll be spending a lot of time in your car, what with visits to the diabetes nurse educator, the dietitian, your doctors, and so on. (Ian advises his patients with pregestational diabetes to expect to see health care providers over 50 times during the pregnancy.) So when you fill up, look at the bright side: You're earning points toward that holiday you will so richly deserve (even if you have to delay taking it).

- **Have your diet adjusted.** Your dietitian will work with you to devise an appropriate meal plan designed to ensure adequate nutrition while assisting with blood glucose control and appropriate weight gain. Your carbohydrate intake will be moderately restricted and you will be advised to eat three meals and three snacks per day (one of which will be a bedtime snack).

- **Monitor your blood glucose levels frequently.** Our preference is for a *minimum* of six tests per day (before and after every meal). Testing at bedtime and, occasionally, overnight is also advised. After-meal tests can be done either one or two hours after you've started eating so long as the appropriate target value is taken into account as the following list of CDA-recommended target blood glucose levels illustrates:

  - Fasting and before meals: 3.8 to 5.2 mmol/L

  - 1 hour after meals: 5.5 to 7.7 mmol/L

  - 2 hours after meals: 5.0 to 6.6 mmol/L

- **Have your A1C checked monthly.** Target A1C is 6 or less (that is, in the normal range). Keeping your blood glucose under excellent control will help your baby develop normally. Bear in mind, however, that obtaining uniformly normal values for blood glucose or A1C may simply not be possible (for example, if it's leading to excessively frequent or severe episodes of hypoglycemia). Though you should strive for perfect control, the truth of the matter is that achieving it is rarely, if ever, possible. Fortunately, occasional mild hyperglycemia is not likely to lead to any harm to your baby. Equally fortunately, if you experience hypoglycemia, it will not hurt your baby.

✔ **Adjust your insulin.** Because the placenta releases hormones that increase insulin resistance (see Chapter 3), your insulin requirement will rise substantially during your pregnancy. It will level off (or even fall somewhat) only during the last few weeks of pregnancy. By the time you deliver, you may be on three (or more) times the amount of insulin you were taking before you got pregnant. Every time you visit your diabetes specialist or diabetes educator, be sure to bring your logbook because they will want to review your readings and insulin doses. They will assist you with insulin adjustment; however, you will almost certainly be able to make most day-to-day changes in dose yourself. (If you have type 2 diabetes and did not require insulin *prior* to your pregnancy, you will, nonetheless, almost certainly require insulin *during* your pregnancy.)

✔ **Test for urine ketones.** Urine ketone testing is typically done once daily, first thing in the morning. You should have hardly any ketones in your urine. (If you have type 1 diabetes, then you're likely familiar with the importance of testing your blood for ketones when DKA is suspected. We discuss blood ketone testing in Chapter 5.)

✔ **See your eye doctor regularly.** The CDA recommends that women with pregestational diabetes see an eye specialist "before conception, during the first trimester, as needed during the pregnancy, and within the first year postpartum." (Because seemingly minor eye damage can progress rapidly during pregnancy, Ian likes to err on the side of great caution and, hence, recommends that *all* his patients with pregestational diabetes — even those with no observed retinopathy — meet with the eye specialist not only before conception and during the first trimester, but routinely *every* trimester and then again *three months* after delivering. Better one eye exam too many than one too few!)

If you reside in a community with access to genetics counselling, your doctor may refer you to this service. A geneticist will review your particular situation to assess your risk of having a fetus with a problem and, moreover, will arrange sophisticated ultrasound and laboratory studies to determine if the fetus is developing normally.

Knowing what to expect during labour and delivery

Congratulations once again. You've made it through nine months of pregnancy and you're now ready to have your baby.

When you are brought into the hospital, if you have been giving yourself insulin injections, they'll likely be replaced by insulin given through an intravenous as this allows for minute-to-minute fine tuning of the dose. If you have been using an insulin pump (we discuss this form of therapy in Chapter 13), we recommend that, unless something precludes it, you continue with using your pump throughout your labour and delivery.

Until recently, insulin pump therapy was not commonplace and neither physicians (except for diabetes specialists) nor hospital staff were comfortable having their labouring patients use them. As a result, as soon as a woman on a pump went into hospital to deliver, the pump was discontinued and replaced with intravenous insulin, and use of the pump did not resume until a few days post-delivery. Fortunately, this is now changing and most women using pump therapy continue it during their labour and delivery. Speak to your obstetrician well in advance of your delivery about this option. Also, in case you are not up to the challenge of doing your own blood glucose testing and insulin pump adjustment during labour, ensure that your partner is pump-savvy and can assist you. (The odds are overwhelming that you — and possibly your partner — will know much more about pump therapy than most of the staff looking after you.)

During labour, your blood glucose level should be checked often — as often as hourly — and your insulin dose adjusted to keep your blood glucose levels between about 3.8 and 6.6.

As soon as you've delivered, your insulin requirements will plummet. If you have type 2 diabetes, and if you didn't require insulin before your pregnancy, you're not likely to require it after you've delivered. If you have type 1 diabetes, your insulin dose once you deliver will be immediately back to where it was before you got pregnant or, for a day or more, even less (sometimes considerably less).

Mark down in your blood glucose logbook (see Chapter 9) what your insulin doses were prior to your pregnancy. You may find this a helpful reference after you've delivered and are trying to estimate your new insulin requirements. This, however, will be just an estimate, and you'll need to adjust your doses based on your blood glucose values. If you're using insulin pump therapy, you can pre-program a second set of basal rates using your pre-pregnancy doses, and then, once you've delivered, you can easily change your pump over to these settings.

Shortly after you deliver, the hospital staff will check your baby's blood glucose level, and, if it's low, he or she will be given some sugar water to drink. A pediatrician will thoroughly examine your baby to make sure everything is all right.

Nine months of appointments — a lifetime of joy

When Leanne, a newly married woman with type 1 diabetes, asked Ian what would be involved if she were to get pregnant, she was expecting a simple answer. The answer she got, however, was complicated. Leanne was surprised to hear about all the things she would have to do leading up to and then during pregnancy, but she was sure she was up to the challenge and was willing to do "whatever it takes" to have a healthy baby.

During her subsequent pregnancy, what with visits to doctors, the diabetes nurse educator, the dietitian, and so on, at times she felt as if she was "doing nothing but going to appointments," but she persevered. Although her nine months of pregnancy seemed to Leanne to "take forever," all recollection of the hassles she had gone through instantly disappeared the moment she first cradled her newborn infant lovingly in her arms, her only thought being "how lucky" she was to have experienced this joy.

We have looked after hundreds and hundreds of pregnant women with pregestational diabetes. And although you need to be aware of the important issues that we discuss during this chapter, you must know that if you look after yourself properly, your likelihood of having a successful pregnancy is excellent. It may not be easy, but it can be done. As we say at the outset of this chapter, we see it all the time.

Handling your diabetes for the first few months after having your baby

Unless you are unable to do so, breastfeeding is far and away the preferred way for you to supply your newborn with nutrition. Because you'll be providing your baby's nutritional requirements, you'll need to ingest an additional 300 calories or so per day.

If you have type 2 diabetes and were being treated with oral hypoglycemic agents prior to your pregnancy, when you have delivered, your doctor will likely advise you to resume these medications and discontinue your insulin. If, on the other hand, you were taking insulin prior to (and during) the pregnancy, you should expect to continue doing so. Although definitive data are lacking, recent research suggests that metformin and glyburide can be safely taken during breastfeeding. (We do not have studies to tell us if other types of oral hypoglycemic agent therapy — which we discuss in Chapter 12 — can be taken safely in this situation.)

By now, you're likely very familiar with all the reasons that excellent blood glucose control is so crucial to maintaining your good health. And in almost all cases you should be striving for optimal glucose control. Recall, however, that the (terribly unfair) price to be paid for so-called tight blood glucose control is a much higher risk of severe hypoglycemia (which we discuss in Chapter 5). Hypoglycemia is a bad enough problem to begin with, but it is even more of a concern if you are going to be home alone with your newborn. Therefore, if you are prone to frequent or severe hypoglycemia, speak to your diabetes specialist to determine if it would be best for you to have somewhat looser blood glucose control for the first few months after you are home with your baby. Ian also routinely advises "his moms" to not bathe the baby unless another capable person is home to assist in the event that the mom experiences a bad episode of hypoglycemia.

Because, soon after delivering, women with type 1 diabetes are prone to a temporary form of thyroid disease called *postpartum thyroiditis,* the CDA recommends that women with type 1 diabetes have a thyroid blood test (called a TSH; short for thyroid stimulating hormone) done 6 weeks after giving birth. Very few doctors are aware of this new recommendation, so it would be a good idea for you to bring this up with your doctor. You can discover more about postpartum thyroiditis at Dr. Dan Drucker's Web site, www.my thyroid.com/postpartum.html.

Part III
Rule Your Diabetes: Don't Let It Rule You

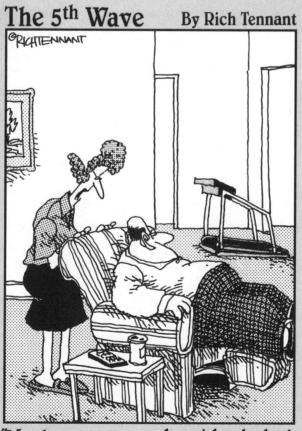

The 5th Wave   By Rich Tennant

"You know, anyone who wishes he had a remote control for his exercise equipment is missing the idea of exercise equipment."

In this part . . .

Is it possible to have diabetes without it dominating your life? You bet! In this part we look at the most effective strategies you can use to control your diabetes and to stay healthy. You'll find out who the members of your health care team are and what roles they play. We also examine the important issues of proper nutrition, exercise, and other therapies available to you, including pills, insulin, and alternative and complementary treatments.

Chapter 8

Meet Your Diabetes Team

. . . .

In This Chapter

▶ Presenting *you*, the star and centre attraction of your diabetes team

▶ Understanding the role of your family physician

▶ Meeting your diabetes specialist

▶ Learning from your diabetes educator

▶ Getting the inside scoop from your dietitian

▶ Looking at your eye specialist

▶ Dispensing knowledge about your pharmacist

▶ Knowing what your foot doctor does

▶ Being supported by family and friends

. . . .

*T*o the best of our knowledge, no hockey team has ever won a medal at the Olympics by sending only one player onto the ice. Nor do we know of any team that ever made it to the podium without having a coach, a general manager, and a slew of fans rooting along the way. And if an Olympic hockey team ever played without a trainer and an equipment manager, it surely must have been way back before Don Cherry put on his first red-checkered sport jacket (with matching lime-green tie, of course!). Heck, it must have been before Howie Morenz notched his first hat trick.

Now it may not be easy to make it onto an Olympic hockey team, but *you* can be the star of *your own* team. Indeed, you should be the star of your own diabetes health care team, because for you to succeed with your diabetes, you must not only be the captain of the team, you must have all the other players working with you. Nothing's second rate about coming home from the Olympics with a silver or bronze, but when it comes to our health, we should always be after the top prize.

In this chapter we look at the different players on your health care team, starting with the first, second, and third star of each and every game. That would be — you guessed it — you. (The only hockey player we can recall who came close to matching your selection as first, second, and third star of the game is Maurice "the Rocket" Richard, who was awarded all three stars back in 1944 after scoring all five Habs' goals in a 5–1 Montreal Canadiens playoff victory. Clearly, you are in rarefied company.)

You Are the Captain of the Team

You may not have wanted to be captain of the team; heck, you didn't want to be on a diabetes team to start with, but here you are, the star of the team, and as you might imagine, with stardom come certain responsibilities. Leadership, for example. This is where diabetes differs from almost any other illness. If you have appendicitis, it isn't very likely that you'll be the one to deliver the anesthetic, hold the scalpel, and put in the stitches. No, your role would be relatively passive as the experts around you tend to your needs. Diabetes is not like that.

When you have diabetes, *you* have to take charge. *You,* after all, live with you. Day and night. Night and day, too, we suspect. *You* are the one who ultimately decides what you will eat, when you will exercise, when you will test your blood glucose levels, when you will take your medicines, and so forth. Other people can offer advice, other people can prompt or even cajole you, but in the end, the decisions are yours. And with your keen and ongoing involvement in your health care, you'll be helping yourself to receive the best possible therapy to achieve and maintain good health.

It may seem rather daunting for you to have so much responsibility placed upon your shoulders. And at times you may simply want people to tell you to "do this" and "do that." But with time and support, you will grow into your role and become comfortable with it.

Here are *your* responsibilities as captain of your health care team. This list may seem intimidating, but you'll be surprised at how quickly these responsibilities can all become part of your normal day-to-day existence:

  ✔ **Follow your lifestyle treatment plan.** This means knowing what foods you should eat, how much, and how often; what exercises you should do and how often you should do them; how much weight — if any — you should lose and the best strategy to achieve this; how much alcohol you can safely drink; and if you smoke and want to quit, what cessation strategies are available to you. (See Chapter 6 for more.)

✔ **Monitor your blood glucose.** You should become familiar with how to test your blood, how often you should test, what your target blood glucose levels are, and, importantly, what you should be doing to achieve these targets. You should also make sure that you have your A1C checked every regularly *and* that you find out the result. (We discuss blood glucose and A1C testing in Chapter 9.)

✔ **Keep track of your blood pressure.** Anytime someone checks your blood pressure, ask what it is and write it down. Become familiar with what your target blood pressure is, and if your readings are too high, ask your doctor how he or she can help you reduce it. (We talk more about high blood pressure in Chapter 6.)

✔ **Keep track of your lipid levels.** As with your blood pressure, anytime someone tests your lipid levels (see Chapter 6 for a discussion on lipids), you should write them down. Also, find out from your doctor what your target levels are, and if you aren't within those targets, ask your doctor how he or she can help you meet those goals.

✔ **Determine if you are at high risk of a heart attack.** Many people with diabetes are at high risk of heart attack and stroke, and, therefore, need to take special precautions to avoid these diseases. In Chapter 6, we look at how you can determine if you have this high risk and, if so, what can be done to help you avoid running into these problems.

✔ **Schedule visits to each member of your health care team.** How often you see each member of the team depends on many circumstances, including your state of health.

Anytime you meet with your health care providers (be it your family doctor, diabetes specialist, eye specialist, diabetes educator, or other member of your health care team), ask them when they want you to return. Book the return appointment *before* you leave the office *and* write down the details on your calendar as soon as you get home (or, for the technologically savvy, in your PDA before you leave the office).

✔ **Know about your medicines.** Every time you see a physician or diabetes educator, bring *all* your medicines with you (both prescription and non-prescription). At the very least, bring a list of your medicines, making note of your drugs' names, dosages, and how many times per day you are taking them. Telling your doctor that you are "on a small blue pill once a day" and a "red capsule twice a day" tells your physician more about the state of your colour vision than the nature of your drugs. Indeed, Ian has seen more than one patient who became very ill because the drugs they *thought* (from memory) they were taking differed significantly from what they were *actually* taking. (For the detailed scoop on medicines, check out *Understanding Prescription Drugs For Canadians For Dummies* — a book Ian co-wrote.)

✔ **Ask questions.** For you to function as an effective captain of your health care team, you must know how you're performing. And you can't know this without your teammates giving you feedback. So, before you leave an appointment, make sure you have a good understanding of what your health care provider has concluded. Don't accept vague phrases like "your blood pressure is okay" or "your cholesterol isn't bad" or "your sugars are reasonable." As diabetes specialists, we can tell you that these terms are meaningless. Meaning*ful* would be to hear that your blood pressure is 125/85, your LDL is 2.4, and your A1C is 7.4.

Your physician deals with many patients each day, and even the most conscientious, well-meaning doctor can easily forget some of the specific issues of your particular situation. Therefore, be sure to bring up any concerns or questions you have about your health. Tell your doctor if you're having a problem such as chest pain, numbness in your feet, sexual dysfunction, and so forth. Otherwise, a potentially serious problem may end up being overlooked.

When it comes to your health care, never accept the old adage that no news is good news. Sometimes, no news means the lab lost your blood sample! If you have had tests done, follow up with your doctor (in person, by phone, by fax, by e-mail, or some other means) to obtain and discuss the results.

The remainder of this chapter looks at the responsibilities of the other members of your health care team. As you see what their roles are, you'll further understand how you can help *them* help *you*. After all, as the old expression says, knowledge is power.

Dress for success

You might normally think that power dressing is something that is done on Bay Street, not in your doctor's office. Well, you may be amazed at how much more power you can have in making sure you get the attention you need by dressing for the occasion. We're not talking business suits here; we're talking easy access.

On the day of a doctor's appointment, you would be well served to dress in such a way that you can easily expose your arm (for a blood pressure measurement) and your feet (for assessment of skin health, circulation, sensation, and so on;

see Chapter 6). Even better, taking off your shoes and socks while you're waiting for your doctor to come into the examining room will ensure that your feet will get looked at. (Of course, you won't want to do this if the doctor you're seeing is your eye doctor!)

You may reasonably conclude that none of this dressing (and undressing) strategy should be necessary, and we would agree completely. But in truth, if this technique makes it more likely your blood pressure or feet get checked, it may be a life- and limb-saving measure.

The Family Physician: Your Coach

Your family physician has a major role to play on your diabetes team; indeed, even if you have a diabetes specialist whom you see from time to time, if you have type 2 diabetes (and, possibly, if you have type 1 diabetes), your family doctor will still provide the great majority of your diabetes medical care. For this reason, if you're fortunate enough to live in one of the few communities remaining in Canada where you can actually choose your doctor, find a family physician who has a particular interest in and expertise with diabetes. If you're unsure about this, simply ask him. If he doesn't feel that diabetes management is his forté, he may be able to recommend another doctor to help you.

Your family physician's responsibilities are far too numerous to list in their entirety (it would take many pages to itemize all the many tasks that these hard-working, dedicated doctors must do), but in terms of your diabetes, here are just some of the things your family doctor will do:

- **Review any symptoms you may have developed.** In most cases, your family doctor should be your first point of contact if you have developed symptoms (for example, such things as mood problems, vaginal discharge, diarrhea, or numbness in your feet).

- **Review your blood glucose control.** You should record your blood glucose readings in a logbook (see Chapter 9 for a detailed discussion of blood glucose record keeping) and review your numbers with your family doctor on a regular basis.

- **Examine you.** Routine components of your physical examination should include checking your blood pressure and pulse, feeling your thyroid, listening to your heart and lungs, and examining your feet for problems with your skin, circulation, or nerve function (see Chapter 6 for a more detailed discussion on testing for nerve problems).

- **Order screening studies.** Your doctor should do a number of tests from time to time, including checking your A1C, cholesterol, urine albumin/creatinine ratio, and so on. See the Cheat Sheet for a detailed list of what tests should be done and how often.

- **Help organize your visits to other team members.** This includes things such as reviewing with you when you are due to see other team members — for example, your diabetes educators and your eye doctor @md and, if necessary, arranging for visits to other providers, including your diabetes specialist and podiatrist.

Please note again that this list is not meant to be exhaustive and does not include the numerous things your family doctor helps you with, independent of your diabetes.

The Diabetes Specialist: Your General Manager

Family physicians provide the great majority of diabetes care in Canada. Nonetheless, seeing a diabetes specialist from time to time is usually a good idea if you have type 2 diabetes (especially if you have known complications from your diabetes) and is essential if you have type 1 diabetes.

Defining the term *diabetes specialist* is exceedingly difficult. Sure, we can say it is a doctor who specializes in diabetes, and although that would be accurate, it would still be incomplete. We can arbitrarily classify diabetes specialists into three groups:

- ✔ **Endocrinologists** (such as Alan): These are doctors who, after medical school, trained in internal medicine and then did additional training in endocrine (hormone) disorders such as those affecting the pancreas (diabetes, for example), thyroid, and adrenal glands.

- ✔ **Internists** (such as Ian): These are doctors who, after medical school, trained in internal medicine and then usually tailored their practice to a particular area. In Ian's case this was diabetes. For other internal medicine specialists, it is, for example, heart disease or high blood pressure.

- ✔ **Family physicians:** This one may surprise you. Not many family physicians are diabetes specialists, but some are. These are doctors who, after medical school, trained in family medicine and then, because diabetes was a particular interest of theirs or because their community may not have had ready access to a diabetes specialist, or both, focused their practice on diabetes. We have given lectures to such family physicians and must admit we have felt that *they* could just as well have been the ones giving the talk.

The main reason to see a diabetes specialist is the greater likelihood that they will be — by virtue of the time they devote to this one topic — "on top of the literature," that they will know about new research findings and new and innovative forms of therapy.

Your diabetes specialist can assess your diabetes-related issues and develop a treatment plan that he or she can then share with other members of your health care team.

Your family physician, your diabetes, and you

As diabetes specialists we are indebted to family doctors. They provide the overwhelming majority of diabetes care in this country. Regrettably, the number of physicians choosing to make a career of family medicine is rapidly dwindling, making it harder and harder for Canadians to obtain basic medical care. Fewer family doctors means that those in this field have to look after more and more patients, which makes it that much harder for them to spend additional time with each individual in their practice. Diabetes specialists are also in short supply, which puts additional work and responsibility on the shoulders of family physicians. The result is that numerous Canadians with diabetes (and people without diabetes too, of course) aren't receiving all the care they require. All the more reason, therefore, that it's crucial for you to be an informed consumer and take on the responsibility of knowing what your health care requires.

Dr. Stewart Harris of London, Ontario, is a family physician. He is also a previous Chair of the Canadian Diabetes Association's Clinical and Scientific Section. Dr. Harris is a perfect example of why a label (be it "family physician," "internist," "endocrinologist," or whatever) does not necessarily tell the whole story. Indeed, given the realities of diabetes care in Canada, Dr. Harris says, "All family doctors are going to have to be diabetes specialists."

Your specialist should send copies of your *laboratory test results* to your family physician. The great majority of specialists do this routinely, but some, alas, do not. Whenever you see your diabetes specialist, make a point of asking him or her to be sure to send these results to your family physician. At the same time, ask them to send a copy of their *letters* not only to your family doctor, but to your diabetes educators, too. Otherwise, using our previous hockey analogy, you and your specialist will be the only players on your team that are handling the puck. And that will make your other teammates less effective.

The Diabetes Educator: Your Trainer

A previous president of the American Diabetes Association once said, "Diabetes education is the single greatest advance ever made in diabetes care." (Ian loves him for having said it and quotes him widely!)

The expanding roles of the diabetes educator

Diabetes educators' roles are progressively expanding. In addition to their traditional teaching role, many educators now have the authority — as well they should — to test your A1C level (see Chapter 9), to help you adjust your insulin dosages, to adjust the dose of your oral hypoglycemic agents, to test your urine for evidence of kidney damage, and to measure your cholesterol levels. Some extraordinary (and extraordinarily *rare*) educators even carry pagers so that they can be contacted 24 hours a day if you're having problems. (Ian works with such educators and feels blessed to have this good fortune.)

Although every member of your diabetes team is, in some way, shape, or form, an educator, a diabetes educator is typically the health care team member who provides the bulk of your initial and ongoing teaching. In Canada, diabetes educators generally have the initials *C.D.E.* (certified *d*iabetes *e*ducator) after their names; however, many excellent educators do not have such certification. Diabetes educators are typically registered nurses (in which case they are referred to as *diabetes nurse educators* or, for short, *nurse educators*), dietitians, or, increasingly, other allied health care professionals such as pharmacists, who, after completing college or university and entering the workforce, have then gone on to do further training to teach people about diabetes.

A diabetes educator teaches you how to take your insulin or pills, how to test your blood glucose, and how to acquire many of the other skills you need. And that's just the beginning. They are invaluable resources, and if you haven't met with a diabetes educator, you're truly missing out.

If you haven't met with a diabetes educator, ask your doctor to refer you to one. If you haven't seen your educator for some time, call to arrange a follow-up visit. What health professionals know about diabetes keeps changing, so why should you be left behind? Stay current; see your educator regularly. (If this sounds like a sales pitch, we offer no apologies. We think diabetes educators are wonderful — in case you hadn't noticed.)

The majority of doctors are fully aware of the essential role that diabetes educators play and make a routine practice of referring their patients to them. (Trust us; it makes life a lot easier for the doctor to have other members of the health care team sharing the work!) Regrettably, there is the occasional doctor who feels that diabetes educators are superfluous and, therefore, won't send their patients to them. If you're placed in this unfortunate situation, ask your doctor to refer you anyhow. If he or she still refuses, call your local diabetes education centre and ask if you can make an appointment — as is typically allowed — without a doctor's referral. (Usually you can find out where your local diabetes education centre is by calling your local hospital.)

The Dietitian: Your Energizer

Registered dietitians are the pros when it comes to assisting you with your nutrition (hence, registered dietitians are sometimes referred to as nutritionists). To be called a registered dietitian in Canada, a person must have official certification establishing that he or she has the appropriate credentials. In Canada, the initials *R.D.* appear after the name of certified dietitians. As we discuss in the previous section, many registered dietitians are also certified diabetes educators. In this book, whenever we refer to dietitians we are referring to *registered* dietitians.

What you eat (and drink) is central to your success with your diabetes. Eat poorly, and you will render many of the pills you're taking less effective. Your oral hypoglycemic agents will be less useful. Your blood pressure pills won't work as well. Your cholesterol medicine will be fighting an uphill battle. And so on.

Your dietitian is the most knowledgeable person when it comes to advising you about what you should eat. It would be a terrible disservice to them — and, more important, to you — to think of the dietitian's role as simply putting you on a diet to lose weight. Sure, if you need to lose weight, they can help you determine the number of calories that your body requires and develop an appropriate nutrition plan, but they do so much more than that, too. Most importantly, they can help you determine the best choice and quantity of foods to help keep you healthy and your diabetes under control.

If you have diabetes and are on an *intensified insulin* program, your dietitian can teach you how to measure the number of grams of carbohydrates you consume with a meal and determine the amount of insulin that this will require you to take. This is called *carbohydrate counting* and is a highly effective means of achieving excellent blood glucose control; particularly if you have type 1 diabetes. We discuss intensified insulin therapy and carbohydrate counting in Chapter 13.

A good dietitian will help you to create a nutrition plan that does the following:

- ✔ Stays flexible
- ✔ Takes into account your particular ethnic and cultural background, and meets your particular religious requirements (if any)
- ✔ Fits with your lifestyle

The importance of tailoring a diet to fit the individual can be no better demonstrated than by the tale of two brothers that Ian met a few years ago. They were both teenagers and both also had type 1 diabetes. Bob was athletic and was captain of his hockey team. David, a year younger than his brother, couldn't have been more different. David could dismantle (and reassemble!) a car or a computer, but the only red line he knew about was the one on the tachometer. For the sake of convenience, the first time they were to meet with their dietitian they went together. The advice they received and the meal plans they took home were as different from one another as night and day. But the plans worked. To each his own (diet, that is!).

If you feel that the treatment plan your dietitian gives you is too rigid, is too out of keeping with your tastes, or is in some other way simply not realistic or practical, *do not* give up on the idea of proper nutrition therapy. Let your dietitian know of your concerns and he or she will be happy to work with you at creating a more appropriate meal plan.

The Eye Specialist: Your Cameraperson

An eye doctor has special expertise in the detection and treatment of eye disease. There are two types of eye doctors — ophthalmologists and optometrists. In Chapter 6 we look at the differences between them and how often you should see one of them. We also look at the various types of eye disease for which you are at risk.

Eye damage from diabetes seldom causes symptoms until it's very advanced, so it's *absolutely essential* that you see an eye doctor routinely — even if you have no problems with your sight!

Although your family doctor and your diabetes specialist may examine your eyes, an eye doctor has additional skills that you should take advantage of.

Although spending inordinate time in doctors' waiting rooms is the stuff of legend, eye doctors' offices are particularly famous for this. Make sure you bring something to read when you go. Hmm . . . how about *Diabetes For Canadians For Dummies?* And you had best plan on doing your day's reading prior to going into the examining room, because when you see your eye specialist, he or she will dilate your pupils using eye drops. This can affect your vision for a few hours and may make it difficult for you to read and, more important, may make it impossible for you to drive yourself home from your appointment. Bring someone with you to drive you home.

The Pharmacist: Your Equipment Manager

If you have diabetes, it's very likely that you're going to be taking medications to assist with the ultimate goal of keeping you healthy. Now, when you go to the pharmacy, your first thought may be, "Oh heck, another errand." Okay, so going to a pharmacy isn't the highlight of your day (thankfully!). But what a great resource you have at your disposal in the form of your pharmacist.

Pharmacists have expertise in medicines, so when you pick up your prescriptions, you have a golden opportunity to become an informed consumer. Here are some of the things that your pharmacist should review with you:

✔ The names of your medicines

✔ The dosages of your medicines

✔ How often you are to take your medicines

✔ What time you should take your medicines (for example, many cholesterol medicines work best if taken in the evening)

✔ What route you are to take your medicines (oral, vaginal, topical, and so on)

✔ Whether you should take your medicines with food or on an empty stomach

✔ Whether it is safe for you to consume alcohol (Some people have bad reactions if they ingest alcohol while on sulfonylurea oral hypoglycemic agents. We discuss oral agents further in Chapter 12.)

✔ What adverse effects (side effects) the medicines can cause

✔ Whether there are any possible interactions between your different medicines (For example, thyroid pills don't get absorbed as effectively if you take them at the same time as calcium or iron pills.)

You can also look up for yourself whether your medicines may potentially interact adversely with one another. Two good Web sites that provide this information are Epocrates (www.epocrates.com) and Drug Digest (www.drugdigest.org).

A good pharmacist will not simply hand your pills to you with a piece of paper (listing 50 side effects!) stapled to your bag and say goodbye. A good pharmacist will sit down with you and not only explain the items listed above, but also review with you *how likely* it is that you will experience the different side effects. Without a pharmacist's help, as you read through the lengthy list of all the bad things that the medicines can do, you won't be truly informed. You'll simply be scared. And *that* is not effective counselling.

Increasing numbers of pharmacists are now also certified diabetes educators. This means that not only can they fulfill their traditional roles as pharmacists, but can also provide you with other aspects of diabetes education.

If you're on several different medicines, ask your pharmacist to prepare a list of your medications that you can keep in your wallet or purse. This list should include the names, doses, and frequency of your drugs. Keeping track of when to take medicines can be very difficult. Your pharmacist can help you out by packaging your medicines in a container (a seven-day pill organizer) where they are laid out by day of week and time of day.

The Foot Doctor: Your Sole Mate

The foot doctor *(podiatrist)* is your best source of help with the minor and some of the major foot problems you may encounter. He or she can assist you with such problems as toenails that are hard to cut, bothersome corns and calluses, and difficulties with excessively dry or cracked skin. If areas of your feet undergo excessive pressure as you walk, a foot doctor can also help fit you with special insoles called orthotics, which more evenly distribute the forces upon your feet.

The longer we are in practice as diabetes specialists, the more we have come to rely on and use the expertise that podiatrists have to offer. They truly are the experts when it comes to helping you keep your feet healthy.

Not all podiatry services are covered by provincial health care plans. Before you meet with your podiatrist, you might want to call ahead to find out what charges you may expect.

Your Family and Friends: Your Fans and Cheerleaders

Okay, so the 1985 Oilers likely would have done just fine, thank you very much, even if they didn't have a single fan in the stands. But they were the exceptions. The rest of us need people rooting for us as we deal with the trials and tribulations of life. And this is especially true if you are living with a health issue such as diabetes.

Your fans and cheerleaders are the people you live with, eat with, and play with. Your family and friends can be a tremendous source of support, but for them to help you, they will need your guidance. For example, you can teach them what to look for if you become hypoglycemic (see Chapter 5). And you can ask them to avoid eating indiscriminately in your presence. Following your diet is challenging enough; you certainly don't need your family exposing you to constant temptation. Your family or friends can also become your exercise partners. Sticking to a program is a lot easier when a partner is counting on you to show up to work out.

Have someone accompany you when you see a member of your health care team — especially if you are meeting the dietitian and you're not the main food preparer at home. A lot of information is going to be communicated, and an extra set of ears is helpful.

If you do plan to bring an extra set of ears with you to your doctor's appointment, be sure to discuss it with your physician ahead of time to be sure it's okay to bring this person in. On occasion, your doctor may want to discuss some issues with you in private before your friend or relative joins you. (You likely wouldn't want to have important conversations with your doctor about, say, sexual dysfunction with your daughter or son in the room.)

Let people who are important to you know about your diabetes. Showing them this chapter might be a good way to introduce them to their important supporting role.

Remembering the rest of the roster

In this chapter we look at the central players on your diabetes team, but many other teammates may be asked to take a face-off from time to time. These include, among others, hospital emergency room staff, cardiologists, neurologists, gastroenterologists (stomach doctors), social workers, dentists, psychologists, and psychiatrists.

Chapter 9

Monitoring and Understanding Your Blood Glucose Levels

*I*n earlier chapters we discuss the bad things that can happen if you're exposed to elevated blood glucose. And because *bad* things can happen if your blood glucose levels are *bad,* you might suspect that *good* things can happen if your blood glucose levels are *good.* And you'd be exactly right. Many diabetes complications — such as blindness and kidney failure — are directly influenced by your blood glucose control. The better your blood glucose levels, the more likely you are to maintain your eyesight and avoid kidney failure. But how will you know if your blood glucose levels are good? Ah, we're so glad you asked. Because that is exactly what we look at in this chapter.

Understanding the Importance of Measuring Your Blood Glucose Levels

Have you ever gotten dressed in the dark only to find out as you were heading out the door that your socks were mismatched or the blue pants you put on were actually black or your red purse was actually brown? You probably either made a mad dash back inside to re-dress, or you just headed out, hoping that your gaffe wouldn't be noticed. Well, not monitoring your blood glucose levels is like getting dressed in the dark every day.

If you are not testing your blood, you will never know if your

- ✔ Nutrition (diet) plan (see Chapter 10) is helping your blood glucose control
- ✔ Exercise program (see Chapter 11) is improving your blood glucose levels
- ✔ Oral hypoglycemic agents (see Chapter 12) or insulin doses (see Chapter 13) need to be changed
- ✔ Recent illness, such as a chest infection, is making your glucose readings dangerously high

Basically, you'll be in the dark, without guidance and, equally important, without feedback.

But what if your readings are poor? "Why do I want to be frustrated by always seeing crummy readings?" you might ask. And you would be perfectly justified in asking this. At least, you would be perfectly justified if you couldn't improve your blood glucose control. But you can *always* improve it. If your readings aren't good, it is time for you to meet with your diabetes educators to see if your lifestyle plan needs adjusting. And to call your family doctor (or diabetes specialist if you're in regular contact with one) to have your oral hypoglycemic agents or insulin therapy reviewed.

People with diabetes tend to look at a record of their glucose readings as a report card, keeping constant score and noting whether they have passed or failed. That is understandable, but terribly inappropriate. Your glucose readings aren't meant to judge you or your efforts. Your readings are being done to serve as an aid — a tool — to help you and your team know when changes to your therapy are in order. And if your readings are good, they serve as a nice source of positive feedback.

ANECDOTE

Testing your blood, not you

Ian recalls his very first meeting with Bill, a 25-year-old man who had had type 1 diabetes for several years. When Ian asked Bill how his blood glucose readings were doing, Bill told him they were excellent and pulled out his blood glucose logbook (we discuss logbooks later in this chapter) which showed his past two months' readings — all of which were within target — consistently and neatly noted. "That's great," Ian said, "why don't I borrow your blood glucose meter for a moment so that we can download your values to keep a computerized record of them in the chart?"

"Ah," Bill replied, hesitantly, "actually, I don't have my meter with me today."

"No problem," Ian replied, "maybe you could drop it off tomorrow."

"Don't think so," Bill went on, "*I lost it months ago.*"

Bill expected recrimination, but got none. Instead, both Bill and Ian shared a knowing smile. Like having homework conveniently chewed by the household dog, people "losing" their blood glucose meter is very common. It's also common for people to make up blood glucose numbers. The reason? Because many people with diabetes have never been sufficiently taught that measuring and recording blood glucose levels are a guide — not a report card or, worse, a disciplinarian's rod. Similarly, many people with diabetes have never been sufficiently taught that their diabetes educators and doctors are more akin to guidance counsellors than truant officers. Ian made sure Bill knew this, and from then on, like Little Bo' Peep, when Bill came to his appointments, his blood glucose meter and logbook were sure to follow.

Testing with a Blood Glucose Meter

You can know if your blood glucose control is where it should be through several different ways:

- Testing your blood glucose using your own portable blood glucose meter.

- Having a blood glucose test performed at a laboratory.

- Having your A1C tested at a laboratory (or, if they have an A1C testing machine, at a diabetes education centre). (See "Testing for Longer-Term Blood Glucose Control with the A1C Test," later in this chapter, for more.)

- Having your *fructosamine* level performed at a laboratory. This is a seldom-required test that indicates what your average blood glucose level has been over the preceding two weeks.

✔ Using a continuous glucose monitoring system (CGMS). (See "Using a Continuous Glucose Monitoring System," later in this chapter, for more.)

Of the various ways of determining your blood glucose control, far and away the easiest, most convenient method is for you to use a blood glucose meter. In this section we look in detail at how blood glucose testing with a blood glucose meter can help you manage your diabetes. (*Urine* glucose testing, by the way, is of no value in monitoring your glucose control.)

Reviewing the supplies you need

Just like any test, a blood glucose test requires some basic supplies:

✔ **Lancet:** If you happen to be like us, the notion of intentionally wounding yourself is most definitely not your idea of a good time. Well, you need not despair because obtaining a blood sample is a nearly painless procedure. In order to prick yourself you use a small, sharp, disposable *lancet*.

✔ **Lancet holder:** Your lancet fits into this spring-loaded holder, and when you push the release button, the lancet springs out and pokes your finger. Lancet holders are typically adjustable so that you can vary the depth the lancet will penetrate your skin. That way you can set it to the minimum depth necessary to get blood (and minimize discomfort).

✔ **Test strip:** This is the small disposable strip onto which you place your drop of blood.

✔ **Blood glucose meter:** This is the device that determines how much glucose is in your blood sample. We talk more about these in a moment.

✔ **"Sharps" container:** This is a small box into which you place your used lancets. You can pick up a sharps container from your drugstore. When the container is full, seal it and bring it back to the drugstore for proper disposal.

Also available is a lancing device (the ACCU-CHEK Multiclix Lancing Device — visit the Web site at www.accu-chek.ca), which contains a cylinder that holds several lancets. An advantage to this device is that you have less to fiddle with and it doesn't require disposal in a sharps container; when used up, it can be placed in the regular garbage. (Another new — and way cool — type of lancing device, currently available in the U.S. and, likely, soon in Canada, is made by Pelikan Technologies (www.pelikantechnologies.com) and, using computerized technology, figures out an optimal lancing depth, velocity, and so on.)

Performing a blood glucose test

Here's how you obtain a blood sample and perform a blood glucose test:

1. **Wash your hands (or at least your finger).** Although you do not need to prepare your site — or your psyche — with alcohol, you need to make sure your finger (or arm if you are using an alternate-site meter, which we discuss in the next section) is clean.

2. **Obtain a blood sample.** Insert a lancet into the lancet holder, press it against the *side* of your fingertip, and activate the trigger. In an instant, you will see a tiny drop of blood appear. It does not hurt much at all, but to make it hurt even less you can

   • Use a lancet holder that allows you to adjust the depth of penetration. An example is the Softclix Lancing Device.

   • Avoid re-using your lancets because they dull quickly. (It's okay to use the same one a few times, but not more than that.)

   • Use the side — not the fleshy pad — of the end of your finger.

   • Change fingers often or — quite the opposite — stick to the side of the same finger and you will find that after you have built up a small callus it hurts less to draw blood from that site.

   • Take blood from an alternate site such as your forearm. (To do this you will need an alternate-site meter.)

3. **Apply the end of the glucose-measuring strip to the blood.** Only a tiny drop of blood is required, but it still has to be sufficient to cover the marked area on the strip. Most strips are designed to draw up the blood in the same way that a strip of paper towel, when dipped into water, draws up the water (a process called *capillary action,* in case you were wondering).

4. **Presto, you're done!** Your meter will display your result in a matter of seconds.

If you have difficulty obtaining a sufficient quantity of blood, try one or more of the following:

✔ Warm your finger with warm water.

✔ Let your arm hang down at your side for a minute before you test.

✔ Hold your finger about 1.5 centimetres (about half an inch) from the tip and squeeze — but only once, as repeated squeezing can interfere with the test's accuracy.

How a blood glucose meter works

Earlier glucose meters relied on a colour change that appeared on the test strips and that was proportional to your blood glucose level. The new meters use a different process to analyze your blood. They measure an electrical potential that is created when the glucose in your blood sample reacts with reagents (glucose oxidase and potassium ferricyanide) on the electrode of the test strip. This reaction generates electrons that produce an electrical current. The higher your glucose level, the greater the current.

Because blood glucose test strips can be damaged (and thus, provide inaccurate results) if exposed to the elements, be sure to look after your unused strips as per the instructions the manufacturer provided. In particular, keep them stored in the airtight container that they came in.

If ever you find that your test result is far lower than you expect, it may be because you had insufficient blood on the strip (this can give falsely low readings). If your blood glucose meter tells you that your reading is, for example, 2.8 mmol/L and you had expected 12.8 mmol/L, retest yourself.

Incidentally, when it comes to used lancets, remember the old adage: Neither a borrower nor a lender be. The only time you should share your blood is when you are donating to Canadian Blood Services (which, incidentally, we discuss further in Chapter 13).

Knowing how often to test your blood glucose

How often you test is determined by three factors: the kind of diabetes you have, the kind of treatment you are using, and the level of stability of your blood glucose. As you can tell, this is not a one-size-fits-all issue. The Canadian Diabetes Association (CDA) recommends different amounts of testing depending on what therapy you're taking to control your blood glucose (we share our take on this following this list):

✔ **If you aren't on medications to control your blood glucose (that is, you're being treated with lifestyle measures alone):** The frequency of testing should be determined (in discussion with you, your diabetes educators, and your physicians) based on your specific situation. Tests should include both before-meal and (two hours) after-meal tests.

✔ **If you take oral hypoglycemic agents, but not insulin:** The frequency of testing should be determined (in discussion with you, your diabetes educators, and your physicians) based on your specific situation. Tests should include both before-meal and (two hours) after-meal tests.

✔ **If you take insulin, but not oral hypoglycemic agents:** Test at least three times daily. Tests should include both before-meal and (two hours) after-meal tests.

✔ **If you take insulin once per day and also take oral hypoglycemic agents:** Test at least once daily. You should test at variable times.

"Two hours after meals" means two hours after you take the first bite of your meal.

The CDA also notes that "in many situations, for all individuals with diabetes, more frequent testing should be undertaken" because this will provide needed information to allow you and your health care team to adjust your treatment to best control your blood glucose.

The CDA recommendations are based, as they should be, on the existing science (or as Joe Friday would say, "The facts ma'am, just the facts"). However, the existing science — especially when it comes to how often testing should be done if you are not taking insulin — is pretty darn shabby. Which means, in the absence of definitive data, that patients and health care providers need to use their collective judgment in deciding how often testing is necessary. In our experience, the more you test, the more information and feedback you have, and, ultimately, the better you do. For this reason we would encourage you to focus on the "at least" wording of the CDA guidelines and aim to test considerably more often than the minimum recommendations.

We have found the following schedule to work very well (note that this schedule assumes your overall control is both very good and very stable; if it isn't, you should be testing *even more*):

✔ **If your treatment consists of lifestyle measures alone** (see Chapters 10 and 11), test *once* daily, varying the timing of your reading so that over the span of a week or two you'll have values from before and after each of your meals and at bedtime. (If your readings are uniformly within target, testing only two or three times weekly may be suitable.)

✔ **If you're taking oral hypoglycemic agents** (see Chapter 12) or **you are an adult taking insulin once or twice daily** (see Chapter 13), test *twice* daily:

• Before breakfast, *and*

• Vary the time of the other test (sometimes do it before your other meals, sometimes two hours after your meals, and sometimes at bedtime).

✔ **If you are an adult taking insulin three or four times a day (or a child or adolescent taking insulin any number of times a day),** test four to seven times daily:

- Before each meal, *and*

- Two hours after some meals (you may wish to rotate so that one day you test after breakfast, the next day after lunch, and the next day after dinner), *and*

- *Every* night at bedtime, *and*

- *Occasionally at about 3 a.m.* (to make sure you aren't having low overnight readings that haven't been awakening you).

✔ **If you have gestational diabetes** (see Chapter 7) **treated with lifestyle measures alone,** test before and two hours after your breakfast, two hours after your lunch, and two hours after your dinner. If readings are consistently within target, you can reduce the frequency of your two hour after-meal testing to once daily (but continue your *daily* before-breakfast testing).

✔ **If you are pregnant and have pre-existing diabetes ("pregestational diabetes")** or **if you have gestational diabetes treated with insulin,** test *six to seven* times per day (before and two hours after each meal, and again at bedtime if your bedtime is four or more hours after your dinner, and periodically overnight).

Never fall into the trap of assuming that if you feel well, your blood glucose levels *must* be good and therefore you don't need to test. The truth is, your blood glucose level can be significantly higher than normal and you may not have a single symptom, even though your body is being irreversibly damaged.

As you can tell from this list, the frequency of testing is directly related to how often you need the information to make decisions about your care. If you're being treated with lifestyle measures alone, getting feedback once per day is usually enough to let you know how effective your treatment plan is, whereas if you're on an intensified insulin program (see Chapter 13), you should test much more often to know what insulin dose to administer.

Almost everyone has times when they get fed up with testing, testing, testing. Don't feel guilty if you feel this way; it's perfectly normal. And if you do happen to go through times when you aren't testing nearly as much as you should, don't berate yourself about it. Just grab hold of your meter and get back into the routine.

Mr. Pereira was a middle-aged man with type 2 diabetes who had come to Ian's office for a consultation. Ian asked him how his blood glucose control was, and Mr. Pereira replied, "It was 7.4 today." Ian asked him if he had any other readings to share. "Sure; it was 9.3 last month so it's getting better." Ian explained to his patient that glucose control varies not only month to month, but day to day and even meal to meal, so knowing two readings taken a month apart tells us virtually nothing about how control is or what trend it's following. Hearing this explanation, Mr. Pereira, a math teacher, asked if he could borrow Ian's calculator, and, a moment later, announced, "Gee, Doctor, now I get it. I've told you what my readings were for a total of 2 minutes out of the past 43,200 minutes. That's not even five one-thousandths of 1 percent of my readings. *No wonder* that doesn't tell you much." Couldn't have said it better ourselves.

Understanding what to do with your test results

If you test your blood glucose readings and don't share the results with your health care team and/or the results don't influence anything you do (such as adjusting your diet or exercise, or adjusting your insulin dose), you're likely to ask yourself, "Why am I bothering to test my blood?" Our answer would be, "We wonder the same thing!"

Testing your blood glucose levels is only of value if it results in some further action (even if this is only to reassure yourself, if your control is excellent, that it remains excellent). If you have a blood glucose meter, speak to your health care team about why you are testing and, importantly, what to do with the results. Without this information, we suspect you'll be likely either not to test very much or to abandon testing altogether. And we wouldn't blame you one bit.

Choosing a Blood Glucose Meter

So many meters are on the market that you may be confused about which one to use. One consideration that should play little or no part in your choice of a meter is the cost. With rebates, promotions, and trade-ins, you'll find almost every meter you look at to be quite inexpensive and competitively priced. Because the meters are so cheap and because the manufacturers replace them with better ones so frequently, you can get a new meter every year or two, to make sure that you have the latest and greatest device.

Another non-consideration is the accuracy of the various machines. All are accurate to a degree acceptable for managing your diabetes. Keep in mind, though, that they don't have the accuracy of laboratory equipment. (If ever you're experimenting with your machine and test your blood twice within a minute or two, you may find that your readings vary by 10 to 15 percent. This is not because your blood glucose level has changed that much in a matter of seconds; it's simply because the machines aren't perfect.) To make sure your blood glucose meter is sufficiently accurate, once a year your doctor (or diabetes educator) should have you do a finger-prick test with your meter at the same time as the lab is testing your glucose by drawing blood from your arm. Once the lab result is available, the two values should be compared. They should be within 20 percent of each other.

Although glucose meters are cheap, the test strips are anything but. Typically they are about a dollar per strip (ouch!), regardless of which meter you are using. If you shop around, however, you will find that some drugstores sell them for less than others.

Some provinces and territories will subsidize the cost of your blood glucose strips. For more information you can contact your provincial or territorial government or the CDA (visit their Web site at www.diabetes.ca/get-involved/helping-you/advocacy/financial-coverage).

Because the machines are similar in price, accuracy, and costs for their strips, base your purchase decision on other factors:

✔ Whether you like products with bells and whistles or prefer those that are plain and simple.

✔ If your eyesight is poor, make sure the display is easily readable. If that is not sufficient, you can purchase a voice synthesizer that connects with a meter or, alternatively, a single device that integrates both a meter and a voice synthesizer. There are two of the former devices available in Canada: the Digi-Voice Contour (currently available only through Danielle Desroches Pharmacy in Montreal; 450-447-9280) and the ACCU-CHECK Voicemate Plus (available through Accu-Chek Customer Care; 800-363-7949). There are also two of the latter devices: The Prodigy Voice meter (www.prodigymeter.com) and the Oracle blood glucose meter.

✔ If you're likely to be testing in the dark, select a meter that has backlighting.

✔ You need to calibrate some meters (by entering a code into the machine) each time you open a new package of test strips. This is typically a fast and simple procedure, but if you think you might find it a hassle, obtain a meter that doesn't require this step. (These heavily promoted meters are referred to as requiring "no coding.")

✔ If you want to test from alternate sites such as your forearm, buy a meter designed to allow this.

✔ Make sure the meter is not too bulky (seldom an issue with current meters), or, conversely, too small to fit comfortably in your hand.

- Some strips are larger than others. If you have a hard time holding onto very small objects, choose a meter that uses larger strips.

- You'll have to decide how much memory you need in a machine. We never recommend a specific blood glucose meter for the simple reason that they're all very good and the one that's best for you will depend on your personal tastes. The one exception to this is the OneTouch UltraSmart, which, because of its excellent ability to display multiple readings at a glance, we recommend for those people who don't keep a written log of their readings. (However, we still far prefer a written log compared to *any* meter's memory. We discuss logbooks later in this chapter.)

- If you have type 1 diabetes, have a meter that tests for ketones. (See Chapter 5 for more on ketones.) The only such meter available in Canada is the Precision Xtra. This meter also tests for blood glucose; however, you may elect to use a different meter for this purpose.

- You may find a device that can hold multiple test strips more convenient.

- If you like the idea of being able to download your readings onto your computer so you can graph (and print) them, buy a meter that has this capacity. Bear in mind that you'll likely encounter an additional charge for the connecting cable.

The Canadian Diabetes Association offers a Consumers Guide to Diabetes Products. This excellent publication, updated annually, is available online at `www.diabetes.ca/about-diabetes/literature/consumer-guide`.

Alternate-site glucose readings are not reliable if they're obtained when your blood glucose level is rapidly rising or falling. For this reason, don't rely on alternate-site tests if you're doing a blood glucose test within two hours of eating, and don't use an alternate site test if you suspect you are hypoglycemic.

You'll save much time, energy, and aggravation by speaking to your diabetes educator before you buy a meter. Not only can he or she show you the latest meters and point out their pros and cons, but also, more important, your educator *knows you* and will able to help you select a meter that meets your particular needs.

If you would like to do some of your own research, you can find (far from impartial) information regarding meters by going to the different manufacturers' Web sites or by calling them. Table 9-1 lists the main manufacturers in the Canadian market, their Web sites, and phone numbers.

Table 9-1	Main Meter Manufacturers	
Company	**Web Site**	**Phone Number**
Abbott Diabetes Care	www.abbottdiabetescare.ca	888-519-6890
Auto Control Medical	www.autocontrol.com	800-461-0991
Bayer Healthcare	www.bayerdiabetes.ca	800-268-1432
Lifescan Canada	www.lifescancanada.com	800-663-5521
Roche Diagnostics	www.accu-chek.ca	800-363-7949

Recording Your Results

Ian recalls going for a haircut a few years back (when he used to have to go more often) only to find his barber profoundly upset. "What's the matter?" Ian asked, to which his barber replied that he could not find his scissors. "Why not just use somebody else's?" Ian innocently asked. His barber immediately stopped his searching and looked at Ian with disbelief. "Use somebody else's? Would you use somebody else's wife?" And that just about sums up most diabetes specialists' opinions about how glucose readings should be recorded. We're very particular and we each have our own preferences.

So then, we *could* show you many different ways of recording your results, or we could just show you the best way, which, ahem, just happens to be Ian's way!

The first thing you need to do is to obtain a logbook. You can find these at your pharmacy, at your diabetes education centre, and at your diabetes specialist's office. Each page in your logbook should be laid out like Figure 9-1 (of course, if you're not on insulin you won't use the right hand side of the page).

Date	Blood Glucose Levels							Insulin Injections					Notes
	Breakfast		Lunch		Dinner		Bedtime	Other	Insulin Type	Units Taken				
	Before	After	Before	After	Before	After				Breakfast	Lunch	Dinner	Bedtime	

Figure 9-1: Ideal logbook format.

Most logbooks, alas, do not have this particular format. If you can't find a book with this layout, you can download similar pages from Ian's Web site (www. ourdiabetes.com/log-book.htm).

The one shortcoming with this layout is, potentially, insufficient space for you to write in the Notes column (where you might want to write things such as "birthday party" or "missed snack" to remind you later of some past event that might explain a high or low reading). If you need more space, you can always create your own sheet on a piece of paper (which you could photocopy) or with a spreadsheet program such as Excel.

Using this layout enables you to quickly assess your overall blood glucose *patterns, trends,* and *averages* for a given time of day. To illustrate what we mean, have a look at two different ways of recording your readings.

Table 9-2 is the typical way that a log is kept or that a machine's memory displays results (although a machine would usually display the time of day, not the meal of the day). The readings in this table are before-meal values.

Table 9-2	Blood Glucose Readings Listed Chronologically
Time of Reading	*Blood Glucose Level*
Breakfast	12.6
Lunch	4.1
Dinner	14.7
Bedtime	5.6
Breakfast	11.7
Lunch	5.2
Dinner	12.1
Bedtime	7.0
Breakfast	10.0
Lunch	5.9
Dinner	11.9
Bedtime	4.0
Breakfast	9.9
Lunch	4.2
Dinner	14.4
Bedtime	4.4

(continued)

Table 9-2 *(continued)*

Time of Reading	Blood Glucose Level
Breakfast	11.1
Lunch	6.3
Dinner	12.2
Bedtime	5.1

If you were to record your readings like this, you would likely feel that your glucose values were all over the place (or, as Ian often hears, "my sugars are up and down like a toilet seat") and you would likely be feeling frustrated by what you concluded were very inconsistent values. Although your conclusion would be perfectly understandable, you might be surprised to see that if we look at your readings from a different perspective, they could be thought of as being remarkably consistent. Table 9-3 takes those same readings and charts them differently.

Table 9-3 **Blood Glucose Reading Listed by Time of Day**

Breakfast	Lunch	Dinner	Bedtime
12.6	4.1	14.7	5.6
11.7	5.2	12.1	7.0
10.0	5.9	11.9	4.0
9.9	4.2	14.4	4.4
11.1	6.3	12.2	5.1

Now, scan the columns from top to bottom. Aha! Your readings at any given time of day are remarkably similar. You're consistently too high at breakfast, consistently normal at lunch, consistently too high at dinner, and consistently normal at bedtime.

The memory on a blood glucose meter does not allow for this type of instant overview, and hence is almost always inferior to using a logbook. (The only meter that comes close is the OneTouch UltraSmart, but even that one does not give as complete a picture as those old and trusted tools: pen and paper.)

Record keeping is of great importance because when you have identified your blood glucose patterns, your health care team can adjust your therapy accordingly. In the preceding example, if you were on insulin therapy, we would know that you need more bedtime insulin to bring down your breakfast blood glucose and, depending on the type of insulin you are taking, more lunchtime or breakfast insulin to reduce your suppertime readings (see Chapter 13 for a detailed discussion of insulin adjustment). We could have figured this out from Table 9-2, but it would have been much more difficult and time-consuming. We discuss how to interpret blood glucose log readings in the section "Interpreting Your Blood Glucose Results," later in this chapter.

If you're using an insulin pump (see Chapter 13) you may need an even more detailed logbook; ask your diabetes educator for their recommended one.

Bring your logbook with you to *each and every* appointment with your diabetes educator and diabetes specialist. Ask your family doctor how often he or she would like you to bring your logbook to your appointments (if you see your doctor only occasionally, he or she will want you to bring it routinely, but on the other hand, if you're seeing him or her very frequently for other health issues — such as, for example, allergy injections — your doctor likely won't need to review your readings at each of these visits).

Discovering Your Blood Glucose Targets

The Canadian Diabetes Association (CDA) guidelines recommend that most adults with type 1 or type 2 diabetes (we look at children's targets in Chapter 15 and targets for pregnant women in Chapter 7) aim for the following readings:

Before Meals	*Two Hours after Meals*
4–7 mmol/L	5–10 mmol/L

However, if your A1C is above 7.0 (we discuss A1C later in this chapter in the section "Testing for Longer-Term Blood Glucose Control with the A1C Test"), the CDA recommends aiming for a lower two-hour after-meal target of 5–8 mmol/L.

Not everyone can safely achieve these targets. Here are some of the things that might make it unsafe or inappropriate for you to aim for these levels:

- You have other health problems that make it too dangerous to risk any hypoglycemia.

- You have *irreversible* problems with hypoglycemia unawareness (see Chapter 5).

- When you try to bring your blood glucose into this range, you experience excessively *frequent, unpredictable, and unavoidable* hypoglycemia.

- Your life expectancy is such that you're at low risk of developing diabetes-related, long-term complications.

No one with diabetes has glucose readings that are always within target. Indeed, having two-thirds of your readings within target is a wonderful accomplishment. Remember that to achieve your targets requires a concerted and ongoing effort by you and your diabetes team. (And also remember, *you* are the first star on this team.)

Consistently achieving target blood glucose values can be very difficult and, for some people, it may simply not be possible. If you and your health care team have worked hard at reaching these goals but have not been able to achieve them, don't feel that all is lost. The reason for this is simple; although fantastic blood glucose readings are our goal, as we discuss in Chapter 6, *any* improvement in your blood glucose control will help reduce your risk of microvascular complications (such as blindness and kidney failure) and, possibly, macrovascular complications (such as heart attack and stroke).

Interpreting Your Blood Glucose Results

In the section "Understanding the Importance of Measuring Your Blood Glucose Levels" earlier in this chapter, we mention that testing your blood glucose (and recording your results) is only of value if something is then done with the results. Otherwise, it's a waste of your time — and an expensive waste at that.

Because your diabetes educators and physicians know you and are aware of your particular circumstances (including your medications), they can provide you with advice that is specific to you. (That is, they can help you determine what your specific blood glucose targets are and how you can best go about achieving them.) Nonetheless, certain basic principles can help guide you. The most important of these is to look for patterns in your blood glucose levels, and the first step in doing this is to record your values in the format we show in Table 9-3. In this section we look at three particularly common problematic patterns you might spot in your results and how you can improve these problems.

When your before-breakfast readings are high (and other readings good)

As we discover in Chapter 13, one particularly common scenario is for people with diabetes (regardless of their treatment) to have higher readings first thing in the morning than later in the day. A typical logbook might look like Figure 9-2.

Date	Breakfast		Lunch		Dinner		Bedtime
	Bef.	After	Bef.	After	Bef.	After	
	8.5	7.2					
	9.0		6.1				
	7.8			5.2			
	6.1				4.4		
	8.2					7.9	
	9.9						8.2

Figure 9-2: High before-breakfast (fasting) blood glucose readings.

The reason for this pattern is that overnight your liver produces and releases glucose into your blood (this is called the *dawn phenomenon*). Often, the best way to treat this increased before-breakfast glucose level is by taking a dose of insulin (NPH, Levemir, or Lantus) before you go to bed (sometimes these insulins are given at other times instead) or, if you are already taking one of these insulins, by increasing the dose (under the guidance of your diabetes educator or physician).

When your after-meal readings are high (and other readings good)

You may observe that your readings are good before your meals but two hours after your meals your values have climbed unduly. Your logbook might look something like Figure 9-3.

In this case, the first thing to do is to review your diet with your dietitian, because your choice of foods may be responsible. Alternatively, if you're taking oral hypoglycemic agents, you might benefit from using one (such as GlucoNorm) that specifically targets after-meal blood glucose spikes. Another very effective measure is to take rapid-acting insulin (Apidra, Humalog, or NovoRapid) before your meals. If you're having this blood glucose problem despite already taking one of these medicines, then your dose(s) may need to be adjusted. (We discuss insulin adjustment in greater detail in Chapter 13.)

Date	Breakfast		Lunch		Dinner		Bedtime
	Bef.	After	Bef.	After	Bef.	After	
	5.5	10.2					
	6.0		6.1				
	7.0			10.8			
	6.1				6.9		
	4.2					11.5	
	5.9						7.2

Figure 9-3: High two-hour after-meal blood glucose readings.

When your readings have no pattern

Perhaps your blood glucose readings are inconsistent, and really have no discernable pattern at all. High then low, up then down; resembling (and making you feel like you're on) a roller coaster. Your logbook may look something like Figure 9-4.

Date	Breakfast		Lunch		Dinner		Bedtime	Other
	Bef.	After	Bef.	After	Bef.	After		
	4.1	8.2						3.5
	12.5		4.2			19.9		7.7
	3.2			14.7				
	16.5				24.4	5.4		
	6.7		13.4			9.9		
	11.2			2.6	7.2			

Figure 9-4: Inconsistent blood glucose readings.

Fortunately, some correctable or at least modifiable factor is almost always present that, when addressed, can improve this situation.

If you're having wide and unpredictable swings in your glucose levels, get in touch with your diabetes specialist and your diabetes educators. They will be able to help sort out the reasons for the problem. It is rare indeed that erratic glucose control cannot be improved.

These are possible causes of erratic blood glucose levels:

✔ **Your nutrition plan isn't optimal for you.** If your nutrition program isn't working out the way it should, it's time for another visit to the dietitian. It could be that your food selection or amount might need to be changed, or it could be that you would benefit from carbohydrate counting (see Chapter 13) or using lower glycemic index foods (see Chapter 10).

✔ **Your adherence to your nutrition plan needs some work.** Are you eating *in*consistently? Do you eat almost nothing all day and then consume the bulk of your calories at suppertime? Do you graze from the time you get home in the evening until you go to bed? All these patterns can adversely affect glucose control. Also, eating disorders are not uncommon for teenage girls and young women with diabetes and can wreck havoc on blood glucose control. We discuss this further in Chapter 10.

✔ **Your exercise pattern needs to be revised.** Are you exercising for 10 minutes one morning and then 30 minutes the next evening and then 15 minutes the next afternoon and then not at all for two days? Consistent duration and timing of exercise is often helpful in maintaining consistent glucose control.

✔ **You have diabetic gastroparesis or celiac disease.** (We discuss these conditions in Chapter 6.) These conditions cause erratic absorption of nutrients into the body, and as a result can cause overly variable blood glucose readings.

✔ **You are under undue stress.** Stress does not cause diabetes, but it can certainly influence it. Stress causes the release of certain hormones in your body, including cortisol and adrenaline, both of which can make glucose levels rise. If you're on an emotional roller coaster, your glucose readings may be too.

✔ **Your menstrual cycle.** For some women with diabetes, where they are in their cycle can influence their glucose control. Some women find their glucose readings are higher around the time of their period and some find their readings are lower. Most women don't find much difference.

✔ **Your work schedule.** If you work a variable shift, you may find your readings are also variable. As most people with diabetes quickly find out, diabetes loves consistency. Nonetheless, working variable shifts does not make excellent glucose control impossible, just more difficult. If you work variable shifts, we recommend basal-bolus or pump therapy (see Chapter 13).

Another very important reason for inconsistent blood readings, as seen in Figure 9-4, is that your insulin therapy isn't working sufficiently well for you. You may need to

✔ **Change to a different type of insulin or a different insulin regimen.** Different insulins have different properties and, like the expression, "different strokes for different folks," you need to take the insulin that most closely matches your needs and works best for you. For example:

- If you're taking NPH insulin and have inconsistent blood glucose readings, switching to Lantus or Levemir may be helpful because both are absorbed more consistently than NPH and as a result can give more consistent blood glucose control.

- If you have type 1 diabetes but are only on twice-daily insulin, your blood glucose control is almost guaranteed to be erratic, and switching to basal-bolus therapy (this is closer to normal insulin release from the pancreas; see Chapter 13) is recommended. (This is also often helpful if you have type 2 diabetes.)

- If you're having erratic readings despite basal-bolus injection therapy, switching to insulin pump therapy may provide you with much more consistent blood glucose control.

✔ **Not miss insulin doses.** If you're missing insulin doses due to forgetfulness, set reminders for yourself when your insulin is due or ask others to remind you. If you are omitting insulin doses by intention (as is not uncommonly done by teenage girls to help them lose weight), this is very, very dangerous and must not be done. If this applies to you, speak to your diabetes educator or physician urgently to see what other, safer measures can help you keep your weight in check.

✔ **Better mix your insulin.** Cloudy insulins such as NPH need to be properly mixed before you inject them (see Chapter 13).

✔ **Make sure your insulin hasn't lost its potency.** If your insulin has been exposed to excessive cold or heat, or is beyond its expiry date, it will have lost its potency and should not be used.

✔ **Change the place you are injecting your insulin because of problems with insulin absorption.** You may give yourself the same dose of insulin every day (something, by the way, that's seldom a good idea, as we discuss earlier in this chapter), but that doesn't mean that your bloodstream sees the same dose. Factors that can affect the rate of absorption of insulin from your injection sites include the following:

- Whether your injection sites have scar tissue. You shouldn't inject insulin into these areas.

- Whether your injection sites have fat build-up (lipohypertrophy; see Chapter 6). Insulin absorption will vary considerably injection-to-injection if given into these areas. Also, injecting into them makes the lipohypertrophy worse. You shouldn't inject insulin into these areas.

- Which part of your body you are injecting into (regular insulin will begin to work more quickly if injected into the abdomen than into the arms or legs). Speak to your diabetes educator about the best locations to inject your insulin and how often you should change the sites you use.

- Whether you exercise a certain part of your body after you inject there. If, for example, you inject regular insulin into your leg and then go for a run, the rate of insulin absorption will speed up. It's best not to inject insulin into a limb that is about to be exercised.

- Whether you're accidentally injecting into muscle. (This would cause the insulin to be absorbed faster.)

The list of possible causes of overly variable blood glucose readings is lengthy indeed. One term, however, that is missing from the list is *brittle diabetes.* We consider this, in general, to be a four letter word. *Brittle diabetes* can be defined as erratic and disabling blood glucose variability occurring for no known reason and defying improvement. Although we often are referred patients with erratic blood glucose readings (some of whom have been labelled as having brittle diabetes), there is *almost always a cause* and *almost always a way to make it better.* For a doctor (or other health care provider or, indeed, for a person with diabetes) to simply attribute erratic blood glucose control to brittle diabetes without first carefully looking for (and treating) any and all possible causes such as those in the preceding list is, in our opinion, not only a shame, but a travesty. (Not that we feel strongly about this or anything.)

Testing for Longer-Term Blood Glucose Control with the A1C Test

Individual blood glucose tests are great for telling you how you're doing at a specific moment in time, but they don't give you the big picture. Frequent blood glucose measurements help, but even then, they only provide a series of snapshots of your glucose levels. So what you need is a test that gives an estimate of your *overall* control over a longer period of time. And that's precisely what can be determined from a test called an A1C. Your *A1C* is a measure of how much glucose has become attached to your red blood cells over approximately the preceding three (to four) months.

Knowing your A1C is crucial because the likelihood of your developing microvascular complications (that is, eye, kidney, and nerve damage, as we discuss in Chapter 6) is directly related to your A1C. A normal A1C reading is 6 or less. An A1C of 7 or less is very good and puts you at quite low risk for microvascular damage. An A1C of 9 or higher is poor and puts you at much greater risk. An A1C that is too high is an alarm to you and your health care team that you need to improve your control. If you can drop your A1C by even 1 percent, you'll substantially decrease your risk of microvascular complications. One landmark study found that reducing the A1C by just 1 percent (equivalent to a reduction in average blood glucose of only 2 mmol/L) resulted in an astounding 37 percent lower risk of microvascular complications.

You may come across other terms for A1C, including *hemoglobin A1C, glycosylated hemoglobin,* or *glycohemoglobin.* You may also come across it abbreviated as HbA1C or HgbA1C. These all mean the same thing. Also you may find an A1C written as a number (9, for example) or as a percentage (9%, for example); both of these are correct and mean the same thing.

After you have had your A1C tested, be sure you contact your doctor (or diabetes educator, if he or she is the one who requested the test) to find out the result. If your A1C is above target (we discuss targets later in this section), be sure to ask your diabetes educator, diabetes specialist, and/or family physician what steps you can take to improve your result.

The A1C test doesn't replace blood glucose meter testing; it's *complementary* to it. Because the A1C represents an overall estimate of your blood glucose control, it doesn't express how many highs and lows you may be having. Your average glucose level may be good even though half your readings are too low and the other half too high. It's sort of like having one foot in ice water and the other in boiling water and saying, "On average, I feel fine."

Table 9-4 shows what the average blood glucose levels are (over the preceding three to four months) for a given A1C.

Table 9-4	A1C with Corresponding Average Blood Glucose Level
A1C	*Average Blood Glucose (in mmol/L)*
5	5.4
6	7.0
7	8.6
8	10.2
9	11.8
10	13.4
11	14.9
12	16.5

As the table demonstrates, the higher your A1C, the higher your blood glucose levels have been running. The lower your A1C, the lower your recent blood glucose levels.

How A1C works

Within red blood cells is a protein called *hemoglobin*. Hemoglobin carries oxygen around the body, delivering it to where it is needed to assist with various chemical reactions that are taking place. Hemoglobin is constantly exposed to the glucose within the blood and becomes permanently attached to it. It attaches in several different ways, and the total of all the hemoglobin attached to glucose is called *glycohemoglobin*. The largest fraction, two-thirds of the glycohemoglobin, is in a form called hemoglobin A1C. This is the easiest form to measure. The rest of the hemoglobin is made up of hemoglobins A1a and A1b. The more glucose in the blood, the more glycohemoglobin forms.

Hemoglobin is destroyed when the red blood cell that contains it dies. This occurs after the red blood cell has been in existence for about 120 days or so. Because glycohemoglobin remains in the blood for that length of time, it is a reflection of the glucose control over that entire time period and not just the second that a single glucose test reflects.

As you can see, your A1C reading is *not* the same as your average blood glucose reading. This is commonly misunderstood. (For example, an A1C of 8.0 does *not* mean that your average blood glucose level is 8.0 mmol/L; it actually corresponds to average readings of 10.2 mmol/L.) (To help alleviate this confusion, a new way of looking at average blood glucose is on the horizon: the estimated average glucose. To learn more about this new measurement, have a look at the sidebar "Estimated average glucose.")

The Canadian Diabetes Association recommends that most adults with diabetes have their A1C tested every three months; the target A1C for most adults with diabetes is 7 or less. (If you are pregnant it will need to be checked more often, and your goal is lower, as we discuss in Chapter 7. We discuss the target A1C for children in Chapter 15.)

As long as you use your blood glucose meter frequently, your A1C result will likely be as anticipated. When it isn't (for example, if your meter's average was 7.0 mmol/L yet your A1C was 10), you and your health care team will need to figure out why. The most common reason for this is that your readings are up when you aren't testing and therefore you wouldn't be aware of the elevations. If your readings have this sort of discrepancy, try testing more often and at times you haven't been testing (including overnight). On occasion, an A1C is affected by other substances in the blood or by anemia. If your physician suspects this, he or she can contact the laboratory to discuss this possibility.

Estimated average glucose

As of August 2008, the American Diabetes Association has adopted a new way of looking at average blood glucose control, called *estimated average glucose (eAG)*. We expect that over the next few years this term will become increasingly adopted and the term A1C will become less and less often used (except in scientific discussions).

In the future you will no longer be told, for example, that your A1C is, say, 7.0. Instead you will be told — in this particular example — that your estimated average glucose is 8.6. Estimated average glucose, as the name suggests, is the estimate of your average blood glucose for approximately the preceding three months. It's a value derived from the A1C using a simple formula. You can find both the formula and, even better, an online A1C-to-eAG calculator at http://professional.diabetes.org/glucosecalculator.aspx.

Apart from going to the lab to have them take blood from your arm, you can check your A1C in two other ways. Some diabetes centres have a desktop machine that can process a finger-prick sample in six minutes so that you (and they) will know your result while you are there for your visit. The cost is usually about $10 per test. A disposable test kit for home use is also available, but it is expensive and isn't covered by most provincial or private health plans, and thus, isn't often used.

Using a Continuous Glucose Monitoring System

One of the neatest things to come along over the past few years in the world of diabetes management is continuous glucose monitoring (CGM), performed using a continuous glucose monitoring system (CGMS). We expect this technology will, sometime in the not-too-distant future, revolutionize the way that diabetes management is performed, initially for people using insulin pump therapy and, ultimately, for most people with diabetes.

Continuous glucose monitoring is, as its name suggests, the continuous measuring of your glucose level. Because it is continuous it is also referred to as real-time glucose monitoring. We discuss the different aspects of CGM in this section.

Understanding continuous glucose monitoring

A CGMS consists of three components: a sensor, a transmitter, and a receiver (or display; see Figure 9-5). The currently available CGMS in Canada has two types of receiver: one that is solely dedicated to this role, or one that is integrated into an insulin pump.

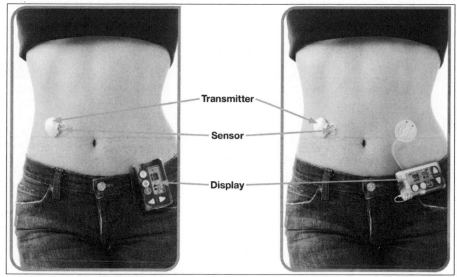

Figure 9-5: Guardian REAL-Time Continuous Glucose Monitoring System.

Transmitter

Sensor

Display

© 2008 Medtronic, Inc.

Here's how the different components of a CGMS work:

- **Sensor:** A sensor is a disposable device with an electrode-containing tiny tail that's inserted under the skin — typically on the abdomen or buttock, but you can also put it on your arm or leg. Like your blood glucose test strips, the sensor measures your glucose level; however, unlike your blood glucose test strips, it measures your glucose level in your *interstitial* fluid, not your blood. The sensor then passes this information along to the transmitter.

- **Transmitter:** The sensor is directly connected to the transmitter. The transmitter receives your glucose level reading from the sensor and, using radio frequency technology, sends this data to the display (receiver).

✔ **Receiver (Display):** The display, well, displays. It shows your current glucose level, your glucose levels over the past number of hours, and whether your glucose level is going up or down (this is indicated by arrows pointing — as you might imagine — up or down), and it also has an alarm that will alert you if your glucose level is too low or too high. (The alarm thresholds are adjustable.)

The display updates every five minutes; that means you will have a total of 288 measurements displayed per 24 hours. (Imagine doing 288 finger-prick samples per day!)

Because the display is wireless, it can be kept anywhere up to several feet from the transmitter. This means that at night, for instance, you can put it on your bedside table and it'll still work. The receiver's data (your glucose levels) can also be downloaded to a computer for reviewing or uploaded to a Web site where both you and your health care team can review it.

Checking out the benefits of continuous glucose monitoring

No matter how often you test your blood, you won't know what your glucose levels are for much of the day. This could mean you're not aware of significant periods of time when your glucose level is outside of the target range (we discuss target blood glucose levels earlier in this chapter). This is especially concerning if you have hypoglycemia unawareness (see Chapter 5) and, thus, don't recognize when you have low blood glucose.

The inside scoop on how a CGMS works

The sensor component of a CGMS doesn't, in and of itself, determine your glucose level. Rather, every 10 seconds, the sensor captures, in the form of an electrical signal, raw data from the interstitial fluid (similar to the way Environment Canada weather balloons capture raw data from their measuring devices in the atmosphere). The sensor's raw data is passed to the transmitter, which, every five minutes averages the data and then sends packets of this raw data to the receiver. The receiver then takes this raw data and converts it into a glucose level result (similar to the way a TV meteorologist takes Environment Canada's raw data and interprets it and then displays it as the beautiful illustrations we see on television).

A CGMS helped Martha, a patient of Ian's, who was testing her blood frequently using a blood glucose meter. (Her test results are marked as *x*'s in Figure 9-6.)

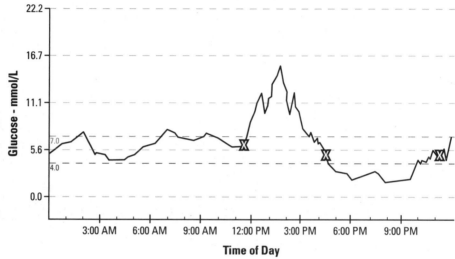

Figure 9-6:
Results from
a continu-
ous glucose
monitor.

Martha's blood glucose levels, measured using her blood glucose meter, were excellent and, indeed, consistently within target. Her A1C was also excellent (6.5). However the continuous line in the graph — which represents the data obtained from her CGMS — reveals that she had elevated blood glucose from about noon until 3 p.m., and low blood glucose from about 5 p.m. to 10 p.m. If Martha and Ian relied exclusively on her blood glucose meter results, they would have mistakenly thought everything was fine, whereas, in fact, her levels were often high and often low. Using the information from the CGMS, Ian, Martha, and her diabetes educators were able to adjust her insulin doses and diet, and her glucose levels were much more consistent thereafter.

Here are some of the ways that CGM can help you:

✔ By providing you with a continuous display of your glucose levels, it gives you immediate feedback to tell you how something you eat or some exercise you do is affecting your glucose control. This will then allow you to modify your diet, your exercise, or your insulin dosing if necessary.

✔ Up and down trending arrows will alert you to an impending high or low blood glucose level so you can take corrective action before your glucose level gets too far out of whack.

- By having an alarm that sounds (and vibrates) if your glucose level is too low (you can adjust the alarm setting; most people set it at about 4.5 or so), you will be alerted to an impending episode of hypoglycemia before it happens. This is especially helpful for people who experience hypoglycemia during their sleep or who have hypoglycemia unawareness.

- By having an alarm that goes off if your glucose level is too high (again, you can adjust this), you will be alerted when you might need to take extra insulin.

Looking at the drawbacks of continuous glucose monitoring

Like all technology — especially new technology — CGM has some shortcomings. These include the following:

- **Cost:** Only one brand of CGMS is currently available in Canada. (Others are available in the United States.) The available sensors cost about $50. The one sensor currently available in Canada is approved by Health Canada for use for no more than three days, at which time it's supposed to be replaced. There is, however, little (if any) significant risk of using it for longer periods of time and, being the frugal souls that people are, most all CGMS users (uneventfully) use their sensors for six days or even longer. The available transmitter (which needs to be replaced every nine months or so) is about $700. The cost of the receiver/display unit is another $1,000 or so, but is much less expensive if integrated into an insulin pump (a sensor augmented pump).

- **Discomfort:** Some people find that inserting the sensor is uncomfortable or even somewhat painful. This is typically fleeting.

- **Inaccuracy:** Sensors are very accurate, but not perfectly so. Indeed, on occasion a value can be way off. For this reason, if you get a value that's low enough or high enough that you would need to take corrective action (for example, say your sensor tells you that your glucose level is 20 mmol/L), you must first do a blood glucose meter test to verify that you are truly this high before, in this example, giving yourself extra insulin. (Just imagine if the sensor told you your glucose level was 20 — and you gave extra insulin — but in reality your glucose level was only 4. This would be very dangerous.)

- **Time lag:** Sensors measure the glucose level in your interstitial fluid (just under the skin surface), not in your blood. Most of the time the source is not important because interstitial fluid and blood have similar glucose levels. However, when your blood glucose level is quickly rising (such as immediately after eating) or quickly falling, your interstitial glucose level is different from your blood level. (It takes about 15 minutes for the interstitial fluid glucose level to catch up to the blood glucose level.) For this reason, you may notice symptoms of hypoglycemia, for example, even though the number you see on the display is not low because the interstitial fluid glucose has yet to catch up. When you suspect your glucose level differs from what you see on the display, you'll need to test your blood to be certain what your level truly is.

✔ **Calibration:** The sensors need to be taught how to interpret interstitial glucose readings. The way you teach them is by, typically twice per day, doing a blood glucose test and entering the result into the CGMS. For this and for the other reasons detailed in this list, having a CGMS does not mean you can throw away your blood glucose meter and lancets.

Despite its shortcomings, CGM can be a life-altering and life-enhancing technology. One of Ian's patients had such severe problems with recurring severe hypoglycemia that an ambulance was visiting her house three times per week. She obtained a CGMS, and thereafter, whenever her levels were heading low, her alarm went off so that she could treat her impending hypoglycemia before it got out of hand. She didn't require a single ambulance visit once she started using the device.

CGM is far from perfect, but every year the technology improves and ultimately this will lead to the development of a feedback loop (essentially, an artificial pancreas) wherein your glucose sensor will continually and reliably measure your glucose level and automatically instruct your insulin pump to give just the right amount of insulin to match your needs. As one of Ian's patients said, "I'll simply have my pancreas outside of my body instead of inside my body."

Finding out more about CGM

You can learn more about CGM by checking out the Web sites of the three companies that sell these devices (note that currently the only CGMS available in Canada is the one sold by Medtronic):

✔ **Abbott** (`www.freestylenavigator.com`) makes the Freestyle Navigator Continuous Glucose Monitoring System.

✔ **DexCom** (`www.dexcom.com`) makes the SEVEN Continuous Glucose Monitoring System.

✔ **Medtronic** (`www.minimed.ca`) makes the Guardian REAL-Time Continuous Glucose Monitoring System and the MiniMed Paradigm REAL-Time Insulin Pump and Continuous Glucose Monitoring System.

Chapter 10

You Are What You Eat: Staying Healthy with Good Nutrition

- -

In This Chapter

▶ Adjusting your diet to enhance your health

▶ Looking at the elements of a healthy diet

▶ Making sure you get sufficient vitamins, minerals, and water

▶ Adding alcohol

▶ Using sweeteners other than sugar

▶ Eating smart when dining out

▶ Losing weight healthfully

▶ Dealing with eating disorders

- -

*I*an has always believed that his power to help someone with diabetes gain control of their blood glucose (indeed, their health in general) pales in comparison to the unbridled power and influence emanating from another source — you (the person living with diabetes)! Time after time, patient after patient, when someone who has not customarily looked after their health begins to take charge of the way they live, what foods they eat, what liquids they drink, what exercise they do, what weight they shed, Ian smiles in awe because he not only gets to put away his prescription pad, but, often, advises someone that their new lifestyle is so potent that some of their current medications can be withdrawn.

In this chapter we look at the key nutrition (diet) strategies you can follow to achieve and maintain good diabetes health. We also look at effective ways that people who are overweight (as most people with type 2 diabetes are; indeed, as most Canadians with or without diabetes are) can safely and effectively lose weight. (In Chapter 11 we explore the important ways that exercise can help you manage your diabetes.)

The Key Ingredients

Our diets are made up primarily of carbohydrates, proteins, and fats. These basic groups are rounded out by the other things we need to consume to survive, including minerals, vitamins, and, of course, water. And, for most of us, our diets also include some amount of alcohol and, often, non-nutritive sweeteners.

The Canadian Diabetes Association (CDA) recommends that people with diabetes follow *Eating Well with Canada's Food Guide* (you can find it online at www.hc-sc.gc.ca/fn-an/food-guide-aliment/index-eng.php). This very helpful guide recommends that you do the following:

- ✔ Enjoy a variety of foods.
- ✔ Emphasize cereals, breads and other whole grain products, fruits, and vegetables.
- ✔ Choose lower-fat dairy products, leaner meats, and food prepared with little or no fat.
- ✔ Achieve and maintain a healthy body weight by enjoying regular physical activity and healthy eating.
- ✔ Limit salt, alcohol, and caffeine.

The CDA also recommends that you divide your diet (based on energy, or calories) as follows:

- ✔ Carbohydrate: 45–60 percent
- ✔ Protein: 15–20 percent
- ✔ Fat: less than 35 percent

Carbohydrates and proteins provide a different amount of energy (measured in calories) than fats. The number of calories contained in 1 gram is

- ✔ Carbohydrate: 4 calories
- ✔ Protein: 4 calories
- ✔ Fat: 9 calories

Of course, you and your dietitian will have to determine the best diet for you based on your particular needs. Your diet will include not only the best food choices for you, but also the appropriate number of calories you should consume. With unrestricted calories, you could limit your carbohydrates to 60 percent of your diet and still have enough energy to power a Boeing 747.

Technically speaking, there is a *calorie* and there is a *Calorie* and there is a *kilocalorie* (1,000 *c*alories equals 1 *Calorie equals 1 *kilo*calorie). However, almost no one speaks of kilocalories in normal, day-to-day discourse, and it's a chore to capitalize the *c* every time, so we use the conventional term *calorie* whenever we talk about nutrition issues. Sure, it's not perfectly scientific to do so, but we won't tell if you won't. (Also, you may come across the term *kilojoules*. One Calorie is equal to about 4.2 kilojoules. Once again, few people use this unit of measure, so we forgo it also.)

Carbohydrates

Carbohydrates do much more than just fuel our bodies. They also fuel debate. Indeed, probably no other area of diabetes management offers quite the same degree of controversy. In this section we look at the important issues for you to be aware of, including the pros and cons of low versus higher carbohydrate diets.

Although *glucose* gets most of the attention, within our bodies we also have other forms of carbohydrate, including glycogen (which is stored in the liver and muscles). Dietary carbohydrates include starches, cellulose, and gums (not the chewing type, although, come to think of it, we can think of more than one occasion when chewing gum has made its way into someone's stomach, but we'll chew on that one some other time).

Food sources of carbohydrate are found primarily in things grown in the ground and in dairy foods. Some of the common dietary sources of carbohydrate are bread, potatoes, grains, cereals, rice, dairy products such as milk and yogurt (cheese has very small amounts of carbohydrate), fruits, and some sweet, usually fleshy vegetables (such as parsnips and squash).

These are some important roles that carbohydrates play in the body:

- Carbohydrates are the main source of energy for muscles.
- Carbohydrates cause the triglyceride (fat) level to rise in the blood.
- Glucose is the carbohydrate that causes the pancreas to release insulin.
- When your body doesn't have enough insulin or your insulin doesn't work sufficiently well, ingesting carbohydrates raises the blood glucose above normal.
- Sugars (as present in sweet items such as candy) are not directly harmful (except, perhaps to your teeth) as long as your total number of calories ingested is not excessive.

Consuming sugar does *not* cause diabetes. Furthermore, don't let any well-meaning friend or relative tell you that because you have diabetes you cannot eat sugar. You can. Tell them Ian and Alan said so. (We'll leave it up to you if you also want to tell them that you recognize that you have to eat appropriate amounts and types of sugar.)

A few years ago an elderly man was referred to Ian after having had type 2 diabetes diagnosed a few months earlier. He was a charming gentleman and clearly was working diligently to maintain his traditionally good health. As they spoke, Ian couldn't help but get the impression that something was bothering his new patient. Finally, because the gentleman was not volunteering anything in this way, Ian asked him point-blank if there might be something on his mind. "Well, Doctor," he said, "I guess I'm just feeling kind of sad that I had my 80th birthday yesterday and everyone got to eat my birthday cake except for me. And it was my favourite, too. Chocolate. I wasn't allowed to have any because I have diabetes." Whatever reply this gentleman was expecting, it was clearly not the one that Ian supplied. "Well, sir," Ian said, "I have a prescription I want you to fill. Right after you leave this office I want you to go *not* to the drugstore, but to the *bakery*. Buy the biggest chocolate cake they sell and cut yourself as big a slice as you want. And if anyone tells you that you 'can't eat it because you have diabetes,' you tell them that your diabetes specialist *ordered* you to." The patient left the room literally singing.

Cake is not a four-letter word! If you have diabetes, you can eat not only cake, but other sweets too. The point is, nothing is forbidden, it just has to be consumed in moderation and, most importantly, not at the expense of other, healthier foods that you need. So long as your total number of carbohydrates and calories is appropriate, there is nothing wrong with having occasional treats. Happy birthday!

A greater percentage of Canadians are overweight now than at any other time in our history. This is due primarily to two things: We aren't as physically active as we once were, and we are consuming, on average, about 200 calories more per day than we did a generation ago. These extra calories are derived almost exclusively from unneeded carbohydrates in supersize soft drinks, extra-large candy bars, and excessive consumption of breads, pastries, and the like. Within our bodies, these extra carbohydrates are turned into fat and stored in our fat cells. This ability to store extra calories as fat was great when everyone lived in caves and got little food for prolonged periods of time, but it doesn't fit today's lifestyle, consisting as it does of abundant food (and minimal foraging for it — unless you count hunting through the supermarket aisles).

Because carbohydrate is the food that raises the blood glucose — and high glucose is responsible for many of the complications of diabetes — it's important to consume the proper amount of carbohydrates.

If you are on a 2,000-calorie diet and are consuming 50 percent of your calories as carbohydrate, that would work out to 1,000 calories of carbohydrate per day. Because a gram of carbohydrate is 4 calories, you could eat 250 grams of carbohydrate in a day. Most people with diabetes do very well on this amount of carbohydrate, but for others a lower percentage works best. In Appendix A we look at the number of grams of carbohydrate contained in a variety of foods and how this information can be used to help you come up with a healthy menu.

Glycemic index

All carbohydrates aren't alike in the degree to which they raise the blood glucose. This fact was recognized some years ago, and a measurement called the *glycemic index* was created to quantify the amount each food raises blood glucose. The glycemic index (GI) uses oral glucose (less often, white bread) as the standard (or indicator) food and assigns it a value of 100. Another food containing an equal amount of carbohydrate is rated according to its ability to raise blood glucose and is assigned a value in comparison to oral glucose. A food that raises glucose one quarter as much as oral glucose has a GI of 25, while a food that raises glucose three quarters as much has a GI of 75. A glycemic index of 70 or more is considered high; 56 to 69 is medium; and 55 or less is low. The point of the index is to select carbohydrates with low GI levels to try to keep the glucose response as low as possible.

Like most things in life, the GI has its supporters and its detractors. Its supporters point out that relying on foods with a low glycemic index has these advantages:

- ✔ May help improve blood glucose control.
- ✔ May help improve lipids. (Following a low GI diet often produces a reduction in levels of triglycerides and LDL cholesterol.)

On the other side of the food fence, GI detractors point out these problems:

- ✔ The GI of a carbohydrate-containing food may be different when it is eaten alone than when it is part of a mixed meal.
- ✔ The GI of a food may differ depending on how it's processed and prepared.
- ✔ Some low-GI foods contain a lot of fat.
- ✔ Figuring out the GI can be difficult and can lead to confusion.
- ✔ Research has not yet proven long-term health benefits of a low-GI diet.

We can think of no better illustration of the controversy regarding the glycemic index than the point that Alan is a supporter and Ian is not yet convinced. Alan notes that he has observed improved glucose control in his patients who follow a low-GI diet, and Ian points out that a Snickers candy bar rates better on the GI than does a bowl of cornflakes. (We are not making this up!) Is it possible that some people might mistakenly believe this means that candy bars are a healthy food choice? What a disastrous error that would be!

The Canadian Diabetes Association, quite appropriately, feels that the decision to implement a low-glycemic-index diet should be individualized based on a person's particular interest and ability.

Because we don't yet have proof that a low-glycemic-index diet is the way to go, the most prudent course would be to initiate your nutrition therapy with the standard Canadian Diabetes Association recommendations, as you will learn from your dietitian. If you have been working with this meal plan and not succeeding the way you should, speak to your dietitian and your family doctor (and diabetes specialist if you are seeing one) to see if they feel you would benefit by switching to a low-GI diet.

Should you elect to proceed with a low-glycemic-index diet, you can easily make some simple substitutions in your diet, as shown in Table 10-1.

Table 10-1	Simple Diet Substitutions
High-GI Food	*Low-GI Food*
Whole-meal or white bread	Whole-grain or multigrain bread
Processed breakfast cereal	Unrefined cereals like steel-cut oats, large-flake rolled oats, or processed low GI cereals like muesli
Plain cookies and crackers, puffed rice cakes	Cookies made with dried fruits or whole grains like oats
Cupcakes and doughnuts	Cakes and muffins made with fruit, oats, and whole grains
Potatoes	Pasta (cooked al dente) or legumes
White rice	Basmati, brown, wild, or parboiled rice

Because bread and breakfast cereals are major daily sources of carbohydrates, these simple changes can make a major difference in lowering your glycemic index. Foods that are excellent sources of carbohydrate but have a low GI include legumes such as peas or beans, pasta, grains like barley, parboiled rice, and whole grain breads.

You can discover more about the glycemic index on the Web at www.diabetes.ca/for-professionals/resources/nutrition/glycemic-index.

Glycemic load

Just because a food has a high GI does not necessarily mean that it will unduly raise your blood glucose. For example, although cantaloupe has a GI of about 70, the amount of total carbohydrate is so low that it does not raise your blood glucose significantly when you eat a normal portion. This concept is called the *glycemic load* (GL). Each food is given a number that takes both glycemic index and total carbohydrates into account. A GL of 20 is high; 11 to 19 is medium; and 10 or less is low.

Carbohydrate counting

Glucose levels rise after you eat mainly because of the carbohydrates in your meal (or snack). Also, in general, the greater the number of grams of carbohydrate, the more your blood glucose level will rise. People who are on an insulin program that includes frequent administration of rapid-acting insulin can gauge the amount of insulin to be given based on the number of grams of carbohydrate they are about to ingest. (We discuss carb counting further in Chapter 13.)

Fibre

Fibre is the part of the carbohydrate that is not digestible and therefore adds no calories. It is found in most fruits, grains, and vegetables. Fibre comes in two forms:

- **Soluble fibre:** This form of fibre can dissolve in water and has a lowering effect on blood glucose and lipids, particularly cholesterol. Soluble fibre gets gooey and sticky when mixed with water. An example is oatmeal.

- **Insoluble fibre:** This form of fibre cannot dissolve in water and remains in the intestine. It absorbs water and stimulates movement in the intestine. Insoluble fibre also helps prevent constipation and possibly colon cancer. This is the fibre called *bulk* or *roughage.* Insoluble fibre doesn't change much when mixed with water. An example is the skin of an apple.

Before the current trend to refine foods, people ate many sources of carbohydrate that were high in fibre. These were all in plant foods, such as fruits, vegetables, and grains. Animal foods contain no fibre.

The Canadian Diabetes Association recommends you ingest 25 to 50 grams of fibre daily.

Because too much fibre causes diarrhea and gas, you need to increase the fibre level in your diet fairly slowly.

Proteins

Protein in your diet is usually in the form of muscle of other animals, such as chicken, turkey, beef, or lamb. Vegetable sources of protein include soybeans, legumes, nuts, and seeds. The main role that protein has in your diet is to maintain the health of tissues such as your muscles. For these reasons, people used to believe that you could build your own muscle by eating lots of another animals' muscle. (The truth is that you can build up your muscle only by exercising or weightlifting.) You need little protein to maintain your current level of muscle or increase it for that matter. Unlike carbohydrates, proteins do not raise blood glucose levels significantly.

Your choice of protein sources is very important because some also contain very high quantities of fat while others are relatively fat-free. The following lists give you an idea of the fat content of various sources of protein.

About 30 grams (1 oz.) of **very lean** meat, fish, or substitute has 7 grams of protein and 1 gram of fat. Examples are

- Skinless, white-meat chicken or turkey
- Flounder, halibut, or tuna canned in water
- Lobster, shrimp, or clams
- Fat-free cheese

About 30 grams (1 oz.) of **lean** meat, fish, or substitute has 7 grams of protein and 3 grams of fat. Examples are

- Lean beef, lean pork, lamb, or veal
- Dark-meat chicken without skin or white-meat chicken with skin
- Sardines, salmon, or tuna canned in oil
- Other meats or cheeses with 3 grams of fat per 30 grams (1 oz.)

About 30 grams (1 oz.) of **medium-fat** meat, fish, or substitute has 7 grams of protein and 5 grams of fat. Examples are

- Most beef products
- Regular fat pork, lamb, or veal
- Dark-meat chicken with skin or fried chicken
- Fried fish
- Cheeses with 5 grams of fat per 30 grams (1 oz.) such as feta and mozzarella

About 30 grams (1 oz.) of **high-fat** meat, fish, or substitute contains 7 grams of protein and 8 grams of fat. Examples are

- Pork spareribs or pork sausage
- Bacon
- Regular cheeses such as cheddar and Monterey Jack
- Processed sandwich meats

You'll find a huge difference in the number of calories depending on whether you choose a high- or low-fat-containing protein source. For instance, 30 grams (1 oz.) of skinless white meat chicken contains about 40 calories whereas 30 grams (1 oz.) of pork spareribs has 100 calories. Because most people eat a minimum of about 120 grams (about 4 oz.) of meat at a meal, they're eating from 160 to 400 calories depending upon the source. That's why it's so important to look carefully at the food you are about to eat: The company your protein source keeps can make the difference between you successfully losing weight or not.

If you're on a 2,000-calorie diet of which 20 percent is protein, 400 calories would come from protein sources. Because a gram of protein is 4 calories, you could eat 100 grams of protein in a day.

Fats

When we think of fat, we tend to think of the fat we see on a steak or in hamburger meat. But there are actually quite a variety of fats and fat-like substances. Although many of these are unhealthy and to be avoided, some, in fact, help to protect our health. This section looks at these different issues.

Cholesterol is the fat-like substance everyone knows. It has been shown to be a major contributor leading to atherosclerosis (such as coronary artery disease, as we discuss in Chapter 6). It is recommended that no more than 300 milligrams a day of fat come from cholesterol. (One large egg has about 210 mg of cholesterol.) Other sources of cholesterol include organ meat such as liver or kidney, whole milk, and hard cheeses such as Monterey Jack and cheddar.

Most people do not realize the extent to which our bodies (our livers in particular) contribute to our cholesterol levels. In fact, the majority of our body's cholesterol is made by our livers. That's why so many people with diabetes, even if faithfully following a low-fat diet, end up requiring medication anyhow to achieve optimal blood cholesterol levels.

The other kind of fat is triglyceride, which we classify into two groups:

✔ **Saturated fat** is the kind of fat that comes from animal sources. The streaks of fat in a steak are saturated fat. Butter, bacon, cream, and cream cheese are other examples of foods rich in saturated fat. Eating a lot of saturated fat can make your bad (LDL) cholesterol level go up. And that's not a good thing. The Canadian Diabetes Association recommends that saturated fat be less than 7 percent of your total calorie intake.

✔ **Unsaturated fat** comes from vegetable sources such as olive oil, canola oil, and margarine. It comes in several forms:

- **Monounsaturatcd fat** raiscs HDL (this is the good cholesterol) and does not affect LDL (bad cholesterol). Avocado, olive oil, and canola oil are examples. The oil in nuts, such as almonds, and pea-nuts is also monounsaturated.

- **Polyunsaturated fat** lowers LDL, but, depending on the level of consumption, may also lower HDL. Examples of polyunsaturated fats are soft fats and oils such as corn oil, mayonnaise, and marga-rine. Polyunsaturated fats should be less than 10 percent of your total calorie intake.

You may have read recently about trans fatty acids. Trans fatty acids also raise LDL levels. They are formed when liquid oil goes through a process of hydroge-nation, turning it into a semi-solid form, like shortening and many margarines. These fats are used widely in the food industry in many commercially baked goods such as cookies, cakes, potato chips, doughnuts, pastries, French fries, and breaded foods. You can significantly reduce your intake of these fats by avoiding commercially fried foods and high-fat bakery products. Looking at the Nutrition Facts table on a food label will also tell you how much trans fat your product contains. The goal is to minimize the amount of trans fat you consume.

Lest you think that everything with the word *fat* in it is bad, here's some good news about fat. Some fats are actually good for you. Mounting evidence suggests that a fat called *omega-3 fatty acids* can help protect you from ath-erosclerosis. These are found in certain fish such as salmon, tuna, mackerel, and trout. Omega-3 fatty acids also help reduce blood pressure and protect against the formation of blood clots in the coronary arteries (thus reducing the likelihood of your getting a heart attack). It's recommended that you eat fish rich in omega-3 fatty acids at least once (better still, two or three times) per week. If you don't like fish, we can't help but think that it must mean you have never tasted salmon cooked on a barbecue or in a dishwasher. (True story: Ian's mom makes marvellous dishwasher salmon, and no, the fish does not swim around in the water; it is wrapped in tinfoil and put through the entire wash and dry cycle — without soap! Readers can find a variety of dish-washer salmon recipes on the Internet.)

If we go back to your hypothetical 2,000-calorie diet — lest you slowly starve while waiting for us to figure out how much fat to feed you so that you get your final 600 calories — fat has 9 calories per gram, so you can eat about 67 grams of fat daily. Seeing as you may have consumed much of this with your protein source, you may not have much fat left to add.

Getting Enough Vitamins, Minerals, and Water

Your nutrition plan must contain sufficient vitamins and minerals. If you eat a balanced diet that comes from the various food groups, you'll generally get enough vitamins for your daily needs. Table 10-2 lists the vitamins and their food sources.

Table 10-2	Vitamins You Need	
Vitamin	*Function*	*Food Source*
Vitamin A	Needed for healthy skin and bones	Milk and green vegetables
Vitamin B1 (thiamine)	Converts carbohydrates into energy	Meat and whole grain cereals
Vitamin B2 (riboflavin)	Needed to use food properly	Milk, cheese, fish, and green vegetables
Vitamin B6 (pyridoxine)	Needed for growth	Liver, yeast, and many other foods
Vitamin B12	Keeps the red blood cells and the nervous system healthy	Animal foods (for example, meat)
Folic acid (also called folate)	Keeps the red blood cells healthy	Green vegetables
Niacin	Helps maintain healthy metabolism	Lean meat, fish, nuts, and legumes
Vitamin C	Helps maintain supportive tissues	Fruit and potatoes
Vitamin D	Helps with absorption of calcium	Dairy products, and is made in the skin when exposed to sunlight
Vitamin E	Helps maintain cells	Vegetable oils and whole grain cereals
Vitamin K	Needed for proper clotting of the blood	Green, leafy vegetables

As you look through the vitamins in Table 10-2, you can see that most of them are readily available in the foods you eat every day. In certain situations, such as if you are pregnant or breastfeeding, elderly, a strict vegetarian, or on a very low calorie diet, you should take a multivitamin daily. (In pregnancy you should also take a folic acid supplement. We discuss vitamin therapy and pregnancy in Chapter 7.) The CDA recommends taking 400 IU of vitamin D daily if you are older than 50. Apart from these special circumstances, taking vitamin supplements is seldom helpful (except for the people selling them!).

Minerals are also key ingredients of a healthy diet. Most are needed in tiny amounts, easily consumed from a balanced diet. These are the main minerals you should know:

- ✔ **Calcium:** We need calcium primarily to maintain strong bones. Insufficient calcium intake can be a factor in developing osteoporosis. Milk and other dairy products provide plenty of calcium. It's important to ingest between 1,000 and 1,500 milligrams of calcium per day. If you aren't consuming enough calcium in your diet, you should take calcium supplements. This also applies if you're growing up (adolescents) or out (pregnant women).

- ✔ **Chromium:** We require chromium for certain internal chemical reactions to take place normally. In areas of the world where there is a severe deficiency of chromium in the diet, people are more likely to develop diabetes. Regrettably, people in areas of the world where we get perfectly adequate quantities of chromium in our diets (this includes Canada) have been inundated with pseudo-scientific and misleading claims that taking chromium supplements will either reduce your blood glucose levels or cure your diabetes. We have no convincing evidence of the former, and as for the latter, it is simply false. Once again, the only people benefiting from this promotion are the people selling the products.

- ✔ **Iodine:** Iodine is necessary for our thyroid glands to work normally. You may have noticed that boxes of salt in Canada are labelled "Iodized." Because of this iodine supplementation, Canadians do not develop iodine deficiency (even if you never add salt to your food).

- ✔ **Iron:** We require iron to make red blood cells. A lack of iron leads to anemia. Most of our iron intake comes from consumption of red meat. Menstruating women are prone to iron deficiency (menstrual blood is rich in iron) and often will require iron supplementation. Vegetarians also often require iron supplements.

- ✔ **Magnesium:** Our bodies use magnesium to allow a number of different chemical reactions to occur. Magnesium deficiency can lead to problems with the heart's electrical system. Magnesium deficiency is very seldom a problem, and routine supplements are unnecessary.

- ✔ **Phosphorous:** Phosphorous in our bodies contributes to the maintenance of strong bones. We get ample phosphorous in our diets, and routine supplements are not required.

- ✔ **Sodium:** Sodium (salt) is present in many of the foods we eat — particularly in processed foods such as prepared meats and some cheeses, as well as packaged snack foods such as pretzels and potato chips. Canadians consume many times more sodium per day than we need.

This may be a factor leading to high blood pressure. You would be wise to avoid adding salt to your food, and if you have high blood pressure, make a point of buying foods that are low in salt to begin with.

✓ **Cobalt, Tin, and Zinc:** These minerals are rarely lacking in the human diet, and supplements are unnecessary.

Although we've saved our discussion about water to last, it is by no means the least important. Water makes up of 60 percent or more of your body. All the nutrients in the body are dissolved in water. You can live without food for some time, but you won't last long without water. Water can help to give a feeling of fullness that reduces appetite. You should make a point of drinking at least 1½ litres (50 oz.) of water per day.

Counting Alcohol as Part of Your Diet

Alcohol is a substance that has calories but no particular nutritional value. It has, however, been shown that a moderate amount (a drink or two per day) may reduce your risk of a heart attack.

If you like to have a drink, it's reasonable that you continue so long as you limit yourself to no more than two drinks per day if you're a man, and one drink per day if you're a woman. If you don't normally drink, do not start just because you're at possible risk of developing heart disease down the road. And, of course, if you're pregnant, you should not drink any alcohol at all.

Having two drinks per day is *not* the same as quaffing 14 cold ones on a Saturday evening while you watch *Hockey Night in Canada.* Even if the game goes into overtime.

Because alcohol has calories, you must account for the alcohol you drink in your diet. Depending on the strength of the individual product, 350 millilitres (12 oz.) of beer, 150 millilitres (5 oz.) of wine, and 45 millilitres (1½ oz.) of hard liquor all have similar quantities of alcohol.

Despite what many people think, drinking beer or wine is not better for you than drinking hard liquor. To your liver they all taste the same.

Apart from the consequences of the calories it provides, there are several other important points about alcohol you should keep in mind:

✓ Alcohol — especially if taken without food — can cause low blood glucose if you are on insulin or some forms of oral hypoglycemic agent therapy (see Chapter 12). It does so by reducing your liver's ability to produce glucose. You can lessen this risk by making sure you eat some food when you drink alcohol.

- Alcohol reduces your awareness of symptoms of low blood glucose (see Chapter 5) and, as a result, makes you less likely to take appropriate corrective action.

- Alcohol can interact with some medicines called sulfonylurea oral hypoglycemic agents (see Chapter 12), which causes a variety of unpleasant symptoms, including nausea and flushing (even if you are not inebriated).

- If you're taking insulin or certain medicines that stimulate insulin production, drinking alcohol two or three hours after your supper can result in hypoglycemia occurring as late as the next afternoon.

Artificial and Sugar Alcohol Sweeteners

Unrestricted consumption of sugars doesn't fit with good diabetes management (or, of course, with good health in general). And because there are limits on how much sugar we should consume, artificial sweeteners have a role to play. Of the artificial sweeteners in common use, aspartame (NutraSweet) is the best known. In the amounts commonly used, aspartame provides virtually no calories, yet provides abundant sweetness. In fact, aspartame is 200 times sweeter than sucrose (table sugar). Aspartame has been the subject of many Internet rumours detailing its dangers. These are false. The truth of the matter is that aspartame is completely safe unless you have a rare genetic disease called PKU. The equal truth is that despite common use of aspartame in our society, we as a population are getting larger and larger, not smaller and smaller.

Other approved artificial sweeteners in Canada are

- Acesulfame potassium (trade name Sunett)
- Cyclamate (this is the sweetener used in Sugar Twin)
- Saccharin (this is the sweetener used in Sweet'N Low)
- Sucralose (trade name Splenda)

These sweeteners are safe to use if you have diabetes — unless you're pregnant or breastfeeding, in which case you shouldn't consume saccharin or cyclamate.

Sugar alcohols (maltitol, mannitol, sorbitol, lactitol, isomalt, and xylitol) are another type of sweetener. They are not artificial. They do provide calories and can affect your blood glucose levels to a degree. Examples of products that may contain sugar alcohols are chewing gum, hard candies, some jams, and syrups. Consumption of more than 10 grams per day of sugar alcohols can cause abdominal cramping and diarrhea.

Eating Out

Canadians are eating more and more of their meals in restaurants. This is not necessarily a bad thing (especially if you happen to own a restaurant!), but it does complicate managing your diabetes. At home you know what ingredients you're using, you can measure quantities, you can follow certain steps to avoid weight gain (see the section "Weighty Issues," later in this chapter, for behaviour-changing tips), and, if you're carbohydrate counting, you can reasonably precisely measure the carbs in your food. In a restaurant, many of these factors are, to variable extents, removed from your control. Also, restaurants (including fast-food establishments) tend to serve food that is richer in fat, higher in salt, and bigger in volume than you might normally eat at home (see the section "Weighty Issues" for more about proper portion size). We may not consider *cake* to be a four-letter word, but *supersize me* sure is!

Here are helpful tips you can follow to make eating out a healthful, not harmful, experience:

- ✔ **Make sure you eat foods from the major food groups.** Even fast-food restaurants have healthy food selections if you look hard enough for them: McDonald's doesn't have to be synonymous with McDiabetes.

- ✔ **If a portion size is big (ask the wait staff; they'll know), order one serving and split it with your dinner-mate.** Ian and his wife do this routinely and, as long as you don't tell anyone, we'll even fess up and admit to — egads — being known to pass a plate back and forth across the table.

- ✔ **Avoid buffets.** It is the rare individual who can go to an all-you-can-eat place and leave the restaurant feeling less than stuffed. Also, buffets often serve carbohydrate-rich foods, which will make your blood glucose level go up.

- ✔ **Order foods that are baked, steamed, or broiled rather than deep fried.**

- ✔ **Avoid foods that are heavily battered or breaded or that are served with rich, creamy, or cheesy sauces.**

- ✔ **Make sure the wait staff are paying attention when you order a diet soft drink.** Waiters sometimes bring a non-diet soft drink to the table despite a diet soft drink having been ordered.

- ✔ **If you take rapid-acting insulin before your meals, don't take your dose until you're certain your food is on its way.** Better still, wait until it's in front of you. More than one person has had an insulin reaction because they took their dose only to then find their food was delayed in arriving.

Making sense of nutrition food labels

Prepackaged foods for sale in Canada have nutrition food labels. Understanding these sometimes confusing labels will help you make healthy food selections when you're at the grocery store. In this sidebar we look specifically at those aspects of nutrition food labels that are especially important for people with diabetes.

These are the most important things about nutrition food labels for you to be aware of:

✔ **The serving size:** In theory, this is the amount of the item that one person would be expected to eat during one meal (or snack, and so on). This amount is set by the manufacturer. It is, however, very easy to buy a package and, based on its size, assume it to be one serving size whereas in fact it may contain two or more servings. (It's astonishing to find out how tiny one serving size of a favourite snack may be.) Remember that you may or may not want to eat one serving size. If you eat two servings, for example, you'll be consuming twice as many calories and twice as much fat as what the label lists the product to contain for just one serving size.

✔ **% Daily Value:** This indicates the percent of your daily nutrition requirements you will meet by eating one serving size of the food.

✔ **The amounts, in one serving, of calories, total fat, saturated fat, trans fat, total cholesterol, sodium, total carbohydrates, fibre, sugars, protein, vitamin A, vitamin C, calcium, and iron.**

These are other important things for you to know about food labels:

✔ Prepackaged foods are often rich in sodium, so keep an especially close eye on this part of the label.

✔ If you're carbohydrate counting, note that although fibre is listed on the label, because it doesn't raise blood glucose it should be subtracted from the total amount of carbohydrate listed when you perform your calculations.

✔ A serving size containing no more than 5 grams of sugar can generally be considered to be low in sugar.

If you have questions about a specific product's nutrition food label, remove it from the package and take it with you to your next appointment with your dietitian. An excellent online resource is www.healthyeatingisinstore.ca.

Weighty Issues

If you're overweight and have diabetes (refer to Chapter 4 if you're not sure how much you should weigh), these are some of the benefits you may experience from even small weight loss:

✔ Improved blood glucose control (You may also find that your oral hypoglycemic agents or insulin — which may not have been working sufficiently well for you — work much more effectively. In some cases, lifestyle change by itself results in such a good impact on blood glucose control that — like Wanda, in the sidebar, "Wanda's winning recipe for health" — you'll be able to discontinue your medications. Which, by the way, is our favourite prescription!)

✔ Improved blood pressure

✔ Improved lipids (cholesterol and triglycerides)

✔ Enhanced self-esteem

✔ Better sex life

✔ More energy and more incentive to exercise

✔ Reduced risk of some types of cancer

✔ Increased life expectancy

Weight-loss challenges

Weight reduction is difficult for many reasons, but perhaps foremost among them is the immense challenge of trying to change lifestyle patterns and habits that you may have lived with for decades. No one should ever tell you that the changes you're being asked to make are easy. They are not easy. In fact, for most people they are downright difficult. But *they can be done*. And if you have initial success only to then revert back to old habits, that does not mean all is lost. Just pick up where you left off and try again.

Another obstacle to losing weight is expecting too much too soon. If you need to lose 23 kilograms (about 50 pounds) and after a month you have lost only 2 kilograms (about 4 pounds), you may start to feel frustrated, as if you're never going to get there. But don't think for a second that you haven't had success. You've had great success!

Diabetes is a long-term disease. Achieving your target weight doesn't have to occur overnight, or even over weeks or months. Slow and steady surely does win the weight-loss race. In fact, if you lose weight too quickly you'll be more likely to regain it.

Nothing is as likely to frustrate your efforts to follow proper nutrition therapy as trying to figure it out without professional help. We would strongly recommend that in addition to reading this chapter, you see a registered dietitian who has expertise in helping people with diabetes. If your doctor hasn't referred you to one, as soon as you finish reading this chapter, pick up the phone, call your doctor's office, and ask them to book you an appointment. You'll be glad you did.

If you have loved ones who are overweight, be sure to share with them how weight loss can markedly reduce their likelihood of developing diabetes. Indeed, you and your loved ones can embark together on a journey of healthy eating, weight loss, and good health.

Wanda's winning recipe for health

Wanda B. Thinner (okay, we admit it; we changed the name), age 46, was recently diagnosed with type 2 diabetes. When the diagnosis was made, her doctor put her on oral medicines to reduce her blood glucose, but they weren't helping and she continued to be bothered by excessive thirst and urination. She was, therefore, referred to Alan. At the time of her first appointment with Alan, she had a blood glucose of 13 mmol/L. She was 165 centimetres (5 feet 5 inches) tall and weighed 85 kilograms (187 pounds).

Alan arranged for Wanda to meet with a registered dietitian — and diabetes nurse educator — and Mrs. Thinner started a lifestyle treatment program that included a meal plan based on the principles in this chapter. She worked hard over the next few months and successfully lost 9 kilograms (20 pounds), which she subsequently kept off. Her blood glucose levels came down to the range of 4 to 8 mmol/L and her readings stayed there. Alan had her stop her oral hypoglycemic agents and her blood glucose readings remained equally good. With her weight loss and excellent blood glucose control, Wanda felt the best she had in years. She was yet another prime example of how drugs are second-rate diabetes therapy compared to the impact of lifestyle treatment.

The best strategy for losing weight

The best strategy for losing weight is to combine reduced calorie intake with increased calorie expenditure. Indeed, a successful program of weight loss typically requires a willingness to make exercise a part of your daily life. If, for some reason, you cannot move your legs to exercise, you can get a satisfactory workout using your upper body alone. A recent study showed that 92 percent of people who maintain weight loss exercise regularly. We look in depth at exercise and diabetes in Chapter 11.

If you need to lose weight, you should aim to shed 1 to 2 kilograms (2 to 4 lb.) per month, losing 5 to 10 percent of your initial body weight over 6 to 12 months. You should try to burn off 500 calories more per day than you ingest. (See Chapter 11 to find out what type and duration of exercise allows you to accomplish this.) Also, if you eat lots of high-fibre foods, you'll find that you won't feel as hungry.

Half a kilogram (about a pound) of fat contains 3,500 calories. Therefore, in order to lose this much fat, you must eat 3,500 calories less than you need or you must burn off these calories by exercising.

As we discuss in the section "The Key Ingredients," earlier in this chapter, we advocate healthy eating following the recommendations of the Canadian Diabetes Association and Health Canada. We do not recommend following any of myriad fad diets. Although these diets often provide success, it is almost always just short-lived, with all (or more) of the weight that was successfully lost being regained later. Many of these diets are so restrictive, they can make you feel unwell with constipation, fatigue, muscle aching, hair loss, and so on. (Hmm, a diet that doesn't provide long-term weight loss, can make you feel unwell, and often costs lots of money to boot; not exactly a recipe for success — except for the people selling the books and running the fad clinics.)

Portion control for weight loss

Although many factors help to explain why Canadians (and most others in the world, for that matter) have become heavier and heavier, one unavoidable fact is that supersized food portions — whether consumed in or outside of the home — have been a major factor leading to our supersized waists. No matter how you slice it, your weight is determined by the number of calories you take in, minus the number of calories you use up by exercise or loss of calories in the urine or bowel movements. If you have an excess of calorics coming in and have insulin with which to store them, you gain weight. If you have fewer calories in than out, you lose weight.

Here are examples of healthy portion sizes:

- ✔ 85 grams (3 oz.) of meat is the size of a deck of playing cards.
- ✔ A medium apple or peach is the size of a tennis ball.
- ✔ 28 grams (1 oz.) of cheese is the size of four dice.
- ✔ 120 millilitres (½ cup) of ice cream is the size of a tennis ball.
- ✔ 240 millilitres (1 cup) of mashed potatoes is the size of your fist.
- ✔ 5 millilitres (1 tsp.) of butter or peanut butter is the size of the tip of your thumb.
- ✔ 120 millilitres (½ cup) of nuts is the size of a golf ball.

We hope our analogies in the preceding list to tennis and golf got you in the mood for some exercise! (Feel free to play cards or throw some dice after you get back.)

Medication therapy for losing weight

We're not big fans of medication therapy for weight loss, but in the event that your best efforts at lifestyle change have not produced a significant decrease in your weight, prescription drug therapy is something that you and your physician might consider. Two drugs are available in Canada to assist with weight loss, neither of which tend to be all that successful, but some people do benefit:

✔ **Xenical** (orlistat) is taken three times daily with your meals. It works by blocking your small intestine from absorbing ingested fat into your blood stream. Unfortunately, most people lose only small amounts of weight while taking this medicine, and, significantly, many people run into problems with oily deposits escaping from their rectum and soiling their underclothes. Ugh! We don't want to sound overly negative, however, because some people do benefit nicely, and recent evidence also suggests that Xenical can help reduce blood glucose levels.

✔ **Meridia** (sibutramine) assists with weight loss by acting directly on the hunger centre in the brain. Like Xenical, its benefits are generally fairly marginal and it can have significant side effects, including making your blood pressure go up.

Medicines to assist with weight loss do not, of course, replace or substitute ongoing dietary change and exercise.

Surgery for weight loss (bariatric surgery)

Surgery is sometimes used in the most severe and resistant cases of obesity (BMI 35 or greater; refer to the chart in Chapter 4). As you might imagine, surgery — any surgery — is not to be undertaken lightly. (There's an old expression that minor surgery is surgery that someone else has.) Nonetheless, for select individuals it can be a very effective form of therapy, with multiple health benefits including improved glucose control.

There are several different surgical treatments available including *Roux-en-Y gastric bypass, laparoscopic vertical banded gastroplasty,* and *laparoscopic gastric banding (lap banding).* The last of these is quite novel and involves the surgical placement of a constricting band containing an inflatable balloon that is placed around the upper end of the stomach to create a small upper pouch and a larger lower pouch. It can be inflated or deflated to control the size of the upper stomach.

Each of the aforementioned surgical options has its pros and cons. If you are considering bariatric surgery, you will need to do your homework, including meeting with surgeons who perform these procedures to find out what risks (both short- and long-term) the procedures would pose, the expected benefits, and the costs (health care plans will not necessarily cover these).

Regardless of which procedure you and your surgeon decide upon, you must be committed to lifelong medical follow-up. You must be willing to give up large meals and be determined to lose weight. Severely obese people with type 2 diabetes can lose much weight and achieve remarkable health improvements (better blood glucose, better blood pressure, less need for medications, and so on) through bariatric surgery, but there is a price to be paid — and not just a financial one (which, by the way is very high indeed).

Behaviour modification

In addition to the lifestyle changes we discuss earlier in this section, a number of other strategies are available to help you lose weight. You needn't adopt all of the following tips (though you are welcome to); adopting even a few of them can have a terrific impact.

Here are some behaviour modification tips you may find helpful in your quest to lose weight:

✔ Eat at set times.

✔ Eat your food in a single place.

✔ Slow down your eating.

✔ Put your cutlery down between mouthfuls.

✔ Don't put more food in your mouth before you have finished your last bite.

✔ Concentrate on the taste of each mouthful before you swallow.

✔ Every few minutes, pause and ask yourself if you're still hungry.

✔ Don't finish every morsel on your plate. There's nothing wrong with leaving some behind.

✔ After the food has been served, remove the serving dishes and bread basket from the table.

✔ Don't keep high-calorie snacks visible in the kitchen or elsewhere in the house. Better yet, don't keep them in the house at all.

✔ Remember that seemingly innocent things like salad dressings can be very rich in calories.

✔ Add bulk to your food (adding a vegetable to pasta for example). Hunger is often satisfied by increasing the volume of food even if the number of calories is reduced.

✔ Avoid impulse buying when doing your grocery shopping. Bring a shopping list and walk the aisles specifically looking for the items you have written down rather than just wandering from aisle to aisle.

✔ Get a 5-kilogram (11-lb.) weight and carry it around for a while to appreciate the importance of a loss of even that little.

✔ Incorporate regular exercise into your weight-loss strategy.

✔ Most important of all, remember that there's no rush. As we say earlier, trying to lose weight too rapidly will make it more likely that you'll regain the weight later.

As you go about the difficult task of losing weight and keeping it off, remember to seek the help of those around you. A loving partner provides great help through the roughest days.

Coping with Eating Disorders

You might remember the expression "You can't be too rich or too thin." How much damage has this statement — or at least the sentiment (especially the "thin" part) — done to society? Young people, particularly girls, are often preoccupied with their body weight. When this preoccupation becomes too great, it can result in an eating disorder.

Young girls with eating disorders (and young boys about a tenth as often) either starve themselves and exercise excessively or eat a great deal and then induce vomiting and/or take laxatives and water pills (diuretics). Someone who starves herself has *anorexia nervosa,* while someone who binges and purges has *bulimia nervosa.* These conditions can result in severe illness and, when carried to extremes, even death.

Anorexia is usually found in girls who have a distorted body image and are fearful of weight gain. The prevalence may be as high as 1 in 200 in these girls. The girls may appear unusually thin and may not menstruate. Their malnutrition may be very severe.

Bulimia involves eating large quantities of food and then purging it by vomiting and taking laxatives or water pills. These people are usually not as severely thin as people with anorexia. Because their weight is closer to normal, they usually menstruate normally.

Management of diabetes requires a certain amount of routine from day to day, so if you have an eating disorder — and thus, inconsistent food intake — it complicates matters and makes achieving consistently good blood glucose levels virtually impossible.

It is imperative that a person with an eating disorder receive proper treatment. Eating disorders clinics specialize in providing this necessary care. If you have an eating disorder or if you care for someone who does, we recommend you see your family physician to let them know of the issue. Your doctor will want to assess your health and refer you to the appropriate specialist clinic as necessary.

Chapter 11

Exercising Your Way to Good Health

*I*t may well be that you look back at your high school grad photos and point out to your children or grandchildren how slim and trim you were way back when exercise was not a chore, but a matter of routine. Perhaps it was not long thereafter that family and work commitments appeared, followed in short order by some excess weight around your middle. And after your lifestyle had changed, maybe you were like millions of your fellow Canadians and simply could never find the time or enthusiasm to get on track with exercise and shedding the extra kilograms you had acquired.

But the wonderful thing is, you're not too late. You're *never* too late. Whether you're 25 or 85, you can still make changes in your lifestyle to enhance your health. And you don't have to feel intimidated by this. The changes don't have to occur overnight. And the changes don't have to be *all* or *none,* because any change is a change for the better.

And we can promise you that the changes you have to make are not quite so intimidating as those recommended by Hippocrates, the renowned physician of ancient times, who said "obese people should perform hard work, eat only once a day, take no baths, and walk naked as much as possible."

Simply put, exercise is one of the most powerful weapons you have to stay healthy. In this chapter we look at how exercise can help you and how you can incorporate exercise into your diabetes treatment plan.

How Exercise Can Improve Your Diabetes Health

Exercise is helpful for everyone, but is especially helpful if you have diabetes. Exercise can

- Lower your blood pressure

- Improve your lipids (cholesterol and triglycerides)

- Lower your blood glucose levels (particularly if you have type 2 diabetes) — and may, as a result, reduce your need for medicines that lower your blood glucose (If you need them anyhow, exercise will allow them to work much more effectively.)

- Help you lose weight

- Reduce your risk of a heart attack (and improve your prognosis if you've already had one)

- Increase your energy level

- Reduce your stress level (and improve your ability to handle stress when it occurs)

- Improve your general sense of well-being

- Improve your sex life (more energy, more stamina . . . more merrymaking)

- Provide social interaction (You can spend time with people who are also concerned with health. These people usually share many of your interests. The person who likes to jog often likes to hike and climb. And more than one lifetime partnership began on a tennis court; hmm, maybe that's why tennis players use the terms _love_ and _match_.)

If we haven't convinced you yet, how about this: Studies have shown that if you have diabetes and you exercise regularly, you can reduce your risk of dying in the next ten years or so by over 50 percent! So, do you need to exercise? Well, only as much as you need to breathe. Literally.

As we discuss in Chapter 4, exercise, healthy eating, and weight control can reduce the risk of developing type 2 diabetes by 60 percent. If you have diabetes, let your loved ones know of this benefit and encourage them to exercise with you.

A prescription for exercise

Ian well remembers John Plant. John was a 46-year-old bus driver who had been living with type 2 diabetes for 13 years. John's family physician referred John to Ian because John's blood glucose levels were too high. The doctor had recommended — and John had declined — insulin therapy. John didn't exercise and he was considerably overweight. He had high blood pressure and high cholesterol. "Dr. Blumer," John said, "I'm already on seven different types of medicines. I take 25 pills a day. Geesh, I feel like I've become my father. Heck, I'm a walking drug store. Don't ask me to take insulin, too."

To John's surprise, Ian didn't. "John, it's your call. You don't have to be your father. You can make changes that will help to keep you healthy and, quite possibly, that could get your blood glucose levels down without requiring insulin."

John looked keenly at Ian. "You think so?" he asked.

"You bet," Ian replied, "and this is how to do it." Ian reviewed many of the key points contained in this book, including the importance of diabetes education, healthy eating, exercise, and so forth. John took this to heart, figuratively and literally. He improved his diet, he began and progressively increased his exercising, he lost weight, and, over the next 12 months his blood glucose levels, blood pressure, and cholesterol all improved without additional medicine. Indeed, things improved so dramatically that not only did he not need additional medicine, in fact he was able — under close medical supervision — to come off over half the pills he had been taking.

At the time of John's last visit to Ian he was beaming: "Dr. Blumer, I saw it like this. Either I made the time to exercise now or I made the time to look after my diabetes complications later. I think you can figure out which I chose."

Taking Precautions Before You Start Exercising

Prior to beginning a new exercise program, check with your family doctor (who may recommend — depending on the nature of the exercise you are about to do and other factors listed below — that you visit with other members of your team, including your diabetes specialist, nurse educator, dietitian, eye doctor, and a fitness instructor or exercise specialist). Although exercise is essential, you must initiate it with caution.

How exercise works its magic

As you exercise and your muscles start to work, they require additional fuel. At first, *glycogen,* the storage form of glucose in the liver, begins to break down and release glucose, which provides a source of energy to your muscles. With continued exercise, glycogen is used up and the liver begins to make glucose from other substances in order to continue to provide energy.

With steady, moderate exercise, the body eventually turns to burning fat as the glucose production begins to diminish. This is a wonderful situation, especially because most people with type 2 diabetes have extra fat to offer.

If the exercise is very vigorous (or if you don't have sufficient insulin), the liver actually makes more glucose than the muscles can use immediately, and the blood glucose begins to rise. This explains some of the instances where the glucose is higher after exercise than it is before exercise. Vigorous exercise will not be continued for very long, and the extra glucose will be there to replenish the muscle tissue, once exercise ends.

Consider these factors before you take up exercising:

- **Whether or not you have heart disease:** Before you start exercising, your doctor may choose to send you for an exercise stress test (this is a test where your heart is monitored while you walk on a treadmill) to look for evidence of coronary artery disease (see Chapter 6) — even if you have no heart symptoms.

- **Whether or not you have high blood pressure:** Although exercise is good treatment for hypertension, it can be dangerous if you have severely elevated blood pressure.

- **The state of your blood glucose control:** Exercise is terrific therapy for elevated glucose levels, but it can be dangerous if you have severe hyperglycemia, in which case your blood glucose levels will have to be reduced to a safer level — generally under 15 or so — before you start an exercise program. On the other hand, if your blood glucose control is excellent before you take up an exercise program, when you then begin exercising you may be prone to low blood glucose. Therefore, whether your blood glucose control is poor or excellent or in between, we recommend you review it with your doctor before you begin an exercise program.

- **The state of your eyes:** Some forms of exercise can aggravate retinopathy (see Chapter 6). If you have not been to your eye doctor within the past year, you should have your eyes checked before you undertake any form of vigorous exercise or weightlifting.

✔ **Whether or not you have peripheral neuropathy:** You can still exercise if you have peripheral neuropathy, but it would be wise for you to read the section (in Chapter 6) on foot care and footwear first.

✔ **Physical limitations:** Things such as obesity, arthritis, peripheral vascular disease (see Chapter 6), and amputations may influence the nature of the exercise you undertake.

✔ **The medications you may be on:** Your doctor may need to adjust drugs such as oral hypoglycemic agents or insulin if you're going to be exercising.

The preceding list looks at those things to consider *before* you initiate an exercise program. If you have type 1 diabetes and your fasting blood glucose is higher than about 15 mmol/L with ketones present, you should not exercise *at all*, whether you have been exercising regularly or never a day in your life. It could cause you to develop worsening hyperglycemia and ketone production (we discuss ketoacidosis in Chapter 5). After your metabolic control is back in order, grab your running shoes and head for the door!

Here are some other things to consider as you embark on your life-enhancing (and possibly life-saving) exercise program:

✔ Obtain (and wear!) a medical alert bracelet or necklace. This is important primarily if you are on medications (especially insulin) that can cause hypoglycemia.

✔ Determine (with your diabetes educator) whether you'll need to do more frequent blood glucose monitoring.

✔ Obtain (and wear) proper socks and shoes. (And remember that in order to avoid getting blisters, you need to gradually wear in your new shoes.)

✔ Ensure that you consume sufficient water when you exercise.

✔ Bring treatment for low blood glucose if you're on medication that can bring this on.

✔ For the first few days after you begin (or increase) your exercise program, check your blood glucose more often than usual (including before you exercise, within an hour or two after you've completed your exercise, and, if you are taking insulin, in the middle of the night) so that you can determine how your blood glucose levels respond to the exercise you are performing. (Overnight testing is required because exercise can make your body more responsive to your insulin, which can, in turn, lead to low blood glucose — even hours after you've completed your exercise.)

The Hockey Heart Study

Where else but in Canada could a medical study called the Hockey Heart Study be conducted? This study showed that a significant percentage of men playing recreational hockey had possible heart troubles develop while playing. The players wore portable electrocardiogram-type (EKG) devices that recorded their heartbeats during their games.

When the recordings were analyzed afterward, quite a few abnormalities showed up, suggesting that the players may have been experiencing heart problems — such as impaired circulation to the heart — even though they had not had any symptoms. The full significance of these findings is not known, but they certainly suggest that the typical Canadian pastime of being sedentary for days, weeks, or months on end and then going out for an hour of sprints up and down the ice may not be the best thing in the world to do.

Finding the Right Type of Exercise

People routinely ask us what the best exercise is. Whenever Ian is asked this, he recalls the time he asked the bicycle store owner what the best helmet was for his son. Her wise answer: "The one he will actually wear." So, too, with exercise. The type of exercise you do is far less important than simply finding one that you enjoy and will stick with.

We can classify exercise into two broad types:

- **Cardiovascular** (cardio): During *cardiovascular* exercise (such as when you walk or run), your muscles use oxygen and your heart pumps faster to keep up with your muscles' demands. When we talk about *cardiovascular conditioning,* we are referring to the benefits on the heart and circulation of cardiovascular exercise.

- **Resistance:** *Resistance* exercise uses muscular strength to move a weight or to work against, well, a resistance. Examples of resistance exercise are weightlifting or exercising with weight machines. Resistance training will improve your muscular fitness and energy level and can also increase your metabolic rate.

Because the benefits of cardiovascular and resistance exercise are complementary, you should do both types.

If we still haven't convinced you that you can start exercising regularly, we suggest you consider joining a community centre or YMCA/YWCA that offers exercise programs. These are usually run by excellent fitness leaders who will be sensitive to your needs and can fit you into a class that's suitable for you. These facilities are often far less threatening (and far less expensive) than large, commercial fitness establishments.

The Diabetes Exercise & Sports Association (www.diabetes-exercise.org) is an organization dedicated to "enhancing the quality of life for people with diabetes through exercise and physical fitness." Among their members are both exercise neophytes and world-class athletes. Have a look at their site.

Cardiovascular exercise and you

The most important thing in choosing an exercise is that you like it enough to carry on with it. Another factor that may influence your decision is the number of calories an exercise burns. Table 11-1 supplies this information.

Table 11-1	Exercise and the Amount of Calories You Burn in 20 Minutes at Different Body Weights	
Activity	*Calories Burned (57 kg/125 lb.)*	*Calories Burned (80 kg/175 lb.)*
Running, 11 kph/7 mph	236	328
Skiing, cross-country	196	276
Skiing, downhill	160	224
Football	138	192
Tennis	112	160
Walking, 6.5 kph/4 mph	104	144
Swimming	80	112
Baseball	78	108
Dancing	70	96
Golfing	66	96
Carpentry	64	88
Gardening	60	84
House painting	58	80
Typing	38	54
Writing	30	42
Standing	24	32

Everything you do burns calories. Even sleeping uses 20 calories in 20 minutes if you weigh 57 kilograms (125 lb).

When Rajeev, a 35-year-old dentist, found out that he had diabetes, he decided to start exercising. Since his best friend golfed, he thought he would try that too. A couple of months later, despite playing golf several times a week, his glucose control and his weight hadn't shown much improvement. As it turned out, he had joined one of the few golf courses in Canada that require you to use a cart. He switched clubs (so to speak) and was soon walking up and down the fairways, burning calories with each and every step. Only 4 percent of golf courses in Canada have rules making cart use mandatory. That leaves you with 96 percent of courses in Canada to choose from. So the next time you are on the links, make sure the only driving you're doing is with your clubs. Fore!

Virtually everyone can do cardiovascular exercise. If you have a limitation that makes it difficult to do some types of exercise such as walking, try a different one, such as swimming.

You do *not* have to go out and spend a whole bunch of money on exercise machines, fitness clubs, and the like (though of course you're welcome to). We wish we had a dollar for every treadmill that now functions as a full-time clotheshorse or dust collector. Some comfortable clothes and shoes are all you need to begin your exercise program.

Starting cardiovascular exercise

Perhaps you have heard the famous Chinese proverb, "A journey of a thousand miles begins with a single step." Proverbs are proverbs for a reason.

In our experience, people face two main obstacles to taking up exercise:

- Feeling overwhelmed by the task
- Inertia

Well, neither of these obstacles is insurmountable. We can assure you — in fact, we can guarantee you — it doesn't have to be too big a task. Set your sights low. Very low. Very, very, low. Get the point? If you never exercise, start your new program by simply walking daily to the end of your block and back. Do that for a few days, then try circling the block daily. A few days later, walk several blocks. Every week try to cover a slightly greater distance, and when you have succeeded with that, increase your pace. Once you have gotten into a routine, you will find that your inertia is a thing of the past.

A good rule of thumb is to increase your daily exercise by five minutes every week. Using this approach, you will be up to half an hour of daily exercise within a month and a half. Not too shabby.

If you think you may want to start getting out for a regular walk but need something else to motivate you, consider buying a dog. Dogs love going for walks. And, just like you, they also need to exercise. Not sure you want the responsibility? Offer to take the neighbour's dog for a daily walk. Both your neighbours and their dog will be thrilled.

Determining the right amount of cardiovascular exercise

The Canadian Diabetes Association recommends that people with diabetes perform at least 150 minutes of moderate-to-vigorous-intensity cardiovascular exercise each week, spread out over at least three days of the week (with no more than two consecutive days without exercise). That's not to say that you have to rest on your well-deserved laurels if you've accomplished this. Indeed, try to build up to at least four hours of weekly exercise. (In other words, about four times as much as your doctor is probably doing! Please don't tell your doctor we said that. We were just kidding; really.)

These are examples of moderate exercise:

- ✔ Brisk walking on a level surface
- ✔ Biking
- ✔ Raking leaves
- ✔ Water aerobics

These are examples of vigorous exercise:

- ✔ Brisk walking up an incline
- ✔ Jogging
- ✔ Aerobics
- ✔ Hockey
- ✔ Fast dancing

Do you eat your entire week's calories in one meal? Do you do your entire week's breathing with one deep breath? No? Then remember, you shouldn't try to do your entire week's exercise in one session either. It's simply not as effective if you do it that way. On the days you are exercising, if you'd like, feel free to divide up your exercise into several ten-minute sessions; it will work just as effectively.

The following are several ways to determine if you are pushing yourself to the right extent:

- ✔ **The talk test:** You should be able to talk while exercising. (See the sidebar.)
- ✔ **The breath sound check:** When you hear yourself breathing (not panting), you are going at the right pace. (Incidentally, this and the talk test were first developed by Dr. Robert Goode based upon pioneering research he did at the University of Toronto. See the sidebar for more information.)
- ✔ **Perceived exertion:** Work at a level that feels moderate to somewhat hard, but not beyond that.

These three techniques are particularly helpful because they allow you to adjust your exercise according to your own needs.

The talk test

The talk test has its origins in the mountain-climbing community, where climbers would say to one another, "Climb no faster than you can talk." Dr. Goode took that phrase and applied it to exercise at sea level. He recognized that at sea level the limiting factor in allowing people to exercise is insufficient oxygen supply to the muscles. He and his team showed experimentally that if you have difficulty talking, you are close to or at your anaerobic threshold (that is, the point at which your muscles can no longer effectively extract oxygen from your bloodstream), which in turn makes your muscles fatigued. This observation allowed Dr. Goode and his team to set a "lid" on how much cardiovascular exercise you can comfortably do.

Do not continue exercising if you have chest discomfort or severe shortness of breath. These can be symptoms of heart problems.

Resistance exercise and you

Weightlifting is a form of resistance exercise. It involves the movement of heavy weights, which can be moved only for brief periods of time. It results in significant muscle strengthening and increased endurance. And, as a nice bonus, pioneering studies by a Canadian researcher, Dr. Ron Sigal, have shown that resistance training also helps improve blood glucose control. (And, though not nearly as important as these other benefits, you may find it a nice plus to discover your more toned appearance as you look in the bathroom mirror.)

Because weightlifting causes a significant rise in blood pressure as it is being done, it has the potential to worsen retinopathy. (This is primarily an issue only if you're selecting weights that are overly heavy.) If you have retinopathy (or if you don't know if you do), we recommend that before you start resistance training, you first check with your eye doctor to ensure it's safe for you.

(*Weight training*, which uses lighter weights, can be a form of cardiovascular exercise. Because the weights are light, they can be moved for prolonged periods of time. The result is improved cardiovascular fitness along with strengthening of muscles, tendons, ligaments, and bones.)

Getting started with resistance exercise

The Canadian Diabetes Association recommends the following for your resistance exercising:

1. **Start with one set of 10–15 repetitions using a moderate weight.**

2. **Progress to two sets of 10–15 repetitions using a moderate weight.**

3. **Progress to three sets of 8 repetitions three times per week using a heavier weight.**

If you choose to do resistance exercise, first meet with a qualified exercise specialist and then keep in touch with him or her periodically.

Checking out some resistance exercises

In this section we look at a variety of resistance exercises you can perform.

Figure 11-1 shows the bicep curl. To do this exercise:

1. **Hold the dumbbells along the sides of your body, palms facing forward.**

2. **Raise the dumbbells until your elbows are fully bent.**

3. **Slowly lower the dumbbells to the original position.**

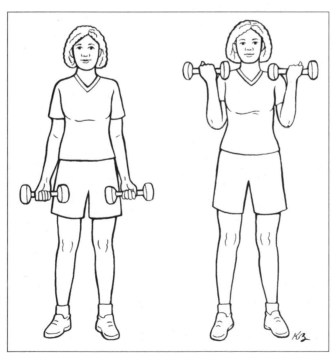

Figure 11-1:
Bicep curl.

Figure 11-2 shows the shoulder press. To do this exercise:

1. **Hold the dumbbells with your palms facing each other and your elbows bent.**

2. **Raise the dumbbells over your head, turning your palms to face forward.**

3. **Lower the dumbbells to the original position.**

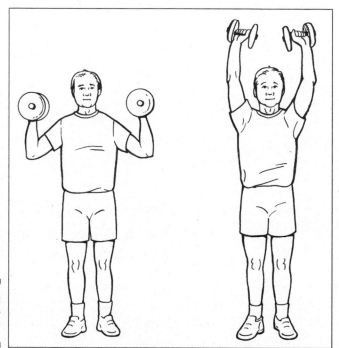

Figure 11-2:
Shoulder
press.

Figure 11-3 shows the lateral raise. To do this exercise:

1. **Hold the dumbbells along the sides of your body, palms facing each other.**

2. **Lift the dumbbells out to the sides, palms facing the floor until they are above your head.**

3. **Lower the dumbbells down to your sides.**

Figure 11-4 shows bent-over rowing. To do this exercise:

1. **Hold a dumbbell in each hand, arms hanging down, legs straight, back bent forward, parallel to the floor.**

2. **Raise the dumbbells up to your chest.**

3. Lower the dumbbells back to the floor.

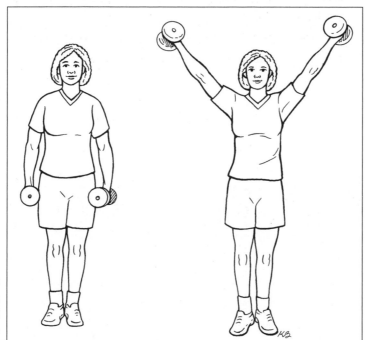

Figure 11-3:
Lateral
raise.

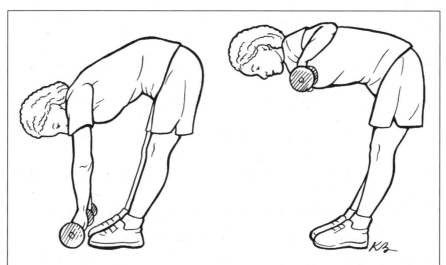

Figure 11-4:
Bent-over
rowing.

Figure 11-5 shows good mornings. To do this exercise:

1. **Hold the ends of one dumbbell above your head, arms straight.**

2. **Lower the dumbbell forward as you bend your back until it is parallel to the floor.**

3. **Raise the dumbbell to the original position.**

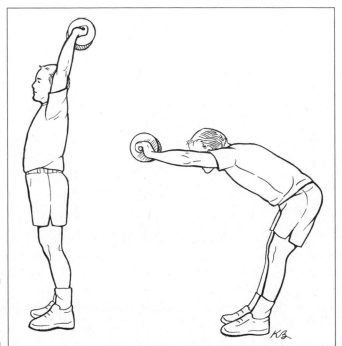

Figure 11-5:
Good
mornings.

Figure 11-6 shows flys. To do this exercise:

1. **Lie on your back and hold the dumbbells out to each side at the shoulder.**

2. **Lift the dumbbells together until they are above your head.**

3. **Lower them to the sides again.**

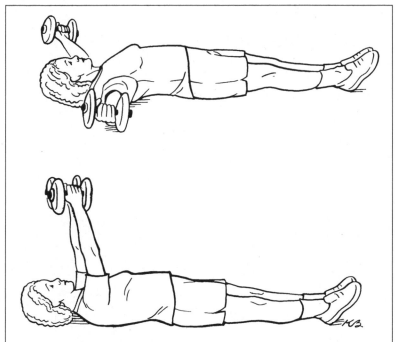

Figure 11-6:
Flys.

Figure 11-7 shows pullovers. To do this exercise:

1. **Lie on your back holding one dumbbell with both hands straight up above your head.**

2. **Lower the dumbbell with your arms straight to the floor behind your head.**

3. **Raise the dumbbell back above your head.**

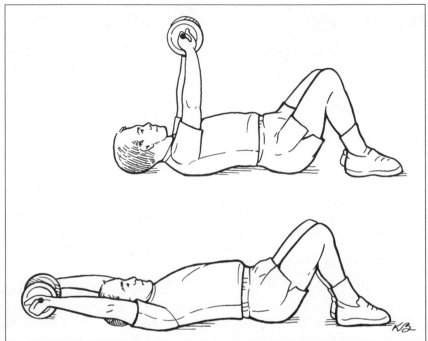

Figure 11-7:
Pullovers.

Exercising If You Are Taking Oral Hypoglycemic Agent Therapy

Taking oral hypoglycemic agent (OHA) therapy (see Chapter 12) need not prevent you from exercising. In fact, your medicines will work *much more effectively* if you exercise regularly. So much so, in fact, that you could be at risk of developing hypoglycemia. In practice this seldom happens, but it's still important for you to carry appropriate treatment with you. (We discuss treatment for hypoglycemia in Chapter 5.) The OHAs that cause hypoglycemia are those (such as glyburide) that stimulate the pancreas to release insulin. If you're on one of these medicines and are running into problems with low blood glucose when you exercise, speak to your physician about either reducing your dose or switching to a different medicine. We can't think of a greater disincentive to exercise than knowing it'll bring on an episode of hypoglycemia!

Exercise and Insulin Therapy

Being on insulin should not stop you from exercising, but you'll likely need to adjust your doses. If you perform vigorous exercise but have insufficient insulin, your muscles will not be able to properly use the glucose in your blood and your glucose level will (temporarily) rise. Conversely, if you exercise and you have too much insulin in your system, you will develop hypoglycemia.

Each person with diabetes has his or her own unique needs, and the way exercise affects your diabetes and insulin requirements will differ from how it affects somebody else's. Therefore, we recommend you meet with your diabetes nurse educator and your dietitian before you take up or significantly modify your exercise program — and then periodically thereafter — so that your educators can develop a nutrition plan and insulin adjustment strategy that will work for you. Things that your educators will review with you will include

- What you eat before you exercise
- When you eat before (during, after) you exercise
- Where you inject your insulin (As we discuss in Chapter 13, some forms of insulin are absorbed much faster if injected into a limb that's going to be exercised.)
- What type of insulin you are taking
- How often to test your blood glucose whilst exercising
- What to do to monitor yourself for (and help prevent) delayed hypoglycemia (Some people experience hypoglycemia many hours after having completed their exercise.)

In almost all circumstances, you should have your insulin and diet adjusted to accommodate your exercise. You should rarely, if ever, have to change your exercise to accommodate your treatment. (As Ian's motto says, "Rule your diabetes; don't let *it* rule *you!*")

Chapter 12

Controlling Your Blood Glucose with Oral Medications

*I*n Chapter 6 we discuss bad things (like blindness, kidney failure, and nerve damage) that you're doing your darndest to avoid (with our help) by maintaining control of your blood glucose levels. In Chapters 10 and 11 we look at the ways that you can improve your diabetes health by making appropriate lifestyle changes. In this chapter we look at how, if you have type 2 diabetes, you can further benefit by taking pills to assist you in your battle to maintain good blood glucose control and avoid diabetes complications.

The pills doctors use to combat high blood glucose are typically referred to as *oral hypoglycemic agents* or *OHAs,* although increasingly they are called oral antihyperglycemic agents. This change in terminology actually makes good sense. After all, your health care team isn't trying to make you have low blood glucose (which is what hypoglycemic means); it's trying to prevent you from having high blood glucose (hence, antihyperglycemic). Nonetheless, because the majority of the time both physicians and patients still refer to them as oral hypoglycemic agents, that's the terminology we use in this book. You may come across yet another term for oral hypoglycemic agents, *oral anti-diabetic agents (OADs).* This isn't our favourite term (in fact we don't like it at all) because it implies that diabetes is purely a problem with glucose, which is far from the case.

You can find additional information about OHA therapy and other prescription drugs in *Understanding Prescription Drugs For Canadians For Dummies* (a book Ian co-wrote with Dr. Heather McDonald-Blumer).

To Take or Not to Take: That Is the OHA Question

If you're like most people, you'd rather not take pills, and who could blame you? Table 12-1 lists some of the possible reasons you may have for *not* wanting to take oral hypoglycemic agent therapy. We take the liberty of quoting some things you might say (even though we probably haven't even met you. How presumptuous is that?), and we even indicate if we agree with your concern or not.

Table 12-1	Reasons Not to Take OHA Medication
I don't want to take OHAs because they:	*Our opinion*
Are chemicals.	We agree.
Can have side effects.	We agree.
Are not as good a treatment as proper nutrition therapy and exercise.	We agree.
Occasionally (depending on the type) cause hypoglycemia.	We agree.
Can interact adversely with other medicines.	We agree.
Can be hard to remember to take.	We agree.
Are a sign that I'm unable to control my blood glucose levels without them.	We agree.

Surprised that you're right (or at least that you're in agreement with us and so must be right!) on each point? But of course you're right. Who wants to take pills if you can avoid them? No one.

But consider the other side of the coin. Table 12-2 lists of some of the possible reasons you may have for *wanting* to take oral hypoglycemic agent therapy.

Table 12-2	Reasons to Take OHA Medication
I'm willing to take OHAs because:	*Our opinion*
They'll help me reduce my blood glucose levels if nutrition therapy and exercise alone can't do the trick.	We agree.
By improving my glucose control, they'll help protect my eyes, nerves, and kidneys.	We agree.
They seldom have serious side effects.	We agree.

I'm willing to take OHAs because:	Our opinion
Minor side effects can usually be easily corrected by adjusting the dose or changing to a different OHA.	We agree.
With the appropriate drug and dose, I can usually avoid hypoglycemia.	We agree.
Serious drug interactions seldom occur.	We agree.
I know diabetes is a progressive disease and that's not my fault. Taking an OHA doesn't mean that *I* have failed, it simply means that *my pancreas* has.	We agree.
Remembering to take pills is a pain in the butt, but it's a heck of a lot better than remembering to go for eye surgery and dialysis appointments.	We agree.
Dr. Blumer and Dr. Rubin are very persuasive.	We couldn't agree more.
Enough already. I give up!	'Nuff said.

Choosing the right medication for you

In recent years, tremendous strides have been made in developing new and innovative medications to help control blood glucose. As a result, your doctor can choose from many different drugs. And over the next ten years you will see a veritable explosion of additional drugs entering the marketplace. This is wonderful; it's great to have additional weapons in our arsenal for helping you stay healthy. But — there's always a *but* — with so many new drugs becoming available, each with their own unique properties (both good and bad), your doctor is going to have an increasingly difficult time knowing which one to choose for you.

That's where you come in. By becoming aware of the different medicines we discuss in this chapter and, in particular, by discovering their pros and cons, you can work with your doctor to find the best medicine for you and your specific situation. (In Chapter 8 we discuss other ways you can be a key member of your health care team.)

Understanding how OHAs work

People develop type 2 diabetes due to two factors: insulin resistance (a condition where your tissues do not respond to insulin properly) and insulin deficiency (wherein your pancreas is unable to manufacture sufficient insulin to keep up with your body's needs). (Refer to Chapter 4 for more.) Many of the drugs doctors use target these specific issues. Some newer drugs also target other areas — such as reducing appetite — to help control blood glucose. In this chapter we look in detail at the different oral hypoglycemic agents and we also discuss some new non-insulin injectable medication.

Figure 12-1 illustrates how the different OHAs work.

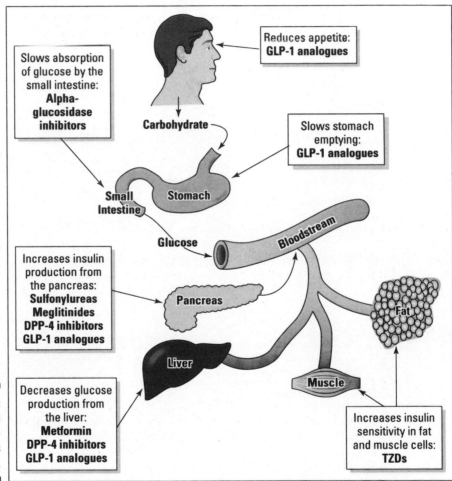

Figure 12-1: How oral hypoglycemic agents work.

Oral hypoglycemic agent therapy (or insulin for that matter) should *never* be considered a substitute for lifestyle treatment. Relying exclusively on pills to keep you healthy, and ignoring proper nutrition, exercise, and weight control, is a sure-fire way to fail with your diabetes management. Medications are *complementary* to what *you* do for you, and how you live your life.

Investigating the Types of Oral Hypoglycemic Agents

All classes of OHAs have at least two things in common:

- ✔ They help to reduce blood glucose (which, as we discuss in Chapter 6, reduces your risk of developing microvascular complications of diabetes).
- ✔ They have unpronounceable names.

In this section we look at the different types of oral agents that are available to assist you.

The label on your prescription drug bottle will have both the trade name *and* the generic name of your medicine; just like Shakespeare's rose, any way you say it, it's the same medicine. In this section we use generic names.

Although most people with type 2 diabetes are treated with oral hypoglycemic agents long before they are treated with insulin, be aware that insulin is a perfectly suitable treatment for type 2 diabetes — at *any* stage of the disease, even as early as when it's diagnosed.

A couple of the types of drugs in this section (metformin and thiazolidinediones) may improve the fertility of women with infertility due to polycystic ovary syndrome (PCOS). Since, as we discuss in Chapter 7, unplanned pregnancy and diabetes should not mix, if you have PCOS, before you begin these types of medicines you should first speak to your doctor about contraception and pregnancy issues.

Metformin

The Canadian Diabetes Association recommends (for reasons we include in the following list) metformin as the preferred OHA for most people with type 2 diabetes. Therefore, if you have type 2 diabetes and you aren't taking metformin, we suggest you discuss with your doctor whether or not metformin would be a good choice for you.

Metformin is available as a single medication and is also available as a combination pill (Avandamet, which contains both metformin and rosiglitazone) and in a long-acting form (Glumetza).

Here's what you should know about this drug. Metformin

- ✔ Lowers blood glucose mainly by reducing the production of glucose from the liver.

✔ Does not cause hypoglycemia, unlike sulfonylureas (which we discuss in the next section).

✔ Does not cause weight gain, unlike almost all other OHAs. Gotta like that!

✔ Reduces your risk of having a heart attack or stroke (if you have diabetes). How metformin provides this benefit isn't clear.

✔ Can improve your lipids.

✔ May improve your fertility if you're a woman with infertility due to polycystic ovary syndrome (PCOS).

✔ Reduces your risk of developing type 2 diabetes if you have prediabetes. (We discuss prediabetes in Chapter 4.)

✔ Tends to cause nausea, abdominal cramping, and diarrhea. These symptoms can be lessened (or avoided altogether) if you take your metformin with food and if you begin taking it in a low dose and slowly increase the dose over a few weeks. The very successful dosing schedule Ian uses is available on his Web site (www.ourdiabetes.com/metformin.htm).

✔ Can make it harder for your gut to properly absorb vitamin B12 from food you've eaten. For that reason you should have your vitamin B12 level checked from time to time; if your level is low, taking an oral B12 supplement typically corrects the problem readily.

Metformin can cause — rarely — a serious adverse effect called lactic acidosis. (Symptoms of lactic acidosis include nausea, vomiting, abdominal pain, poor appetite, and malaise.) For this reason, you should not use metformin if you have significant liver disease, active heart failure, or kidney failure. *Mild* kidney malfunction does *not* prevent you from taking metformin. Your doctor should check your kidney function with a blood test that measures creatinine before prescribing this medication.

If you're having certain types of X-rays where you'll be given intravenous dye, your doctor will likely advise you not to take your metformin for a few days before and after the test. This precaution ensures that if the dye causes kidney problems, you won't have excess metformin accumulating in your body.

Sulfonylureas

Sulfonylurea drugs have similar properties (with some significant exceptions as we discuss below). These are the different types of sulfonylurea medication:

✔ Glyburide

✔ Gliclazide (This drug is also available in a long-acting form taken once daily.)

- ✔ Glimepiride (This drug is also available as a combination pill, Avandaryl, which contains both glimepiride and rosiglitazone. This combination pill is rarely used.)

- ✔ Chlorpropamide (This drug is rarely used.)

- ✔ Tolbutamide (This drug is rarely used.)

Glyburide, for years the most commonly used sulfonylurea, is more likely than the newer sulfonylureas — gliclazide and glimepiride — to cause hypoglycemia or weight gain. For these reasons, gliclazide and glimepiride are preferred. (Unfortunately, they are also more expensive.)

Here's what you should know about these drugs. Sulfonylureas

- ✔ Lower blood glucose by making your pancreas produce more insulin.

- ✔ Can cause hypoglycemia.

- ✔ Can cause weight gain.

- ✔ Can occasionally cause a photosensitive skin rash (a rash that occurs upon sun exposure).

- ✔ Can cause allergic reactions in people who have sulfa-drug allergies. This does not happen often.

- ✔ Can interact with alcohol in some cases, causing unpleasant symptoms such as nausea and flushing (even if you aren't inebriated).

Scientists discovered sulfonylureas accidentally when they noticed that soldiers given certain sulfur-containing antibiotics developed symptoms of low blood glucose.

Meglitinides

We admit to taking liberties here, but practicality trumps fussing over nomenclature, so we're going to do what the whole medical world does and group together two very similar (but not identical) classes of drugs — meglitinides and D-phenylalanine derivatives — and simply refer to them collectively as meglitinides. Do you care? We didn't think so. (Incidentally, meglitinides are also sometimes referred to as glinides for short.)

These are the different types of meglitinide medication:

- ✔ Repaglinide (also called GlucoNorm)
- ✔ Nateglinide (also called Starlix)

Because repaglinide is more potent than nateglinide, nateglinide is seldom used.

Here's what you should know about these drugs. Meglitinides

- Lower blood glucose by making your pancreas produce more insulin
- Are particularly effective at reducing after-meal blood glucose levels, compared with other OHAs
- Can cause hypoglycemia
- Can cause weight gain

Compared with some sulfonylureas, such as glyburide, meglitinides are less likely to cause hypoglycemia.

Thiazolidinediones

Thiazolidinediones (more easily referred to as TZDs, and sometimes referred to as glitazones) entered the OHA marketplace a few years ago and were rapidly gaining in popularity until a highly controversial study came out in 2007, after which use of this class (particularly one member of this class) of medicine diminished. We look at the controversy surrounding TZD therapy in the sidebar, "Does Avandia cause heart attacks?"

TZDs have (with some possibly significant exceptions, as we mention below) similar properties. These are the different types of TZD medication:

- Pioglitazone (which goes by several other names, including Actos)
- Rosiglitazone (also called Avandia)

Here's what you should know about these drugs. TZDs

- Lower blood glucose mainly by helping glucose move from the blood into fat and muscle. They do this by reducing insulin resistance (see Chapter 4).
- Do not cause hypoglycemia.
- Can cause fluid retention leading to swollen ankles. This can be a nuisance but is not serious.
- Typically cause some weight gain. This is partially related to fluid retention.
- May cause mild anemia. (This is important in only one way: If your doctor is not aware that TZDs can cause mild anemia, you could end up having unnecessary tests done.)

- Increase your risk of having a fracture of a forearm, hand, or foot if you're a woman. The reason for this is not yet known. (It may turn out that it's related to loss of calcium from the bones.)

- May improve your fertility if you're a woman with infertility due to polycystic ovary syndrome (PCOS).

- Can affect your lipids. Some evidence suggests that pioglitazone is more favourable than rosiglitazone in this way. (Whether this is a meaningful difference is controversial.)

- Reduce your risk of developing type 2 diabetes if you have prediabetes. (We discuss prediabetes in Chapter 4.)

- Increase your risk of heart failure. This is more likely if you have previously had a heart attack and also if you're taking insulin. The great majority of people taking TZD therapy do *not* develop heart failure; nonetheless, the risk remains real.

If you develop breathing difficulty while you're on a TZD, you may have heart failure and you should seek immediate medical attention. Also, if you have significant heart damage, you should not take a TZD.

It can take a few weeks of treatment before blood glucose levels start to improve. (Patience is a virtue with these drugs.)

Alpha-glucosidase inhibitors

Because of a limited ability to reduce blood glucose levels, alpha-glucosidase inhibitor medication is not often used. On the other hand, it's very safe therapy with virtually no serious side effects. The only member of this class of medicine available in Canada is acarbose, which goes by the trade name Glucobay — as in keeping your *glucose* at *bay* (although we must admit it does bring to mind images of, ahem, a sweet Caribbean beach destination).

Here's what you should know about acarbose. Acarbose

- Lowers blood glucose by slowing the rate of absorption of glucose from the small intestine into the blood. (It does this by blocking the action of an enzyme — alpha-glucosidase — that breaks down larger carbohydrates into smaller ones such as glucose.)

- Is less effective than other OHA medicines at reducing blood glucose levels.

- Does not cause hypoglycemia.

✔ Reduces your risk of developing type 2 diabetes if you have prediabetes. (We discuss prediabetes in Chapter 4.)

✔ Virtually never causes severe side effects and is, therefore, a very safe medicine, but acarbose frequently causes *non*-severe, unpleasant gastro-intestinal side effects (including gas, bloating, and flatulence). An often helpful way to avoid these side effects is to start with a very low dose and then slowly increase it. The dosing schedule that Ian uses is available on his Web site (`www.ourdiabetes.com/acarbose.htm`).

Given acarbose's side-effect profile, you could say that the best candidates for this drug are those people who are "loud and proud."

If you develop hypoglycemia when you're on this medication, you must treat yourself with glucose or dextrose (such as Dextrosol), not sucrose. That is, you should not treat yourself with table sugar, fruit juice, or colas.

Does Avandia cause heart attacks?

The diabetes world was shaken in June 2007 when the prestigious *New England Journal of Medicine* published a study by Dr. Steven Nissen. Dr. Nissen's study reported that people with diabetes who were taking rosiglitazone (Avandia) — the study did not look at piogli-tazone (Actos) — had a 43 percent increased risk of having a heart attack. Following publication of this study, thousands upon thousands of people discontinued taking Avandia and, since then, many thousands of others have opted not to start this medicine. So, is this justified? Is Avandia a dangerous drug?

There are two key points to consider when answering these questions:

✔ Dr. Nissen's study was what is called a *meta-analysis,* meaning that it was actually a compilation of many pre-existing studies. It was not a new study in the sense that he did not take patients and newly enroll them in a research trial. Meta-analyses are subject to many potential shortcomings and can be performed a number of different

ways. The exact same data that Dr. Nissen used, when analyzed using other methods, did *not* reveal an increased risk of heart attack with Avandia.

✔ A number of other studies — including, most notably, the RECORD study, which is an ongoing research trial looking at the specific issue of Avandia safety — have not found evidence that this drug causes heart attacks.

The bottom line: The evidence that Avandia causes heart attacks is very limited, contro-versial, and not supported by other studies. Hopefully, a definitive answer will be forthcom-ing with the publication of future studies.

How controversial is this issue? Suffice it to say that when this topic was debated at the American Diabetes Association annual scien-tific meetings, organizers had to turn people away. The room was filled to overflowing and — we've never seen this before at a medi-cal conference — when one of the speakers got up to give his opinion he was booed.

Another new drug to watch for: Pramlintide

Pramlintide (brand name Symlin) is an extract from the same beta cells of the pancreas that produce insulin. It's not yet available in Canada, but is used in other countries including the United States. It's an injectable medication that reduces blood glucose by reducing appetite (and, therefore, food intake), slowing how quickly the stomach empties food, and decreasing glucagon production by the pancreas.

DPP-4 inhibitors

DPP-4 inhibitors are a new class of medicine. There are two DPP-4 inhibitor drugs available in Canada: sitagliptin (which goes by the trade name Januvia), and saxagliptin (which goes by the trade name Onglyza). DPP-4 inhibitor drugs are becoming increasingly popular in the management of type 2 diabetes and other members of this class of drug will soon also appear on the market.

In your Internet travels, you'll come across two terms for this class of drug: DPP-4 inhibitors and DPP-IV inhibitors. Both are correct, and both refer to the same thing (the IV is simply the Roman numeral equivalent of the number 4). Our preference is to refer to them as DPP-4 inhibitors so nobody thinks the IV means *intravenous* and takes that to mean that this *oral* drug is given intravenously!

Here's what you should know about these drugs. DPP-4 inhibitors

- ✔ Lower blood glucose by increasing insulin and decreasing glucagon production by the pancreas. (As we discuss in Chapter 3, because glucagon causes the liver to release glucose into the blood, reducing glucagon levels reduces blood glucose.)

- ✔ Are given orally, whereas another new and related class of drugs — the GLP-1 analogues (which we discuss next) — are given by injection under the skin.

- ✔ Reduce blood glucose levels only modestly (that is, better than some drugs; not as well as some others).

- ✔ Don't cause hypoglycemia.

- ✔ Don't cause weight gain (a significant advantage compared to many other OHA medications, which often cause weight gain).

- ✔ Don't cause side effects for the majority of patients.

GLP-1 analogues

Now available in the United States and likely soon available in Canada is exenatide (trade name Byetta), the first member of a new class of drugs called GLP-1 analogues. This will likely soon be followed by liraglutide, with many other additions to this exciting new class of drug sure to follow. Because GLP-1 analogues are given by *injection* (under the skin, similar to the way insulin is given), they are, naturally enough, not *oral* hypoglycemic agents. Their properties, however, are otherwise quite similar (with significant exceptions, which we discuss below) to DPP-4 inhibitors, so we discuss them here.

Here's what you should know about these drugs. GLP-1 analogues

✔ Lower blood glucose by a number of different mechanisms including increasing insulin production, reducing appetite (and, therefore, food intake), slowing how quickly the stomach empties food, and decreasing glucagon production by the pancreas. (As we discuss in Chapter 3, because glucagon causes the liver to release glucose into the blood, reducing glucagon levels reduces blood glucose.)

✔ Don't cause hypoglycemia.

✔ Often cause weight loss. As the great majority of people with type 2 diabetes are overweight — and as most other OHA therapies cause weight *gain* — the ability of GLP-1 analogues to help you lose weight is clearly a very nice benefit indeed.

✔ Frequently cause nausea. This typically diminishes with ongoing use of the medicine. Other side effects seldom occur.

When reading about GLP-1 analogues, you may come across the term *incretin* or *incretin mimetic*. *Incretins* are hormones made by the intestine. GLP-1 analogues share many of the properties of incretins and hence are said to mimic them.

Effectively Using OHA Medication: The CDA-Recommended Approach to Treating Type 2 Diabetes

Every few years the Canadian Diabetes Association assembles a group of experts in the field of diabetes who volunteer their time to review all the available medical evidence regarding diabetes management and come up with recommendations on how best to manage this condition. (Ian is one such volunteer.) The entirety of this book is based on these recommendations. In this section we look at the CDA's recommended drug strategy to get your blood glucose control in order.

These are the CDA recommendations (based on what should be done from the day of diagnosis):

1. As soon as your diabetes is diagnosed

   • You should be referred to diabetes educators to receive appropriate diabetes education.

   • You should start lifestyle therapy. All the other recommendations noted in this list are *in addition to* (not instead of) lifestyle treatment.

   • If your A1C is 9 or higher (see Chapter 9 for more on A1C), you should immediately begin taking either metformin or insulin. (Often metformin and another OHA are advised, starting either with both at once or adding the second one soon thereafter.)

2. After two to three months, if your A1C remains above target (that is, it remains above 7.0) and you are not yet taking metformin, it should now be prescribed. If you're already taking metformin, a second OHA or insulin should be added (this is especially important if your A1C is above 9).

   In choosing which OHA to add to metformin, your doctor needs to consider the pros and cons of the different available drug classes (see the section, "Investigating the Types of Oral Hypoglycemic Agents," earlier in this chapter) and select the most suitable drug from the most suitable class for your particular situation. Your doctor should take into account the specific drug's mechanism of action, how the medication may help you, and what kinds of side effects might occur.

Here are the most important messages to take from these CDA recommendations:

✔ From the day you are diagnosed with type 2 diabetes, you should consider yourself racing against the calendar. Your goal is to achieve a target A1C (7 or less) within 6 to 12 months. (See Chapter 9 for more on A1C.)

✔ As you race against the calendar, you may well find yourself requiring more and more medication to achieve your target A1C. This doesn't mean you're sicker than someone who requires fewer medicines. It may well mean that you're wiser than the person who declines taking necessary medicines, runs blood glucose levels that are too high, and develops (what would have been avoidable) diabetes complications as a consequence.

✔ Insulin therapy is never a bad choice. As we discuss in Chapter 13, taking insulin — be it in addition to OHA therapy or instead of OHA therapy — doesn't mean you are less healthy than the person who doesn't require insulin therapy.

> ✔ Achieving target blood glucose control is more important than which drug (or drugs) you use to achieve this goal.
>
> ✔ Lifestyle therapy is *always* a key component of therapy.

Wilson's excellent blood glucose adventure

Wilson Chang, a 49-year-old small-business owner, had recently developed blurred vision and was drinking more water than usual. He saw his doctor and was found to have a fasting blood glucose of 11.2 mmol/L (and A1C of 8.5). Diabetes was diagnosed and he was sent to see Ian. Apart from being overweight (BMI 31 — see Chapter 4 for a discussion of BMI), Wilson appeared healthy. This was how Ian and Wilson decided to proceed:

✔ **Day one:** Wilson was referred to a diabetes education centre, where he met with a diabetes nurse educator and dietitian (see Chapter 8). Lifestyle therapy (see Chapters 10 and 11) was started immediately. Because Wilson was having symptoms and because his glucose was quite high, he needed to be on OHA therapy right away. Ian prescribed metformin because it would not cause weight gain (unlike most OHAs), it could help protect against heart disease, and (unlike sulfonylureas) it would not cause hypoglycemia. Wilson was instructed to gradually increase his metformin as per Ian's usual schedule.

✔ **One month later:** Wilson was working with his diet and had lost 2 pounds (1 kg), but after showing some initial improvement, his glucose levels had plateaued at about 9 to 10 mmol/L. Ian added a TZD to Wilson's OHA therapy.

✔ **Another month later:** Wilson was no longer having symptoms and had been doing some regular exercise, though not as diligently as he had hoped to. He had lost another 2 lbs (1 kg) but was feeling a bit disappointed with his very modest success. His fasting blood glucose levels were now about 8 mmol/L. Ian reassured him that his weight loss, though not dramatic, was promising. As his blood glucose readings were still significantly higher than normal, Ian increased Wilson's TZD dose.

✔ **Another month later:** Wilson's weight had gone up 1 lb (½ kg) and his running shoes were still whiter than Ian would have liked. Wilson's blood glucose readings were somewhat better, with fasting values averaging 7.0. Wilson promised to redouble his efforts at exercise and weight loss. No change was made to his OHA therapy.

✔ **Another month later:** Success! White running shoes no longer white. BMI 29. Blood glucose readings 4 to 7. Wilson happy. Ian happy. Dietitian happy. Nurse happy. Local greasy spoon devastated.

Ian's choice of a TZD was an arbitrary decision; he could just as appropriately have chosen another class of OHA such as a DPP-4 inhibitor. Each OHA class has its advantages and disadvantages, and there is seldom a right or wrong way to do things — with the exception of doing nothing and letting blood glucose readings remain too high on an ongoing basis, which is never right.

Write a note with the date 12 months from when you found out you have diabetes. Stick the note on your fridge and look at it periodically; that's your due date (even if you're not pregnant!), the date by which you and your health care team are striving to deliver a healthy blood glucose level. And this is one delivery that is quite fine if it comes early.

As Time Goes By: OHA Therapy and You

The good news about controlling your blood glucose is that shortly after your diabetes is diagnosed, an excellent chance exists that you can achieve target blood glucose readings (see Chapter 9) with intensive lifestyle therapy and often just one type of OHA. The bad news is that diabetes is a progressive disease, meaning that with time, your pancreas's ability to produce insulin peters out so that the therapy that worked so well initially works less well with time. That's *not* your fault! But it does mean you and your doctor should continually review your glucose control and reassess your treatment.

As doctors have learned more and more over the past few years about the importance of excellent blood glucose control, they are introducing oral agents sooner in the management of diabetes and, equally importantly, they are increasingly recommending *multiple* OHAs early on, sometimes from the day of diagnosis of diabetes (particularly if your blood glucose levels are especially high). Doctors are also using insulin more often.

Though you may hate the idea of taking a whole bunch of pills, consider the alternative. Do you really want toxic levels of glucose poisoning your system day after day after day? Now, we recognize that some people would say that they don't want pills poisoning them either. True enough. All we can say to that is that the pills doctors use have proven themselves safe for the overwhelming majority of the millions of people that have used them, but high glucose levels are dangerous to everyone. And that includes you.

Chapter 13

Using Insulin Effectively

*T*he discovery of insulin over 80 years ago was rightly heralded as a miraculous event. Indeed, since Banting, Best, Macleod, and Collip's famous breakthrough in 1921 (see Chapter 3 for the inside scoop), the lives of tens of millions of people have been enhanced or, often, saved as a direct result of insulin therapy. However, as the years have passed, along with insulin's justified reputation as a *miracle,* so, too has insulin come for many people to be thought of as being something dangerous and scary. In this chapter we look at the many benefits insulin therapy has to offer and we clear up misconceptions surrounding one of Canada's most famous contributions to the world.

What Is Insulin?

If you're a person with type 1 diabetes, insulin is your saviour. Simply put, without insulin you could not survive. And if you have type 2 diabetes, though insulin may not very often be the difference between life and death (not in the short term, anyhow), it frequently is the difference between good health and bad health. As we explain in Chapter 3, *insulin* is a hormone that's produced in the pancreas and released into the bloodstream, where it travels to different parts of your body. Insulin acts on certain cells (such as fat cells and muscle cells) to allow glucose to enter so that they can carry out their normal functions. If you don't have insulin in your body to allow glucose to enter into the tissues, the glucose hangs around in the blood, damages your organs, and starts to spill out into your urine.

We measure injected insulin in units. Nowadays medical science has very scientific ways of determining the strength of insulin with laboratory machinery. We've come a long way from the time that a unit of insulin was based on how much insulin it took to cause a 2 kg rabbit to have severe enough hypoglycemia that it would have a seizure.

Looking at the Types of Insulin

Our pancreas normally functions on autopilot. When we eat, our blood glucose level goes up and our pancreas immediately responds by releasing insulin into the bloodstream, which promptly brings our glucose level back to normal. If your pancreas is malfunctioning and you require insulin injections, the goal is to try to reproduce what your pancreas would normally do if it was healthy. You can consider this "thinking like a pancreas." We're aided by having a variety of different insulins to choose from, each with its own set of properties. When you're prescribed insulin, your doctor should try to match your body's needs with the most appropriate insulin (or, if you have type 2 diabetes, oftentimes, the most appropriate combination of insulin and oral hypoglycemic agents; we discuss oral hypoglycemic agents in Chapter 12). Because each person is different, the type of insulin you first start on may be changed to a different one depending on how your body responds.

Insulins (and their properties) available in Canada are listed in Table 13-1. Note that the times given are approximations and can vary significantly — even for the same person.

ANECDOTE

Moving away misperceptions:
How Dorothy overcame her fears about insulin

Dorothy Strait was 50 when she was diagnosed with type 2 diabetes. Her initial treatment was lifestyle therapy, and she was thrilled when a change in her diet, modest weight loss, and a daily walk brought her glucose levels down to normal. A couple of years later, however, her glucose levels started to climb and she began taking oral hypoglycemic agents. That helped, but only temporarily, and her glucose readings had now risen to 11 and she was feeling fatigued. Her family doctor referred her to Ian to see if she should be on insulin. When Dorothy came to Ian's office, she was sad, angry, and frightened all at once. She felt like a failure. She was terrified of the needle and told Ian, "I would hate jabbing myself. I simply couldn't do it. You can't convince me otherwise." As she spoke to Ian she was on the verge of tears.

"Dorothy," Ian said, "we will do whatever you want. I can't force you to do anything. And I wouldn't want to even if I could. *You* are the boss and *you* will decide what you want to do. But I think you would be unfair to yourself if, whatever you decide, it wasn't an informed decision. So let's make sure you know the most important information to help you make your decision." Dorothy was certainly agreeable to that.

Ian said a few things to Dorothy that day. He remembers telling her, "It is crucial that you know that *you* are not a failure, your *pancreas* is, and that's not your fault. It happens to most people with diabetes. And as for hating jabbing yourself, why would you like it? Who would? But you are *already* jabbing yourself each time you test your blood glucose. And doing a blood finger jab is more uncomfortable than giving insulin.

With the tiny needles we use nowadays, giving insulin is virtually pain free. And as for not being able to do it, look at the other obstacles that you have overcome; you've changed your diet, you've lost some weight, you're exercising regularly, you're taking a whole bunch of pills that I'm sure you'd rather not have to, and you're testing your blood every day. You've managed all those things. And if you can handle all those things, I'm sure you could manage giving insulin also."

Dorothy became more at ease but was still apprehensive. "But, Doctor, when you start insulin, you're on it forever."

"That's usually true, Dorothy," Ian replied, "but not because insulin is addictive. It's because your pancreas is failing and it's not going to be rejuvenated. It can no longer make enough insulin, so we have to supplement it. We're simply giving your body back the hormone it's lacking. One other thing: Medical science is always progressing. Other ways of giving insulin are being developed. Better pills are always coming along. I don't know if you'll be on insulin injections forever. Maybe in a few years you won't have to be."

Well, Dorothy still wasn't thrilled with the prospect of giving insulin. And of course there was no reason for her to be thrilled. But she met with the diabetes educator and was pleasantly surprised to find that giving insulin wasn't nearly as bad as she had thought. It wasn't fun by any means, but it wasn't horrible either. And as her glucose levels returned to normal and her energy improved, she was very glad she had decided to take insulin after all.

Table 13-1	Types of Insulin Available in Canada and Their Properties				
Classification	Generic Name	Trade Name(s)	Onset of Action	Peak Action	Duration of Action
Rapid-acting	aspart	Novorapid	10 to 15 minutes	1 to 2 hours	3 to 5 hours
	glulisine	Apidra			
	lispro	Humalog			
Short-acting	regular	Humulin-R Novolin ge Toronto	30 minutes	2 to 3 hours	5 to 8 hours
Intermediate-acting	NPH	Humulin-N Novolin ge NPH	1 to 3 hours	5 to 8 hours	14 to 18 hours
Long-acting	detemir	Levemir	90 min.	Virtually none	16 to 24 hours
	glargine	Lantus	90 min.	None	24 hours
Premixed (the numbers after the names refer to the ratio of rapid- or short-acting insulin to intermediate-acting insulin)		Humalog Mix25 Humalog Mix50 Humulin 30/70 Novolin ge 30/70 NovoMix 30	Depends on specific type	Depends on specific type	Depends on specific type

One common misunderstanding is equating Humulin with Humulin-N. Humulin is a trade name and refers to a *variety* of types of insulin marketed by one particular company (Eli Lilly in this case). Humulin-N refers to Eli Lilly's brand of NPH insulin. To say you are on Humulin conveys the same degree of information as saying you drive a Chevrolet — helpful, but only part of the story. More specific would be if you said you drove a Malibu or an Impala or a Corvette. Even better would be if you said Ian could drive your Corvette!

You might notice in our discussions of the various types of insulin in this section that we mention basal-bolus insulin therapy a few times. *Basal-bolus insulin therapy* has, as you might guess, two components:

✔ **Basal insulin** (NPH, Levemir, Lantus): Insulin you give once (or, in some cases, twice) a day to prevent your blood glucose levels from climbing between meals.

✔ **Bolus insulin** (Apidra, Humalog, NovoRapid): Insulin you give before each meal to prevent your blood glucose levels from climbing after a meal. For this reason it is also referred to as mealtime insulin. (Although regular insulin can also be used as a bolus insulin, because it less closely replicates normal insulin release from the pancreas it is typically not as good a choice.)

The other way of using basal-bolus insulin therapy is with an insulin pump (see "How to Give Insulin" later in this chapter).

Basal-bolus insulin therapy forms the backbone (so to speak) of managing type 1 diabetes (and is also excellent therapy for many people with type 2 diabetes).

Basal-bolus insulin therapy is also commonly called *intensified insulin therapy.* Although we do use this term, we admit to not being overly fond of it, because *all* people with diabetes need to be treated intensively regardless of whether that means simply with diet and exercise, or oral hypoglycemic agents, or one, two, three, or more doses of insulin.

Assistance obtaining insulin

No one's health should suffer because they cannot obtain insulin due to financial hardship. If you require insulin therapy but have neither the money nor the insurance (governmental or private) coverage for it, you can still obtain insulin (without charge) in several ways.

You can contact the insulin manufacturers directly (all Canadian insulin manufacturers have compassionate care programs for this very purpose):

✔ Eli-Lilly (Lilly Canada Cares Insulin Assistance Program): 888-545-5972

✔ Novo Nordisk: 800-465-4334. (Novo Nordisk doesn't have a specific compassionate care program, but in special circumstances it will provide insulin to your doctor or diabetes educator who in turn can provide it to you.)

✔ Sanofi-Aventis (Lantus Compassionate Care Program): 800-265-7927

Additionally, try your diabetes educators. They will almost certainly have samples they can provide you with in a pinch.

Rapid-acting insulin

Three types of rapid-acting insulin are available: aspart (NovoRapid), lispro (Humalog), and glulisine (Apidra).

Rapid-acting insulin

- Is a mealtime insulin. That is, you take rapid-acting insulin to prevent your blood glucose levels from rising too high after your meal.

- Is a bolus component of basal-bolus insulin therapy.

- Can be taken anywhere between $1/4$ hour to immediately before you eat. (This will depend on how your blood glucose levels respond to the insulin. Some people get the best response taking it as long as $1/2$ hour before a meal.)

- Has its peak effect at the same time as the glucose from your food is being absorbed from your small intestine, so the action of the insulin matches the rise in your blood glucose. That's what a healthy pancreas does, too.

- Wears off within a short period of time (three to five hours).

- Compared to regular insulin, is less likely to cause hypoglycemia, provides better after-meal blood glucose control, and is more convenient to use (it can be given as soon as immediately before a meal). As a result, rapid-acting insulin has largely replaced regular insulin in Canada.

If you have gastroparesis (a condition in which your stomach becomes less efficient at propelling food into your small intestine; see Chapter 6) *and* erratic blood glucose control, you may benefit from taking rapid-acting insulin an hour or so *after* your meal. Your diabetes specialist can help you determine if this would be a good option for you.

For all intents and purposes, all rapid-acting insulins are identical in their actions. Indeed, the only significant way in which they differ is that if you buy one type you help boost the share price of one company, and if you buy the other type you help the other company's valuation.

Regular insulin

Because regular insulin is sometimes referred to as a short-acting insulin (as in the Canadian Diabetes Association 2008 Clinical Practice Guidelines) and is sometimes referred to as a fast-acting insulin (as it was in the 2003 version of the Guidelines), you might get (understandably!) confused. For that reason, unless we forget, we refer to regular insulin as, simply, regular insulin" throughout this book.

Regular insulin is also called Toronto insulin, but it is seldom called that anymore. (Too bad; it reminded people around the world of insulin's Canadian roots.)

These are the most important properties of this insulin. Regular insulin

✔ Is a mealtime insulin, given to prevent your blood glucose levels from rising too high after your meal.

✔ Is a bolus component of basal-bolus insulin therapy. (Although both regular insulin and rapid-acting insulin are bolus insulins, the latter is preferred, as we discuss in the preceding section.)

✔ Does not have much action until 30 minutes after you inject it, so you should take it — you guessed it — 30 minutes *before you eat.* That can be such a hassle, so most people end up taking it immediately before they eat anyhow. It'll still work, but not as effectively.

✔ Has a longer duration of action and is more likely to cause hypoglycemia than rapid-acting insulin.

✔ Is more likely to cause hypoglycemia, provides less effective after-meal blood glucose control, and is less convenient to use (as it needs to be given 30 minutes before a meal) than rapid-acting insulin. Consequently, doctors are recommending regular insulin less and less often.

Intermediate-acting insulin

NPH (sometime simply called *N*) is the only available intermediate-acting insulin. Intermediate-acting insulin

✔ Is given to prevent your blood glucose levels from going up too high between meals.

✔ Is a basal component of basal-bolus insulin therapy.

✔ Is often given at bedtime to prevent your blood glucose level from going up too high overnight. (We discuss this *dawn phenomenon* later in this chapter.)

✔ Does not have much effect until a few hours after it's injected, so it doesn't help to reduce your blood glucose levels immediately after you eat.

✔ Is more likely than long-acting insulin to cause hypoglycemia (including overnight). For this reason, NPH is being used less and less, and long-acting insulin more and more.

Long-acting insulin

Long-acting insulin works for, well, a long time. Two types of long-acting insulin are available: Levemir and Lantus. Long-acting insulins

- Are given to prevent your blood glucose levels from going up too high between meals.

- Are the basal component of basal-bolus insulin therapy.

- Are often given at bedtime to prevent your blood glucose level from going up too high overnight. (We discuss this dawn phenomenon later in this chapter.)

- Don't have a quick action, so they don't help to reduce your blood glucose levels immediately after you eat. For this reason, long-acting insulins are usually supplemented with rapid-acting (or regular) insulin given with meals (or, in the case of type 2 diabetes, sometimes with oral hypoglycemic agents).

- Have a very consistent action — they have pretty well the same effect on blood glucose levels two hours after the injection as they do eight or more hours after the injection. (Lantus has no peak action and Levemir has only a slight peak.)

- Last up to 24 hours, so they are typically taken just once per day. (There are, however, many exceptions to this pattern. Many people — particularly if taking Levemir, but also with Lantus — find they require it twice daily.)

- Result in more consistent blood glucose values (meaning that your blood glucose readings will be less variable) than with intermediate-acting insulin.

- Often cause less weight gain for those people newly starting insulin therapy than intermediate-acting insulin. (This may be particularly true of Levemir insulin.)

- Are less likely to cause hypoglycemia (including overnight) than intermediate-acting insulin. For this reason, long-acting insulins are being used increasingly often and intermediate-acting insulins less and less often.

- Should not be mixed in the same syringe with any other insulin.

- Cause discomfort in a small percentage of people upon injection. With Levemir insulin, an even smaller percentage may develop a sore, red rash at the injection site.

   If you experience more than minimal discomfort when injecting these insulins or if you develop a rash at the injection site, be sure to promptly inform your physician because you may need to change the insulin to a different type.

- Cost much more than intermediate-acting insulin.

Levemir and Lantus insulins are clear (you can see through them). So are rapid-acting and regular insulins. Because of this similarity in appearance, people have mistakenly given themselves one type of insulin when they meant to give the other. Read the label very carefully before administering your insulin. (Because NPH insulin is cloudy, it isn't as likely to be confused with the other, clear types of insulin.)

Premixed insulin

Premixed insulin combines, in a single cartridge (or vial), both a mealtime insulin (either Humalog, NovoRapid, or regular insulin) and a longer-acting insulin (either NPH or another insulin that acts similar to it). The percentage of mealtime insulin and longer-acting insulin differs depending on the specific type of premixed insulin. Determining which of the various available premixed insulins provides the best blood glucose control for a given individual is largely a matter of trial and error. The various types of premixed insulin are listed in Table 13-1, earlier in the chapter.

If you ever need to buy premixed insulin in the United States, be aware that what we call 30/70 insulin here is called 70/30 insulin there.

The advantage of a premixed insulin is that you have to take it only twice per day (before breakfast and before supper). If you were to separately take bolus insulin (three injections per day) and basal insulin (one or two injections per day), you would need more frequent injections.

The huge disadvantage to premixed insulin is that, because it is premixed, you can't independently adjust each of its two insulin ingredients to match your body's specific requirements. Although some diabetes specialists use it often, we find premixed insulin seldom provides sufficient flexibility and blood glucose control, and therefore we don't routinely recommend it for people with type 2 diabetes and we never recommend it to people with type 1 diabetes.

Animal insulins

In very rare circumstances, people with diabetes are treated with animal insulins. The two available products are Hypurin Regular and Hypurin NPH, made by Wockhardt UK. You can find further information on this topic at `www.hc-sc.gc.ca/dhp-mps/brgtherap/activit/fs-fi/qa_qr_insulin_02_2006-eng.php`. (Daunting task indeed to type this Web address into your browser; instead, just type the terms *"Hypurin health Canada"* into your Web search engine and this link to Health Canada's information on animal-sourced insulins will show up.)

Type 1 Diabetes and Insulin Therapy

The best insulin treatment strategy if you have type 1 diabetes is *basal-bolus* therapy, meaning that you either use an insulin pump (see "How to Give Insulin," later in this chapter) or you take intermediate- or long-acting (basal) insulin once (or twice) a day, and rapid-acting or regular (bolus) insulin prior to meals. Of these two methods, pump therapy is the best treatment currently available for type 1 diabetes because it most closely mimics what a normal pancreas does.

If you have type 1 diabetes and aren't being treated with basal-bolus therapy (with or without an insulin pump), contact your doctor to find out if you should change to one of these state-of-the-art forms of diabetes treatment.

Because Levemir and Lantus insulins, compared with NPH insulin, cause less hypoglycemia (including nocturnal hypoglycemia) and less blood glucose variability, they are often the preferred basal insulin for people with type 1 diabetes. On the other hand, long-acting insulins cost considerably more than NPH insulin. If you're doing well with NPH insulin as part of basal-bolus therapy, you don't *have to* change to Levemir or Lantus insulin. On the other hand, if you are having problems with overly frequent hypoglycemia (especially overnight) or inconsistent blood glucose readings, discuss with your doctor or diabetes educator switching from NPH to Levemir or Lantus.

Type 2 Diabetes and Insulin Therapy

Unfortunately, insulin therapy for people with type 2 diabetes has typically been looked at as a sign of failure, a last resort greeted with equal parts doom and gloom. What a shame! Insulin is simply one more treatment option — one that's terribly underused. Goodness knows how many people might have been spared complications if only insulin had been used sooner in the course of their therapy.

The right time for you to start insulin if you have type 2 diabetes is when you cannot achieve appropriate blood glucose control without insulin or when very quick blood glucose lowering is required (for example, if your blood glucose readings are very high and you are having symptoms from this; see Chapter 2). For some people that means starting insulin at the time of diagnosis; for others, after years of combined use of two or more oral hypoglycemic agents. The key point is that you and your health care team must always be looking at ways to optimize your glucose control. If lifestyle change does the trick, great. If oral agents bring your readings into target, terrific. What you want to avoid is the all-too-common scenario where the person with diabetes and their physicians spend month after month, year after year, awaiting a magical improvement in glucose control that simply isn't going to happen without insulin administration.

There is no "best" insulin to be on if you have type 2 diabetes; however, these strategies are particularly effective:

- Taking basal insulin (that is, NPH, Levemir, or Lantus) at bedtime and an oral hypoglycemic agent (particularly metformin; often in combination with a second OHA) during the daytime. (We discuss oral hypoglycemic agent therapy in detail in Chapter 12.) This is our preferred way to begin insulin therapy for most insulin-requiring people with type 2 diabetes. The insulin (if given in sufficient dose) prevents blood glucose levels from rising unduly overnight, and the oral medications keep blood glucose levels under control during the day.

- Basal-bolus insulin therapy (see "Looking at the Types of Insulin" earlier in this chapter).

- Premixed insulin taken twice daily. (Because of the limited flexibility of this strategy, we use it less often.)

- Insulin pump therapy. (This is not often used to treat type 2 diabetes but is a good option for select people with this condition such as those who are very active, are lean, and who have not had a sufficient response to basal-bolus insulin therapy.)

Because metformin therapy complements the action of insulin for people with type 2 diabetes, it's typically used regardless of which of the aforementioned insulin strategies you follow. A TZD (Actos, Avandia) in conjunction with insulin therapy is especially effective in treating type 2 diabetes and therefore is sometimes used, but this combination can increase the risk of heart failure and is not officially approved by Health Canada.

Your diabetes educator, family physician, and diabetes specialist can help you decide which treatment program is best for you.

The importance of adherence to a program of proper nutrition and exercise should never be minimized. Doctors often see people who, despite being on huge doses of insulin and numerous oral hypoglycemic agent pills, are still having problems with glucose control — problems that improve virtually overnight when those people have made appropriate dietary changes and renewed efforts with exercise.

Debunking Insulin Myths

The longer we're in practice as diabetes specialists, the greater is our sadness when we meet patients who have developed diabetes complications that could have been avoided if only they had been made aware that certain beliefs they had about insulin therapy (and which led them to avoid it) were based on incorrect information. Well, in case you, too, have any misperceptions regarding insulin therapy, here we list a few of the most common insulin myths:

✔ **Giving insulin is difficult.** In fact, giving insulin is very, very simple and straightforward. And as a bonus, taking insulin often means you can discontinue a whole bunch of pills you might be presently (unsuccessfully) taking for blood glucose control.

✔ **Insulin needles hurt.** They are virtually pain free.

✔ **It's embarrassing to be seen giving an insulin injection.** With current techniques, such as using insulin pen devices, giving insulin is typically very discrete; indeed, the odds are good that you've sat near — or even right beside — someone in a restaurant who injected insulin and you never noticed.

✔ **Insulin will make me feel like I'm prisoner to my diabetes therapy.** Many people find taking insulin liberating as they discover how it allows greater flexibility (compared to some types of oral hypoglycemic agent they had been on prior to insulin) with meal timing, when they exercise, and so forth.

✔ **Insulin will make me feel unwell.** In fact, on insulin therapy you will likely feel *better* as your blood glucose levels improve — typically after many months (or even years) of suboptimal therapy on oral hypoglycemic agents that are no longer working sufficiently well for you.

✔ **Taking insulin means I've failed.** Taking insulin means your *pancreas* has failed, not you. Indeed, taking insulin means you've succeeded in adopting an excellent form of therapy.

✔ **Once you're on insulin, you're on it forever.** Insulin is used when your own pancreas can no longer sufficiently do its job. And because medical science doesn't have a way of making your pancreas rejuvenate itself, sure, most people who start insulin need to stay on it. But this isn't because insulin is addictive or creates dependency; it's because your underlying diabetes isn't going to go away. However, if you have type 2 diabetes and you're able to make appropriate lifestyle changes, including losing weight, then there is the chance that you could discontinue your insulin (under appropriate medical supervision) and replace it with oral hypoglycemic agent therapy.

✔ **Insulin leads to complications.** Perhaps your Aunt Sally went blind after she started insulin. If so, the insulin didn't cause it; in fact, the delay in starting insulin may have led to this.

✔ **Insulin will likely make me go into a coma.** Although taking insulin can lead to low blood glucose, which has the potential to cloud your thinking and even cause you to lose consciousness, this seldom happens to people with type 2 diabetes. And if you have type 1 diabetes, taking appropriate precautions will minimize this risk.

Insulin therapy has been improving and saving lives for over 80 years, yet it remains very underutilized, and as a result, many people get unnecessarily sick. We think that's a tragedy — and that's no myth.

How to Give Insulin

There is, in truth, only one way to learn how to give yourself insulin, and that's by sitting down with a diabetes educator and having her or him teach you. You can no more learn how to give insulin by reading a package insert (or even this book, we're quite willing to admit) than you can learn how to drive a car without ever getting behind the wheel. This section will therefore address *general* principles of insulin administration.

Insulin delivery devices

Have you ever seen a movie where the actor says, "We can do this the easy way or we can do this the hard way. You decide." Well, the same applies to giving insulin.

Pens and syringes

For decades, the only way to give insulin was with a syringe and a bottle. Giving insulin this way is perfectly acceptable. But so is driving a 1990 Chevy. It may get you where you want to go, but it isn't quite the same as driving a brand-new Lexus. By far the easiest way to inject insulin is with an insulin pen (see Figure 13-1). Pen devices are easy to use and are very reliable. The great majority of Canadians who use insulin give it with pen devices. Of the thousands of patients in Ian's practice, he can count the number of syringe users on the fingers of one hand.

Figure 13-1:
Novolin-
Pen 4® and
Humapen
Luxura.

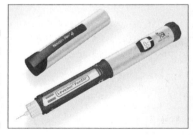 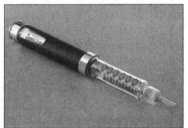

Used with permission of Eli Lilly Canada Inc.

Here's what you need to know about insulin pens:

- Your diabetes educator or pharmacist can provide you with a free pen device.

- When you first start insulin, your diabetes educator will likely provide you with an initial, small, free supply of insulin for your pen device.

- Most pen devices are refillable. As your diabetes educator will demonstrate, you simply remove the used insulin cartridge and pop in a new one.

- Some pen devices are pre-filled with non-removable insulin cartridges. When they're used up, you return the entire pen to your pharmacy for appropriate disposal.

- Insulin pens have a display that tells you how much insulin you are about to inject. If your dose exceeds the maximal amount that can be delivered with one injection, you don't need to remove the needle and inject yourself again. Instead, you can re-dial the pen while the needle is still inserted.

Whether you've been taking insulin for 20 days or 20 years, a time may well come when you accidentally give yourself either the wrong insulin or the wrong dose, or even forget to give a dose altogether. Fortunately, such a slip-up seldom leads to anything serious. Don't feel guilty or stupid if you make a mistake with your insulin; it happens to everyone. The way to deal with this type of oversight will depend on many factors, including the type of insulin you are taking (or, ahem, not taking), the dose, your blood glucose control, and the type of diabetes you have. Because so many factors must be taken into account, it's best that you speak to your diabetes educator to formulate a plan of action if you make an error with your insulin.

Jet injectors

If neither pen devices nor syringes suit your fancy, and if you don't mind spending a whole bunch of money (about $700), you can obtain a jet injection device (such as the AdvantaJet Injector — www.advantajet.com — distributed in Canada by Activa Brand Products; 800-991-4464). The idea behind these is that because they don't have needles, using them to give insulin won't hurt as much. Although that's true for some people, it's not for others, and in any event, giving insulin with a pen device is virtually pain free anyhow. Jet injectors are rarely used in Canada.

Pumps

With each passing day, more and more Canadians with type 1 diabetes are changing from using insulin pens to insulin pumps. This is no surprise. Insulin pumps are reliable, effective, and sophisticated devices that are excellent tools to help manage diabetes. They are, however, definitely *not* the right choice for everyone. We discuss these and other pump-related issues in this section.

What is an insulin pump?

Simply put, insulin pumps are pumps that pump insulin. They are the key component of what we call *continuous subcutaneous insulin infusion* (CSII) therapy. These are the basic components of CSII (see Figure 13-2):

- **An insulin pump:** These are small, pager-sized computerized devices with buttons that you press to program and instruct the pump on how much insulin to give you and when to give it.

- **An insulin reservoir** (which you fill with insulin every few days): The pump has a small motor that controls a cylinder that pushes the insulin from the reservoir into the attached tubing.

- **Tubing and insertion site:** The tubing carries the insulin from the pump to your body. It has two ends: one end connects to the reservoir on the pump and the other end connects to a tiny plastic needle that (using an inserter) you place just under the surface of the skin of your abdomen (or buttocks or arms or legs). The insulin reservoir, tubing, and insertion site are replaced every two to three days.

These are important aspects of pump therapy:

- Pump therapy is most suited to people with type 1 diabetes who are on four or more insulin injections per day. People with type 2 diabetes who are on similar amounts of insulin may also benefit from pump therapy.

- An insulin pump uses only rapid-acting insulin. If you use pump therapy, you no longer administer insulin by syringe or pen and you no longer give intermediate- or long-acting insulin. Rapid-acting insulin most closely mimics insulin from a healthy pancreas.

- Just like a normal pancreas, the pump delivers small amounts of (basal) insulin into your body 24 hours a day. You must program the pump to tell it how much basal insulin to give.

- The pump, again like a normal pancreas, delivers extra (bolus) insulin into your body at mealtimes (and, often, with snacks). You must tell the pump — based on the type and amount of food you are about to eat — how much of this bolus insulin to give (typically, within 15 minutes prior to beginning your meal). For this reason, carbohydrate counting is a crucial element of successful pump management. (We discuss carbohydrate counting later in this chapter.)

- Pumps don't measure your blood glucose levels. If you use a pump, you must continue to do blood glucose meter tests. As we discuss in Chapter 9, one pump is available in Canada (the MiniMed Paradigm REAL-Time Insulin Pump and Continuous Glucose Monitoring System) that combines an insulin pump with a glucose sensor to automatically measure and display your (interstitial fluid) glucose level, which in turn allows you to test your blood glucose level less frequently.

✔ Some pumps are said to be waterproof (indeed; some marathon swimmers successfully and uneventfully use these). Nonetheless, in general we feel it is best to avoid getting *any* pump wet (whether waterproof or not) in case its protective seal has been compromised, which could allow water to get into the pump and interfere with its function. Briefly disconnecting your pump while you take a dip (or shower) is usually a better option than swimming with it.

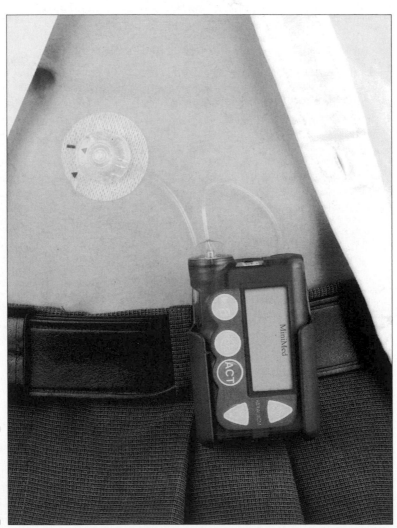

Figure 13-2:
Insulin pump with its infusion set.

If you have diabetes, you already know that no aspect of treatment is perfect and that what is good for your next-door neighbour may not be good for you. This is true of pump therapy as well.

Here are the pros of pump therapy:

- ✔ **It's very convenient.** You have less stuff (syringes, vials, pens, needles, and so on) to carry around with you and it's much easier to bolus (that is, give an extra quantity of insulin) with meals and snacks. It also allows for much greater flexibility regarding meal timing, exercise, shift work, sleeping in, and other routine day-to-day aspects of your existence.

- ✔ **It provides better blood glucose control.** It can help smooth out blood glucose levels — with fewer episodes of hypo-and hyperglycemia — because problems with inconsistent and erratic insulin absorption of longer-acting insulins are no longer an issue. For many pump users, pump therapy also results in improved A1C readings.

These are pump therapy's cons:

- ✔ **It is *very* expensive.** A pump will cost you about $6,800, and supplies will run you about $250 per month (and that doesn't even include the cost of insulin or blood glucose test strips).

- ✔ **You and your pump are virtually inseparable.** You can disconnect your pump for an hour or so, such as when you shower or swim, but just like a teenager and a phone, separations must be kept to a minimum.

- ✔ **Pumps do not think for you.** They are clever computers, but they are still a darn sight less clever than your brain. You need to spend 15 or more hours being trained (by a "pump trainer" diabetes educator) how to operate and adjust your pump based on your glucose levels, your exercise, your diet, and so on. (Within the next few years this may change; rapid progress is being made on closing the loop, wherein a pump, in conjunction with a glucose sensor, would automatically know how much insulin to give you.)

- ✔ **It's lots of work.** If you aren't using a glucose sensor (we discuss these in Chapter 9), you must test your blood glucose 6 to 12 times per day, the pump's insulin infusion rate has to be frequently reassessed, you have to spend many hours with your diabetes educator to learn how to use your pump, and so on. If you aren't up to this type of commitment, then that nearly $7,000 insulin pump you just got will become nothing more than one very, very expensive paperweight.

Many private insurance companies (and, very recently, some provincial/territorial governments) will pay for most (or even all) of the cost of an insulin pump and supplies. Be sure to speak to them about this. They will likely require a supportive letter from your diabetes specialist and, in the case of governments, they will require that you meet a number of criteria. The pump companies themselves often offer interest-free financing as well as a several-month return policy so that if you decide you don't want to stay with a pump you can obtain a full refund. Be sure to find out all these details (in writing) before you commit yourself to a pump purchase.

When we first suggest pump therapy to our patients, the usual response we hear is, "Doctor, I can't imagine having that thing attached to me all the time. It would make me feel like a prisoner." But we must say that these words are seldom spoken by actual pump users; it's pretty well only people that haven't tried a pump who voice this concern. Indeed — and as surprising as this may seem — what we typically hear from our patients on insulin pumps is that they find pump therapy liberating and would never go back to conventional insulin injections. Heck, we'd have to wrestle them to the ground to get them to give up their pumps. And as for the extra work involved with pump therapy, that's a trade-off that pump users are invariably happy to make.

Portrait of a pumper

Tom, a 24-year-old accountant, was a very active man and was exceptionally attentive to his diabetes management. He would test his blood five, six, seven, or more times per day and was giving himself Humalog insulin with meals and Levemir insulin at bedtime. In addition, when he snacked he would take a few extra units of Humalog. Some days he would take a total of seven injections of insulin. Tom's blood glucose readings and A1C were both excellent. "Tom," Ian said to him at the time of an appointment, "I think you should consider getting a pump." Tom was surprised and wondered why he should. "Because you are working very, very hard at managing your diabetes and I think you would find things are much easier for you on a pump," Ian replied. "Not easy, but *easier*."

Tom was hesitant at first but then decided to try the pump. A few months later he was back in the office. "How's it going?" Ian asked. "Well," Tom said, "I must admit I was a bit skeptical of your advice, but I decided to try the pump anyhow." Ian looked on expectantly. "And I have to tell you it was a *fantastic* decision. And like you said, life isn't now *easy*, but it is *easier*. When I need a bolus, presto, it's done. No one even notices when I give my insulin, not that that would bother me anyhow. And guess what; I'm having fewer lows than I was." Ian asked Tom if he would ever go back to his insulin pen injections. "Not on your life. They'd have to shoot me to get this pump from me!"

Tom was an ideal candidate for an insulin pump. He was testing and injecting many times per day. He was motivated and interested in putting in the considerable time and energy necessary to learn how to use a pump. In the absence of this devotion, switching to a pump is no more likely to make your glucose control better than driving a Porsche rather than a Hyundai instantly makes you a better driver.

People often ask Ian why he is such a proponent of pump therapy. To which Ian replies that it is not just that the science shows it to be an excellent option (which it does), but also that his patients have convinced him. When patient after patient after patient tells Ian it's the best thing they've done since they were diagnosed with diabetes and they wished they'd done it sooner, this is not something that can be ignored. In Ian's opinion, for those people *who are appropriate candidates* and have the financial resources, pump therapy is not only the way of the future, it's the way of the present!

If you're trying to decide if a pump is for you — and, if it is, which pump to choose — your diabetes educator is the best person to speak with. Not all educators have studied pumps, so your educator may refer you to an even more specialized teacher called a "pump trainer." Speaking to pump users to hear what they have to say would also be a good idea. Your educator likely can provide you with the name of a "pumper" to contact (pump users are almost always more than happy to spread the word). You can also find more information on pump therapy (and continuous glucose monitoring — see Chapter 9) by surfing over to a video on pump therapy that Ian made (www. drblumervideo.com) or by directly contacting the companies in Canada that sell insulin pumps:

- ✔ Animas Canada: www.animas.ca, 866-406-4844
- ✔ Disetronic Medical Systems Inc.: www.disetronic-ca.com, 800-280-7801
- ✔ Medtronic Diabetes of Canada Ltd.: www.minimed.ca, 866-444-4649
- ✔ Smiths Medical Canada Ltd.: www.cozmore.com, 800-461-0991

In our experience, we find that *all* the pumps currently available in Canada work very well. We also find that the pump companies provide excellent customer support. The decision to buy one brand of pump versus another, therefore, often comes down to which pump has a design you prefer, which display you like the best, and what other bells and whistles suit your fancy. The one other very important consideration is whether or not you want (or might want in the future) a pump that is integrated (or can be integrated) with a continuous glucose monitor (we discuss continuous glucose monitors in Chapter 9). If this last feature is important to you (and it is, appropriately, to most people), then your choices will be quickly narrowed down because only Medtronic presently offers such a combined device.

Caring for Your Insulin

Although insulin is not particularly difficult to look after, you should be aware of some handling issues:

✔ Do not use insulin after the expiration date marked on the label.

✔ Before its first use, store an *unopened* vial or cartridge of insulin in the refrigerator. (Refrigeration helps to preserve the potency of the insulin.)

✔ After you use it for the first time, you can keep your vial or cartridge of insulin either refrigerated or at room temperature (see the tip below).

✔ After its first use, your vial or cartridge of insulin has a limited time (usually about four weeks) before you will need to discard it. The package insert that came with your insulin will indicate the precise time recommended by the manufacturer of the particular insulin you are using.

✔ Insulin doesn't take well to excessive heat (such as being kept inside a car on a hot summer day) or, contrarily, to excessive cold (as Ian's patient found out when he returned to his car after his son's mid-winter hockey practice only to find his insulin bearing a surprising resemblance to a Popsicle). You should not use insulin that has been frozen or subjected to extreme heat.

✔ If you will be travelling to a destination where you won't have access to refrigeration facilities for insulin storage, use an insulated travel pack to keep your insulin protected from the elements. Frio (www.frious.com) makes a particularly good and quite novel line of travel packs that, when dunked in water, automatically start to cool. After a few days the cooling effect diminishes and it's time for another dunk.

✔ Many a person has successfully injected insulin through clothing, but we don't recommend you do it routinely.

✔ Most people reuse their needles, but because needles can get dull so quickly (which can both increase the discomfort of an injection and lead to skin damage including *lipohypertrophy* — which we discuss in Chapter 6), we don't recommend doing this routinely either.

✔ Dispose of used needles in a puncture-proof "sharps" container that is sealed shut before being discarded. Most pharmacies will accept these containers and will dispose of them for you.

✔ If you're using cloudy insulin (some insulins are clear and some are cloudy), roll the vial to mix the contents before you inject it. If clumps are present, do not use the insulin.

You'll find that injecting insulin that is at room temperature is more comfortable than injecting insulin you have just taken out of the refrigerator.

Adjusting Your Insulin Dose

If you're taking insulin, you can pat yourself on the back; you have just been given the right to prescribe your own medicine. Well, not entirely, but to quite a significant extent. Insulin is different from almost any other medicine your doctor will ever ask you to take. Unlike antibiotics, heart medicines, or, for that matter, oral hypoglycemic agents, insulin is *not* designed to be taken in a set dose day to day. If your pancreas was working properly, it would constantly adjust how much insulin it was producing based on your body's requirements at any given moment. When you give yourself insulin, you're trying to mimic what your pancreas would normally do, so that means you, too, should be constantly adjusting your insulin dose. In fact, when we ask patients how much insulin they are taking, it is music to our ears when they reply, "Oh, well that depends. . . ." Precisely right. It depends. It depends on many things, including

- What you are about to eat (This refers to both the *type* of food — particularly the carbohydrate content — and the *amount* of food you're about to enjoy. We discuss the importance of *carbohydrate counting* if you have type 1 diabetes later in this chapter. Some people with type 2 diabetes also benefit from carbohydrate counting.)
- Your current blood glucose level
- Your recent blood glucose levels
- Whether you will be exercising
- Which type of insulin you are using

The common denominator in this list is the need to make *pro-active* insulin adjustments. The single greatest reason for failing to achieve good blood glucose control is making *retroactive* insulin adjustments. To be pro-active, you should be like a soothsayer, trying to predict what your reading is likely to be in a few hours and taking the amount of insulin *now* that will anticipate your needs *later*. Far too often people simply say, "Oh, my reading is high, I need more insulin," or "My reading is low, I need less insulin." These statements are perfectly true, but they take into account far less information than is available and necessary.

 Although insulin adjustment is essential for the great majority of people with diabetes, if you have type 2 diabetes and have excellent blood glucose control on the same daily dose of insulin, it would not be necessary for you to make routine changes.

Many, many people have the mistaken impression that their insulin dose correlates to the severity of their diabetes. In case you're one of those people, we're glad you are reading this paragraph. Your insulin dose tells you (and us) absolutely *nothing* about how good or bad your diabetes is. You can be on 10 units per day and have all sorts of complications and difficulties with your diabetes, or you can be on 300 units per day and sail along very nicely, thank you very much. Just like you should wear the shoe size that your feet require, so should you take the dose of insulin your body requires. That's all there is to it.

Bill was a 65-year-old man with type 2 diabetes. He was taking 10 units of NPH insulin at bedtime. Although his readings were 5 to 7 mmol/L at bedtime, his before-breakfast blood glucose readings were running 10 to 12 mmol/L. Bill blamed the high readings on eating too big a bedtime snack, but when he reduced his snack, it didn't help. Ian suggested to Bill that he increase his bedtime insulin dose by one unit every night until his before-breakfast readings came down to target. Two weeks later, Bill was up to 24 units of insulin daily and his before-breakfast readings were down to 5 mmol/L.

Bill's problem is a very common one. In the absence of sufficient quantities of insulin in your system, your blood glucose level will tend to rise overnight as your liver starts to release glucose into the blood (starting at about 3 a.m.) in response to increasing levels of other hormones (such as cortisol and growth hormone). This is called the *dawn phenomenon*. Intermediate- or long-acting insulin (the former routinely taken at bedtime; the latter usually but not always taken at bedtime) is the ideal way to combat this as the insulin will provide a substantial effect in the middle of the night to combat the liver's tendency at that time to release glucose. To get this benefit from your insulin, however, the dose *has to be adjusted* to meet your body's demands, as Bill discovered.

If you have elevated before-breakfast readings, but you are also having lows in the middle of the night, then you should *not* increase your bedtime insulin. The best solution will depend on what insulin you're taking. If you're having overnight hypoglycemia, we recommend, in consultation with your doctor and diabetes educator, the following options to help you avoid this problem:

- If you're taking NPH insulin at suppertime, change the time you take it to bedtime.

- If you're taking regular insulin at suppertime, discontinue this and take a rapid-acting insulin at suppertime instead.

- If you're taking NPH at bedtime, discontinue this and take Levemir or Lantus instead.

- If you're taking Levemir or Lantus at bedtime, reduce the dose. If that doesn't help, take it earlier in the day.

For generations, health care providers and people with diabetes have believed that high blood glucose readings first thing in the morning were sometimes (or often) a rebound from having had (and slept through) a low in the middle of the night. (This is called the *Somogyi phenomenon* or a *Somogyi reaction*.) With the introduction of continuous glucose monitoring (see Chapter 9), we now know that this type of rebounding seldom, if ever, occurs. So if you have a high blood glucose reading when you wake up in the morning, it's much more likely that your glucose levels have been steadily creeping up overnight; not that they were low (but you were unaware of it) in the middle of the night. The best way to be sure about what's going on is, from time to time, for you to set your alarm for the middle of the night and get up and test your blood glucose at that time.

When you start insulin, you must consider it as just that, *a start.* You'll need to stay in regular touch with your diabetes educator for *ongoing* dosage adjustment guidance. Your educator knows you as an individual and can provide advice specific to you. For example, your educator will help you learn how to adjust your doses based on your blood glucose readings, your diet, your exercise, your travelling, and, for women, where you are in your menstrual cycle. Without the educator's ongoing assistance, very few people ever master insulin adjustment and they typically end up feeling very frustrated. You may find it helpful to have a look at a handout Ian gives his patients who are about to start insulin (www.ourdiabetes.com/insulin-initiation.htm).

Carbohydrate Counting

As we discuss in Chapter 10, carbohydrates are *the* key nutrient in raising blood glucose readings after meals. You can take advantage of this by adjusting your insulin dose to fit with the likely effect on your blood glucose of the quantity of carbohydrates you are about to eat. This is called *carbohydrate counting* (*carb counting* for short) and is an essential part of type 1 diabetes management, especially if you're using an insulin pump. It can also be a helpful component of type 2 diabetes management if you're taking rapid-acting insulin with your meals.

The best way to learn how to perform carbohydrate counting is by meeting with your registered dietitian. They are expertly trained in this field and will likely spend at least an hour with you to go over the basics. Having a follow-up meeting (or meetings) with them to have the principles of carb counting reinforced is often a good idea.

Having a honeymoon — whether or not you're married

The *honeymoon period* is a period of time after the onset of type 1 diabetes when individuals have some recovery of their pancreatic function and are able to stop giving themselves insulin injections (or, at least, require far lower doses than they had been on). Typically this lasts for no more than a few weeks or months. All honeymoons are short, including — with rare exceptions — this one.

You're an award winner

Two companies that manufacture insulin in Canada give out awards to celebrate those individuals who have used insulin for many years. NovoNordisk has the Novo Nordisk Half Century Award Program (recognizing, as you might surmise, 50 years of using insulin) and Eli Lilly has the Lilly Diabetes Journey Awards (of which there are three: one for 25 years of insulin use, one for 50 years of insulin use, and one for 75 years of insulin use). You can find out more about the Novo Nordisk award by calling 800-465-4334 and you can find out more about the Eli Lilly awards by calling 888-545-5972 or on the Web at www.lillydiabetes.com/content/lilly-programs.jsp (click on Journey Awards).

Mary was a 16-year-old girl with type 1 diabetes. She was taking Lantus insulin at bedtime (to prevent her blood glucose from rising overnight) and was taking Humalog insulin with each meal to prevent her blood glucose readings from climbing too high after she ate. Nonetheless, she found that sometimes her two-hour, after-meal readings were excellent and other times they were poor, without any rhyme or reason. Mary met with the registered dietitian and discovered there was indeed a reason: Her consumption of carbohydrate was varying quite a bit from meal to meal, but she wasn't adjusting her insulin dose. Mary learned how to adjust her insulin based on how much carbohydrate she was eating, and soon thereafter her readings were excellent.

The first step in carbohydrate counting is to calculate how many grams of carbohydrate you're about to consume and to then give a certain number of units of rapid-acting insulin based on that. (See the following tip.) Because each person responds differently, adults are typically arbitrarily started on a ratio of 1 unit of insulin for every 10 grams of carbohydrate, but it can range from 1 unit per 5 grams to 1 unit per 20 grams. (And even that's not written in stone.) Bear in mind that not all carbohydrates will raise your blood glucose to the same degree (see our discussion on the glycemic index in Chapter 10). Do not count the fibre you eat when totalling the number of carbs in your diet because, although it's a carbohydrate, it will not raise your blood glucose.

You can find out the carbohydrate (including fibre) content of foods by having a look at the Nutrition Facts label on the food you buy. (See Chapter 10.) Also, some excellent books are available to help you learn and use carb counting. One particularly helpful book is *The Calorie King Calorie, Fat & Carbohydrate Counter* (Family Health). Also, some so-called smart insulin pumps are smart indeed and can perform the required calculations for you; all you have to do is tell the pump how many grams of carbs you're about to eat (and some of these devices make even that step easier by coming with a pre-loaded inventory of foods and their carbohydrate content). Bon appétit!

If you're carbohydrate counting, you'll also benefit from using a *correction factor* (or *insulin sensitivity factor*). A correction factor tells you the amount of insulin you'll need to bring an elevated before-meal blood glucose level down to normal. In other words, your correction factor corrects your elevated blood glucose (and your carb counting–determined dose prevents your level from going up from the food you're about to eat).

ANECDOTE

Yolanda has type 1 diabetes treated with Humalog insulin with meals and Levemir insulin at bedtime. She's about to eat supper. Her before-supper blood glucose is 12 mmol/L. Her about-to-be-devoured scrumptious meal contains 40 grams of carbohydrate. She uses a carbohydrate counting ratio of 1 unit per 10 grams of carbohydrate (a 1:10 ratio) and a correction factor of 1 unit for each 5 mmol/L her blood glucose is above 7. To know how much insulin she needs to take, she does the following calculation:

1. She uses her carbohydrate counting ratio: 40 g of carbohydrate × 1 unit/10 g = 4 units

2. She uses her correction factor: 12 mmol/L – 7 mmol/L = 5 mmol/L × 1 unit/5 mmol/L = 1 unit

3. She adds these two amounts together and determines she needs 4 units + 1 unit = 5 units.

4. She injects 5 units of insulin and smiles to herself as she recalls how the once intimidating notion of carb counting and use of a correction factor came quickly to seem like second nature after she had spent an hour with the wonderful dietitian.

Carbohydrate counting may not be rocket science, but it isn't easy either and it's certainly not for everyone. If you're doing very well without carbohydrate counting, don't feel you have to take on this additional task. If, however, things aren't going sufficiently well for you (and in particular if your glucose control is inconsistent and/or your A1C isn't particularly good), you should contact your dietitian to discuss whether carbohydrate counting would be good for you.

Donating blood

If you're on insulin therapy, Canadian Blood Services' current policy is that you are not a candidate to give blood. We are sure this policy is well intentioned, but we feel it's overly restrictive. (Incidentally, the American Red Cross allows people being treated with insulin to donate blood so long as they have never taken *beef* insulin.) If you are on oral hypoglycemic agents, you are eligible to donate blood unless some other health problem precludes this.

Travelling with Your Insulin

We live in a mobile society, and if you use insulin, then where you go, your insulin goes too.

Breezing through the border

As you well know, airline security is now greater than ever. And this means you will need to take some additional measures when you are planning on travelling by plane.

Transport Canada has issued guidelines for when you are flying with diabetes supplies. The following information is from the Canadian Diabetes Association's reference to these guidelines:

- ✔ Advise the security personnel that you have diabetes and that you're carrying your supplies on board. Have available a letter from your physician indicating that you have diabetes and that you need to carry your diabetes medication and supplies.

- ✔ Organize your medication and supplies into one separate container and take it with you in your *carry-on* (not your stowed) baggage.

- ✔ Ensure that your syringes have the needle guards in place and are accompanied by the insulin.

- ✔ Place your insulin and any other medications in a container with a professionally printed pharmaceutical label identifying the medication. If the pharmaceutical label is on the outside of the box containing the insulin, the insulin must be carried in that original packaging.

- ✔ Cap your lancets. They must be accompanied by a glucose meter imprinted with the manufacturer's name.

- ✔ If you have any difficulty throughout the screening process, request to speak to the screening supervisor.

- ✔ If you are travelling outside of Canada, consult with your airline for applicable international regulations.

If you use an insulin pump, you may wish to pre-emptively notify the screening officer that you are wearing the device. They will probably not bat an eye (insulin pumps are quickly becoming so commonplace they are likely seeing them routinely), but it may spare you some additional time and questions.

An insulin pump–wearing patient of Ian's was recently passing through airport security in an Asian country when the screener yanked her out of line. The patient surmised that the screener was alarmed by the presence of an unfamiliar device. Wrong! The screener smiled broadly as he lifted up his shirt to show Ian's patient that he, too, was a pump user! He then let her continue her otherwise uneventful journey through security.

There are at least three important reasons to take your insulin and supplies (injection devices, blood glucose meter, lancets, and so on) with you as part of your carry-on (not your checked) luggage:

- If you are going to Sydney, Nova Scotia, for example, your *carry-on* luggage is not going to get mistakenly sent to Sydney, Australia.
- The baggage compartment temperatures may not be appropriate for your insulin.
- You will need it!

And although not technically an insulin supply, make sure you take extra snacks with you on board in case your meals are delayed.

And on the subject of insulin supplies, if you will be travelling for any sort of extended period, make sure you have lots of extra insulin, blood glucose test strips, and so on. Better to have too much than to try finding a pharmacy at midnight in an unfamiliar city.

The Canadian Diabetes Association offers travel insurance to its members. We discuss this further in Chapter 18.

Because rapid-acting insulin works so quickly, even if you see the flight attendant moving the food cart down the aisle in your direction, do *not* take your insulin dose until your food has been set down in front of you. We've had more than one patient who, anticipating imminent arrival of his meal, took his rapid-acting insulin only to find the food cart then quickly whisked away when unexpected turbulence interrupted food services. With his mealtime insulin having been given but no meal to go with it, he was at risk of having hypoglycemia. Fortunately, he had wisely taken some snacks with him in his carry-on luggage and substituted the snacks for the missed meal.

Adjusting your doses between time zones

Travelling seldom causes big problems, especially if you're on basal-bolus therapy (we define this earlier in this section). Often the best thing to do is to

✔ Take your *bolus* insulin at your new mealtimes, regardless of when they happen to be.

✔ Take your *basal* insulin at the same hour of the clock you normally take it. For example, if you live in Vancouver and usually take, say, Lantus insulin at 10 p.m. *PST* and you then travel to Montreal — which has a three-hour time difference — you would instead take your Lantus insulin at 10 p.m. *EST*. The first day you would end up taking your injection three hours earlier than usual (and, upon your return, three hours later than usual), but this is seldom a problem with basal insulins. Thereafter you would be taking your basal insulin every 24 hours as you likely do customarily.

If there is going to be a significant delay between meals, take a snack and a small amount of your rapid-acting or regular insulin halfway between those meals.

If your travels will take you beyond more than a few time zones or if you are not taking basal-bolus insulin, we recommend that you be in touch with your diabetes educator before you travel to get advice specific to your situation. Bon voyage!

Was inhaled insulin just so much hot air?

For years, the diabetes world was awaiting the development and availability of inhaled insulin. Many companies were working feverishly to develop such a product as they anticipated a financial windfall. Well, billions upon billions of research and development dollars later, inhaled insulin has come . . . and gone. Pfizer Corporation launched Exubera in the United States in 2006, then, quicker than Harry Potter can say "expelliarmus," withdrew it from the market citing poor sales. Seems like Exubera sales were anything but exuberant. Quickly following suit, pretty well every other company developing inhaled insulin — with the notable exception of Mannkind Corporation — halted their own initiatives to develop similar products.

However, other, novel routes of insulin administration continue to be explored. The Canadian company Generex Biotechnology Corporation has developed Oral-lyn, an aerosol form of insulin that is sprayed onto the inside of the cheek. It's now available for use in Ecuador and India. Whether it will prove to be a safe, effective, and useful product remains to be seen.

Chapter 14

Complementary and Alternative Therapies

Up to half of people with diabetes use some form of complementary or alternative therapy (also known as complementary or alternative medicine; CAM for short). Alternative and complementary therapy refers to non-traditional treatment, typically offered or recommended by people outside of the mainstream medical community. Suffice it to say, a fair bit of controversy surrounds some (but not all) of these treatment options. Some CAMs have been around for many years, while others are fairly recent. In Chapter 10 we look at the role of vitamins and minerals as part of your nutrition plan. In this chapter we look at a variety of other treatments and see what role they may have in helping you with your diabetes.

Cautions Concerning CAMs

The media frequently mentions how this or that nutrient/herb/mineral may help you if you have diabetes. Indeed, we seldom see a day go by when some such mention isn't made. Disappointingly, what we invariably discover is that the evidence of improvement comes not from a research study involving real people or, for that matter, even laboratory animals. Rather, the new "discovery" is typically that a substance, which *theoretically* should help diabetes, has been found to be present in a berry or leaf or root or some such place. Ah, if only theory and reality were the same (or, often, even close facsimiles).

Carefully evaluate non-traditional therapy in the same way that we hope you would consider prescription medication: Know what it's supposed to do, what it's *not* supposed to do (that is, side effects), and, most important, whether certain health problems or other medicines you're taking would make it dangerous to take at all. In other words, you need to be an informed consumer. Never assume that because something is natural it must be safe. After all, arsenic is natural too.

Because some non-traditional therapies can interact with your prescription drugs, let your physician know if you are taking non-traditional therapies. Bring them (in their original bottles) to your doctors' appointments. You can also go online to www.drugdigest.org to check for potential adverse interactions between your CAM and your prescription medicine.

Determining the value of complementary and alternative therapies in managing diabetes is very difficult for several reasons:

✔ Very few scientific studies have investigated these treatments.

✔ Potential side effects have not been adequately assessed.

✔ The strength of non-traditional agents can vary enormously from bottle to bottle, even if the label on the bottle says the same thing.

✔ The purity of non-traditional agents can also vary enormously. One survey of traditional Chinese medicines found potentially toxic substances or potent unlisted ingredients in up to 30 percent of bottles.

✔ Alternative and complementary therapies have not been required to pass much in the way of government scrutiny, so long as they are marketed as foods, not drugs. This is a surprise to most people, who think — quite understandably — that a company could not say its product performs in such and such a way without evidence to back the claim. (The federal government introduced the Natural Health Products Regulations in 2004 in an attempt to improve this situation. You can learn more about these regulations at www.hc-sc.gc.ca/dhp-mps/prodnatur/index-eng.php.)

If CAMs are helpful for diabetes (and, as we discover in this chapter, there is very little evidence for this), most likely they would be of benefit only if you have type 2 diabetes. If you have type 1 diabetes, your problem is lack of insulin, and no CAM is going to change that. If you have type 2 diabetes, a main problem is insulin resistance and it's possible that there exist CAMs that could reduce this.

Because of the limited evidence that CAMs have any helpful role in managing diabetes and because of concerns regarding their safety, the Canadian Diabetes Association Clinical Practice Guidelines do not advocate their use.

We sincerely hope that eventually at least some complementary and alternative medicines are found to be safe and effective to help control blood glucose; the more weapons in our arsenal, the better.

Because of the limited scientific information available to guide our decision making, if you are considering taking an alternative or complementary therapy, you'll have to make your decision based as much (or more) on hope as on science. That's fine, of course, if medical science knows the product has no potential for harm; but in the same way that it doesn't know about all the benefits that some remedies may hold, it doesn't know about all the potential downsides they may have. Thus, caution is required.

Herbs for Herbivores (And Carnivores and Omnivores)

We suspect there are few people who don't routinely include herbs as part of their diet. Although an herb is, technically, a "plant without a woody stem," in this section on CAMs we take some liberties and use it to mean *any* additional nutrient specifically taken to help your diabetes.

Alpha Lipoic Acid (ALA)

Some (not much mind you, but some) scientific evidence suggests that taking supplemental alpha lipoic acid (ALA) — which is an antioxidant — can lower blood glucose levels. Early evidence also suggests that it might be of benefit in reducing symptoms of diabetic peripheral neuropathy (see Chapter 6). Whether it's truly effective in these ways remains to be determined.

Cinnamon

Of all the CAMs purported to help diabetes, Ian had his heart most set on cinnamon. Inexpensive, ubiquitous, colourful, flavourful, and great on a cappuccino . . . what more could one want? Alas, although early evidence suggested a theoretical benefit in controlling blood glucose levels, recent, definitive studies showed no value. Well, no *health* value to you if you have diabetes; lots of *financial* value to the enthusiastic entrepreneurs who had quickly gotten their "medicinal" cinnamon onto store shelves (where we continue to see it).

Fenugreek (Trigonella Foenum Graecum)

Fenugreek is a legume grown in India, the Mediterranean, and North Africa. Its use in treating diabetes goes back many centuries, and some evidence suggests that it may be effective in reducing blood glucose levels. Once again, this is preliminary information.

Garlic

Garlic is used for many purposes. Sometimes, it is even used for cooking! There has been a suggestion that garlic could help lower glucose levels, though the evidence for this is contradictory. We can only hope that garlic does turn out to be helpful at lowering glucose levels; can you imagine the recipe possibilities? Garlic ice cream, garlic cheesecake . . . the list is endless. Anyone for a garlic brownie?

Some evidence indicates that garlic may increase your risk of bleeding during or after surgery. If you're going to be having surgery or if you're on blood thinners, be sure to speak to your doctor before you start taking garlic supplements.

Ginkgo biloba

Ginkgo (more fully titled *ginkgo biloba,* not to be confused with Rocky *Balboa*) is one of the oldest living tree species. Innumerable people take ginkgo to treat dozens of different ailments. There's some very preliminary evidence that ginkgo may offer some benefit in the treatment of diabetic retinopathy. On the other hand, there's also experimental evidence it could make your blood glucose levels go *up.*

Ginseng

Although people usually speak of ginseng as being one product, in fact several different plant species share this name. There is Chinese or Korean ginseng as well as Siberian, American, and Japanese varieties to name but a few. *American* ginseng has been found to improve glucose control to a small but significant degree (of the other varieties, those that have been studied have not been found effective); however, these observations must be considered preliminary.

Glucosamine

Glucosamine, a product derived from the outside skeleton of shellfish (such as crabs and shrimps), is commonly used to treat arthritis pain, not diabetes, but because it is used as an alternative therapy, we thought it opportune to mention it here. A few years ago, concerns arose that glucosamine might worsen insulin resistance and, as a result, could worsen your blood glucose control. Subsequent research offers reassurance that this is unlikely. So, the way things currently stand, it looks like taking glucosamine will have no impact on your diabetes, one way or the other.

Gymnema Sylvestre

Gymnema sylvestre is a tropical plant found in central and southern India. In Hindi, it goes by the name "destroyer of sugar," based on folklore that chewing the leaves results in the inability to taste sweet things. That, of course, would suggest that if it was effective in treating diabetes, it would be because it wrecks your appetite for dessert (maybe even for those garlic brownies we talked about earlier), but no, there is some *preliminary* evidence that, apart from suppressing appetite, it has the ability to reduce blood glucose levels; possibly by improving the insulin-producing beta cell function.

Tea

Three types of tea exist: green, oolong, and black. Some (very limited) evidence suggests that oolong tea might help you control your blood glucose levels. If you are going to try it, however, you had best *really* like the stuff, because the test subjects drank 1.5 litres of it daily. Also, not all oolong tea is the same. In the study they used the variety found in China (because it is more strongly fermented). If further studies find oolong tea to be beneficial in controlling blood glucose levels, doctors may soon be recommending tea for two — 2 million Canadians with diabetes that is.

Investigating Other Alternative Treatments

There are hundreds of other alternative therapies for diabetes (none of which have met the standard of being proven safe and effective). Here, we look at three of the more commonly considered options.

Chromium

A few years ago a whole bunch of excitement arose after a study of people with type 2 diabetes in China found that if they were given high doses of chromium they improved their blood glucose control. After all, if taking chromium supplements helped people living in China, why wouldn't those of us living on this side of the ocean have a similar benefit? Well, as we all know, China and Canada share many differences, chief of which (in this particular case) is that the people studied in China were chromium deficient whereas we here in Canada are not. Indeed, if people with diabetes are not deficient in chromium to start with, we do not have evidence that taking additional chromium is helpful.

Pancreas formula

Pancreas formula is sold on the Internet as a mixture of herbs, vitamins, and minerals that help diabetes. No clinical or experimental evidence shows that pancreas formula does anything of value in the human body. Factual evidence does not support the claims that are made for this "treatment." The true *formula* here may simply be one that allows the sellers to get rich at others' expense.

Vinegar

Ian fondly recalls how the wait staff at Schwartz's deli in Montreal would take the vinegar bottle you used for your fries, turn it upside down, and sprinkle the contents onto the table to clean it. Hmm, edible, hygienic, and — could it be — medicinal, too? Maybe so. A study from 2004 showed that ingesting vinegar may help control your blood glucose levels. In that very small study, consuming 20 grams of apple cider vinegar reduced insulin resistance (which, in turn, may lead to improved blood glucose levels). We don't recommend you start taking apple cider vinegar based on this limited data, but we're going to cross our fingers that more solid evidence emerges to support this form of therapy.

Laughter

We thought we would save the best for last (you know what they say about the person who laughs last). An article in a major diabetes medical journal has shown that doctors should perhaps be prescribing laughter — and we're not just talking Patch Adams here. Japanese researchers looked at a group of people with type 2 diabetes and assessed their blood glucose levels after the participants listened to a 40-minute lecture that was described by the researches as being "monotonous" and "without humorous intent." (Oh my, shades of medical school!) The next day these same subjects' blood glucose levels were measured after watching a comedy show.

Well, you probably already figured out the punch line: the blood glucose levels were lower when the participants watched the comedy show than when they listened to the boring lecture. And that's no laughing matter. Then again, maybe that's exactly what it is.

Miracle cures for diabetes

In your travels — especially of the cyber kind — you've likely come across promotions for products that are said to be a miracle cure for diabetes. Everyone is tempted by come-ons for products that seem to be the magic bullet for what ails us. But these magic bullets are more likely to be poison darts. The fraudulent nature of these false claims is clear if you watch for certain common themes in the promotions:

✔ A reliance on personal testimonials rather than hard science. Anecdotes are not proof of the value of a treatment or test. The favourable experiences of one or a few people are not a substitute for a scientific study. If they did seem to respond to the drug, it may be for entirely different reasons.

✔ References to scientific studies or journals that sound impressive and legitimate, but in fact are pseudo-scientific, obscure sources that cannot be readily reviewed to verify their accuracy.

✔ Lofty claims of benefit far surpassing any other available treatment.

✔ Allusions to conspiracies among the medical community in hiding something from the public.

One day there will be a cure for diabetes. And every person with diabetes will find out about it because every person in the diabetes health care field will be shouting with joy at the top of our lungs. You'll hear us. We guarantee it.

Part IV
Particular Patients and Special Circumstances

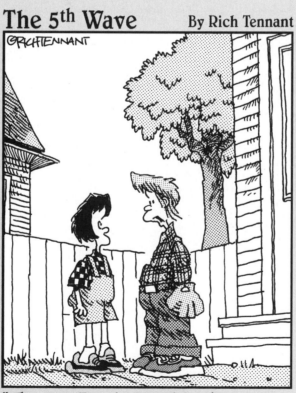

The 5th Wave   By Rich Tennant

"The way I understand it, the reason I was getting cold and tired was because my body wasn't making enough insulation."

In this part . . .

Diabetes in a child or an elderly individual poses special challenges and requires special management. In this part we look at the unique challenges that these groups have to contend with. Aboriginal communities have to tackle some special issues of their own, as you'll discover. We also look at some very practical issues that confront people with diabetes, including employment, insurance, and driving. Those whose preferred means of locomotion is at the controls of an airborne vehicle will find answers to questions about piloting here, too. Lastly, we look at precautions you can take so that you are prepared in the event of a disaster.

Chapter 15

Your Child Has Diabetes

Children with diabetes present special issues that adults with diabetes don't have. Not only are they physically growing and developing, but they also are contending with issues of psychological and social adjustment. Diabetes adds complexity to a period of time that is not exactly smooth, even without it.

When a child has diabetes, it's a concern. When *your* child has diabetes, you may see it as a disaster. If your child has diabetes, in a sense your whole family has diabetes; or at the very least your whole family has to deal with it. If something affects those with whom you share common interests (or, in your case, love), what affects them affects you, too.

In this chapter we look at how you can keep your child healthy and prevent diabetes from ruling his or her life, and yours. You find out how to manage diabetes in your child at each stage of growth and development from infancy up to and including early adulthood. And as we look at these issues, remember that you're not to blame for your child's diabetes. You didn't cause it. And your child didn't cause it either. So neither you nor your child should ever feel guilty about it.

Your Baby or Preschooler Has Type 1 Diabetes

Although type 1 diabetes doesn't usually show up in babies, it can, and you should know what to expect when it does. Obviously, your baby isn't verbal and can't tell you what's bothering him or her. For this reason, you may miss the fact that your baby is constantly thirsty and urinating excessively in his or her diaper. The baby will lose weight and have vomiting and diarrhea, but this may understandably be attributed to a stomach or intestinal disorder rather than diabetes. When the doctor finally makes the diagnosis, your baby may be very sick and require a stay in a pediatric intensive care unit. Do not blame yourself for not realizing that your baby was sick.

After you have the diagnosis, the hard work begins. You must immediately learn to give insulin injections and to test the blood glucose in a child who may well be reluctant to have either one done. You have to learn when and what to feed your baby to satisfy the child's appetite, to encourage growth and development, and to prevent low blood glucose.

At this stage, the goal is not for tight blood glucose control. Rather, for children 5 years of age and less, the Canadian Diabetes Association's recommended target before-meal readings are 6.0 to 12.0 mmol/L and the target A1C is up to 8.5 percent. Also, you must be extremely careful to avoid hypoglycemia. There are several reasons for this. First, the baby's neurological system is still developing. Frequent, severe low blood glucose can damage this development, so the glucose is permitted to be higher now than later on. Second, studies show that changes associated with high blood glucose leading to diabetic complications aren't as critical until just before puberty, so you have a grace period during which you can keep looser control over your baby's blood glucose levels.

A main reason to avoid having your baby's or infant's blood glucose levels run above target is because this can lead to dehydration. A small baby is fragile, and even small losses of water, sodium, potassium, and other substances can rapidly lead to a very sick baby.

Here are some of the things you will need to know:

✔ How to identify the signs and symptoms of hyperglycemia, hypoglycemia, and diabetic ketoacidosis (see Chapter 5)

✔ How to administer insulin (see Chapter 13)

✔ How to measure the blood glucose and ketones (see Chapter 9)

✔ How to treat hypoglycemia, and how and when to use glucagon (see Chapter 5)

✔ How to properly nourish your child (In Chapter 10 we talk about general nutrition principles, but of course with a child this young you'll need to get very detailed advice from a dietitian.)

✔ What to do when your child is sick with another illness (see "Sick Day Solutions for Your Child with Type 1 Diabetes," later in this chapter)

Your responsibilities as the parent of a baby or preschooler with diabetes are extensive and time-consuming, and the list above may seem rather daunting. But you can do it. Indeed, you must. But you should never feel you are in this alone. You should train family members and friends who can help out, even for a short time. Otherwise, you may end up feeling constantly emotionally and physically exhausted (as if being a parent isn't hard enough to begin with!).

Keeping in regular contact with a diabetes education centre is crucial if you have a child, especially an infant, with diabetes. A diabetes nurse educator and dietitian can provide invaluable assistance. Also, these centres may allow you to access additional services such as that of a social worker, if necessary. Not all diabetes education centres specialize in children with type 1 diabetes, so ask them if this is their particular area of expertise; if it isn't, they'll gladly refer you to a centre that has this expertise. You should also have a pediatrician who has particular expertise in looking after young children with diabetes. Your family physician can refer you. If your family doctor isn't familiar with one, your diabetes educator will certainly be able to recommend someone to you and your family doctor.

Your other children may resent the attention that you pay to this one child. If your other children start to misbehave, this may be the reason. Remember to include them in the education (and, if possible, allow them to assist when they can).

Diagnosing diabetes in your preschooler may be just as difficult as diagnosing it in a baby. The child is still running around in diapers and may be unable to tell you how they're feeling.

Preschoolers are beginning the process of separating from their parents and starting to learn to control the environment (by becoming toilet trained, for example). This separation process makes it more difficult for you, the parent, to give the injections and test the glucose. You must be firm in insisting that these things be done. You'll need to do them yourself, of course, because a small child neither knows how to do them nor understands what to do with the information generated by the glucose meter.

Because a child's eating habits may not be very regular, the use of rapid-acting insulin (see Chapter 13) taken after meals is often helpful. You can first see how much of the meal your child ate and then give an amount of insulin based on that. Be sure to speak to your diabetes educators about this option.

Your Primary School Child Has Type 1 Diabetes

In some ways, managing diabetes gets a little easier with a primary school child, but in other ways, it gets more difficult. Your child may now be able to tell you when he or she has symptoms of hypoglycemia, so it's easier to recognize and treat. But you must begin to control your child's blood glucose more carefully because at this stage tighter control becomes necessary.

Your child is still growing and developing, so nutrition remains very important. You must provide enough of the right kinds of nutrients for this process. You will need to remain in ongoing contact with the dietitian as she will need to work regularly with you to adjust your child's meal plan as your child grows.

When children go to school, they interact with other children and want to fit in. Children with diabetes may consider their condition a stigma. They may be very reluctant to share the fact of their diabetes with other children, or they may have told their friends and found that other children didn't know how to handle the information. This is where your newfound expertise with diabetes can be invaluable because you can educate your child's friends about diabetes. You may need to speak to their parents as well.

As time goes on, your child is going to separate from you further. He or she may insist on giving the insulin injections and doing the blood tests. Although you should encourage your child's involvement in these tasks, you should not give full responsibility for them to your child. Your ongoing supervision is mandatory to ensure that things are being done properly. You should also be aware that because your child may feel uncomfortable letting peers know about the diabetes, he or she may avoid glucose testing and insulin administration when friends are around. In this circumstance, fast food may also tend to replace proper, healthy nutrition on a too frequent basis.

Having diabetes should never, ever be a stigma, but, alas, it's sometimes seen this way. Insulin pumps (refer to Chapter 13), on the other hand, are often perceived by children (whether having diabetes or not) as being cool (or, at the least, interesting), whereas insulin injections are sometimes seen as scary. This should not be a main reason for having your child use an insulin pump, but it is something to take into consideration.

For children ages 6 to 12, the CDA target before-meal blood glucose readings are 4.0 to 10.0 mmol/L and the target A1C is up to 8.0. The higher end of this target range is suitable for a 6-year-old, but you should aim for the lower end as your child advances through this age range. Because you are aiming for tighter control for children in this age range, hypoglycemia is more of a risk, especially at night. You can reduce the risk of hypoglycemia by taking any or all of the following steps:

✔ Give your child a bedtime snack. (A snack made with cornstarch is particularly helpful. Because cornstarch breaks down slowly, it provides glucose over a longer period of time. Your child's dietitian can provide you with cornstarch-containing recipes; you can also find some tasty ones in the book *Food and Diabetes,* by Doreen Yasui and Doreen Hatton of the British Columbia Children's Hospital.)

✔ Measure your child's blood glucose at bedtime and increase the amount of the bedtime snack if the glucose level is under target.

✔ Occasionally check your child's blood glucose at 3 a.m.

✔ Ask your child whether he or she has symptoms such as nightmares, headaches, and unexplained sweating, which might be clues to nighttime low blood glucose.

✔ Be sure your child doesn't skip meals or scheduled snacks.

✔ Have your child check his or her blood glucose before exercising and, if below target, take extra carbohydrate according to the planned duration and intensity of exercise.

✔ If your child tends not to finish meals, speak to your diabetes educator about occasionally using rapid-acting insulin *after* rather than *before* meals. (We discuss insulin therapy in Chapter 13.)

Mature siblings and, of course, parents should be aware of symptoms of hypoglycemia and know how to treat it (including knowing how and when to use glucagon). We discuss these issues in Chapter 5.

Seeing as your child spends so much time in school, this environment must be set up suitably. Schoolmates will likely not have much, if any, knowledge of diabetes, and your child's teacher may have only limited experience as well. As most any minority group member knows, overcoming ignorance is the surest way to prevent or undo stigmatization. For this reason as well as for reasons of safety and practicality, we encourage you to meet with your child's teacher and the appropriate administrative people within the school to review issues such as these:

✔ When blood glucose monitoring will need to be done and whether your child will need assistance/supervision with this task. This discussion should also include where testing will take place and where to dispose of lancets

✔ When insulin is to be administered and whether your child will need assistance/supervision with this task (or, if your child uses an insulin pump, whether he or she will require assistance with it)

✔ Supervising a younger child during meals and snacks. (No, not simply to make sure that food fights aren't about to break out! Rather, it is important to make sure the youngster is actually ingesting the wonderful nutrients that are on their plate and in their glass.)

✔ How to recognize and treat hypoglycemia, including, importantly, knowing how and when to use a glucagon kit

✔ How to recognize hyperglycemia and what school staff should do if they suspect it is present (Calling you — the parent — is an appropriate first step if your child is feeling perfectly well. But, if your child is at all unwell — especially if they are vomiting — the safest and best thing for the school to do is to immediately call an ambulance.)

✔ The need to allow your child to have a water bottle at his or her desk and to have permission to freely leave the classroom to go to the bathroom

Your child should participate in any and all school activities, including academics, sports, and field trips. This will require additional expertise, however, on the part of school officials and chaperones. Once again, you, the parent, can help out by teaching them what you have already learned.

The Canadian Diabetes Association, in order to "acknowledge and clarify the essential partnership among parents or caregivers, students and school personnel in the care of students with type 1 diabetes in the school system," has created the helpful and detailed *Standards of Care for Students with Type 1 Diabetes in Schools*. This document can be found on the Web at www.diabetes .ca/files/StandardsofCare.pdf.

Your diabetes educator can serve as an invaluable resource in helping you familiarize your child's teacher and, most important, schoolmates about diabetes and how it affects your child. For example, Ian is blessed to work with wonderful diabetes educators at the Charles H. Best Diabetes Centre for Children and Youth (www.charleshbest.com) who, in addition to their already myriad duties, have developed a school program in which they visit a child's school and give class presentations. It has been an overwhelming success. Ask your child's diabetes educator if they would consider doing the same. If they would like, have them call the Best Centre (905-666-7796) to learn more about the program.

Your Adolescent Has Type 1 Diabetes

Your adolescent with diabetes may provide some of your biggest challenges. (As if adolescence isn't tough enough even when you have perfect health.) The adolescent can achieve tight blood glucose control at this age, but it certainly isn't easy. To have excellent control requires a high degree of adherence to proper lifestyle therapy (nutrition and exercise), and regular attention to blood glucose monitoring and insulin adjustment. As you can imagine, most adolescents, eagerly seeking independence and freedom, would not be thrilled with this. (And who could blame them?) Yet, for all of that, adolescence and the teenage years don't have to mean that diabetes gets neglected.

After your child reaches 13 years of age, the Canadian Diabetes Association–recommended target blood glucose levels for most adolescents are as follows: before-meal 4.0 to 7.0 mmol/L, two-hour after-meal 5.0 to 10.0, A1C 7 or less. (For the minority of adolescents for whom it can be safely achieved, the CDA recommends aiming for even lower blood glucose targets: before-meal blood glucose of 4.0 to 6.0, two-hour after-meal blood glucose of 5.0 to 8.0, and an A1C of 6 or less.)

The hormonal changes that occur in puberty can result in worsening glucose control; however, this can be compensated for by appropriate adjustment of insulin therapy. And speaking of hormonal changes, adolescent girls must be made aware of issues surrounding contraception and sexual health. Unintended pregnancy in an adolescent is always a problem; unintended pregnancy in an adolescent with diabetes is even more of a problem. Appropriate members of the health care team should address these concerns. We discuss diabetes and pregnancy in Chapter 7.

You can help your adolescent children with their diabetes in many ways:

✔ Make sure that they know you have certain expectations — expectations born of love and concern — in terms of their management of the diabetes.

✔ Be supportive and understanding — even when they go through periods when they are less attentive to their diabetes than they should be. On the other hand, you want your child to know that you're far from indifferent to that inattention. Encouragement often works better than being authoritative or dictatorial (though, of course, these measures also have their occasional role, as any parent knows).

✔ Remind them that they need never be ashamed of diabetes. In its very essence, it is a simple shortage of a hormone. What shame is there in that?

✔ Keep an eye out for evidence of insulin omission. Teenage girls not infrequently skip insulin doses (with consequent hyperglycemia) because they have learned that it results in weight loss.

✔ Review, in a non-judgmental way, their blood glucose levels and assist them with insulin adjustment.

✔ As your child grows, gradually transfer responsibility for looking after the diabetes — based on your child's ability and interest — to him or her. This may be the most important way you can help your child in the long term. It's not an abdication of responsibility, but the fulfillment of your ultimate responsibility: creating a responsible, mature individual who is able to look after him- or herself independently. (This is often the toughest task on this list to carry out.)

Up to 10 percent of teenage girls (and some teenage boys) with diabetes have an eating disorder, such as anorexia nervosa or bulimia. These disorders can result in malnutrition and, usually, poor blood glucose control. The child may deny that the problem exists. If your adolescent has erratic glucose control, you should consider the possibility of an eating disorder and discuss it with the child and the child's doctor.

Sometimes, adolescents will share things with their diabetes educator that they may not so readily share with you, even though they know you love them dearly and care about their health. Indeed, diabetes educators often say that children of this age will spend the entirety of their first visit talking about everything in their lives except the specifics of their diabetes. But that is in no way a shortcoming. To help children with their diabetes, it's essential to know them as people first and people with diabetes second. Diabetes is, after all, but one component of their existence (and one they want to be far from front and centre). A diabetes educator who knows "how the adolescent ticks" will be in a far better position to know how best to help with the diabetes.

Your Young Adult Child Has Type 1 Diabetes

By the time children reach their late teens, they are young adults and should be the ones in charge of their diabetes. But even then, your son or daughter shouldn't lack a support system.

Regrettably, what often happens is that teenagers "graduate" from a pediatric diabetes program (where they have started to feel very out of place as they sit amongst the younger — and smaller — children in the waiting room) and fail to hook up with an adult program or with an adult diabetes specialist. They fall through the gaps, and it can take many years (all the while without proper supervision or guidance and without adequately controlled diabetes) before they end up seeking help. The single most important thing you can do to assist your young adult child with diabetes is to find out if he or she has transferred care to an adult diabetes specialist and adult diabetes education centre that has a special program for type 1 diabetes, and if not, to encourage him or her to establish these contacts. (If, despite your encouragement, your young adult child doesn't make these contacts, with your child's permission make them yourself on behalf of your child.)

If your young adult child is heading off to post-secondary school and will have a roommate, your child should teach the roommate

 ✔ How to recognize if your child has hypoglycemia.

✔ How to help your child if he or she has hypoglycemia. This should include knowing where appropriate snacks are kept and how to give glucagon. If the roommate isn't comfortable giving glucagon, at the very least he or she should be reminded what situations require a call to 911.

✔ To be aware that, if your child has been drinking alcohol and is acting drunk, he or she may, in fact, be hypoglycemic, not inebriated. (Or, indeed, may be both inebriated *and* hypoglycemic.)

Sick Day Solutions for Your Child with Type 1 Diabetes

Children with type 1 diabetes are susceptible to all the usual childhood illnesses, but diabetes complicates their care. An illness can affect glucose levels in opposite ways. An infection may increase the level of insulin resistance so that the usual dose of insulin isn't adequate. Or it may cause nausea and vomiting so that no food or drink can stay down, and the insulin may cause hypoglycemia. For this reason, when your child is ill you will need to measure his or her blood glucose and blood ketone levels (see Chapter 9) as often as every two to four hours. If the blood glucose levels are significantly elevated (above 12 mmol/L or so), the child may require additional rapid-acting or regular insulin.

If your child's blood glucose levels are elevated — especially if ketones are present in the blood (0.6 mmol/L or higher) — the safest thing to do is to have your child promptly taken to the hospital emergency department. However, if you're fortunate enough to be working with a diabetes educator that is both trained — and empowered — to deal with diabetic ketoacidosis (DKA) and is *immediately* available, you can first contact him or her for detailed advice regarding the right type of fluids your child should take and how to properly adjust your child's insulin. Often, you can avoid visits to the hospital with this type of intensive management. However, very few educators have this degree of expertise and authority. You should discuss these issues with both your educator and your diabetes specialist before your child gets sick so you'll know what to do if and when your child becomes unwell.

The fact your child isn't eating well doesn't necessarily mean that less insulin is required; depending on blood glucose levels, he or she may need *more* insulin than usual. Some of the sickest patients we've ever seen are those that became sick, had high blood glucose levels, and needed more insulin, but because they weren't eating well, it was mistakenly assumed by the patient (or, in the case of children, their caregivers) that — despite the elevated blood glucose — because they were not eating well, they needed less insulin.

Screening Tests for Organ Injury in Children and Adolescents with Type 1 Diabetes

The Canadian Diabetes Association recommends the following testing schedule for children with type 1 diabetes (see Chapter 6 for a detailed discussion on organ injury and how to test for it):

- **Blood pressure:** Your child's blood pressure should be checked at least twice per year.

- **Celiac disease testing:** Because the risk of celiac disease is higher with type 1 diabetes, your child should be tested (with a blood test taken at a laboratory) if he or she has symptoms of celiac disease. (Whether to test a child with type 1 diabetes who does *not* have symptoms of celiac disease is controversial.) We discuss celiac disease in Chapter 6.

- **Eye testing:** At the age of 15 (then at least annually), your child should have an eye examination by an expert eye professional if your child has had diabetes for at least five years. (Sometimes the frequency of screening can be changed to every two years depending on your child's particular circumstances, such as blood glucose control and eye health.)

- **Kidney testing:** At the age of 12 (then annually), a urine sample should be tested for albumin/creatinine ratio (ACR) if your child has had diabetes for at least five years.

- **Lipid testing:** If your child is less than 12 years of age, lipid testing (including cholesterol and triglycerides) is required only if some additional risk factor for cardiovascular disease is present. When your child is 12 years of age, his or her lipids should be tested, then retested five years later (earlier than that if necessary).

- **Nerve testing:** At the onset of puberty (then annually), your child should have his or her feet tested (by using, for example, a thin nylon rod called a "10 gram monofilament," as we describe in Chapter 6) if he or she has had diabetes for at least five years. These painless tests can be done in the doctor's office and take but a moment to perform.

- **Thyroid testing:** Because the risk of thyroid disease is higher with type 1 diabetes, your child's thyroid function should be tested (by measuring, on a blood sample taken at a laboratory, the child's *TSH* level and *thyroperoxidase antibody*) at the time of diabetes diagnosis, then at least every two years thereafter.

Summer Camps for Children with Type 1 Diabetes

One resource that can be tremendously valuable for you and your child with type 1 diabetes is a diabetes summer camp. Run by the Canadian Diabetes Association (CDA), these camps are located in a number of regions across Canada and provide a safe, well-managed place where your child can go and be in the majority. He or she can learn a great deal about diabetes while enjoying all the pleasures of a summer camp environment. (Certainly not a minor benefit is the opportunity for you to have time off for perhaps the first time in years.) A listing of diabetes summer camps is available on the Canadian Diabetes Association Web site (www.diabetes.ca) or by phoning the CDA (800-226-8464).

All CDA camps offer assistance with camp fees. The CDA advises that you contact the camp nearest you for more information.

Of course, you may be looking at sending your child to a regular day camp program. This is perfectly reasonable, but some advance planning is important. In particular, it would be wise to do the following:

- ✔ Speak to the camp director to make sure the camp can safely accommodate your child.

- ✔ Find out if the camp has a nurse on site.

- ✔ Arrange for your child to have a mature counsellor.

- ✔ Meet with the counsellor before the start of camp to make sure he or she has the necessary knowledge to look after your child. In particular, talk about how to deal with hypoglycemia and, especially, how and when to use a glucagon kit.

- ✔ Make sure that your child will receive the necessary snacks (and, of course, meals) at the appropriate times.

- ✔ Send a kit of important supplies with your child to camp. The kit should include glucose monitoring equipment, snacks, a glucagon kit, and, if your child will need to give insulin during the day, necessary insulin supplies.

- ✔ Make sure other staff — such as swim instructors and lifeguards — know that your child has diabetes.

- ✔ Find out if the camp has had other children in the past — or currently — who have had diabetes. If so, consider speaking to their parents to find out if things went well or, if not, why not.

- ✔ Ensure that your child wears a medical alert bracelet.

Your diabetes educator may have experience with regular day camps that have looked after children with diabetes. Give your educator a call and ask.

Your Child Has Type 2 Diabetes

The epidemic of obesity, which has spread to children in Canada (and elsewhere) in the past few decades, has led to a much higher prevalence of type 2 diabetes in children than has ever been seen before. Indeed, up to 25 percent (or, in some communities, considerably more) of children with diabetes have type 2 diabetes. This was virtually unheard of until recently.

The Canadian Diabetes Association recommends screening children, once they reach ten years of age (or younger if they have reached puberty) for type 2 diabetes (with a fasting blood glucose drawn at a laboratory) every two years if they meet two or more of the following criteria:

- Are obese (Obesity for a child is defined as having a body mass index — BMI — at or above the 95th percentile for the child's age and gender. You can find a pediatric BMI calculator at a variety of Web sites including `pediatrics.about.com/cs/usefultools/l/bl_bmi_calc.htm`.)

- Are a member of a high-risk population group (Aboriginal, Hispanic, South Asian, Asian, or African descent) and/or have a family history of type 2 diabetes and/or were exposed to diabetes while they were inside the mother's uterus (that is, the mom had diabetes while pregnant with the child)

- Have evidence of insulin resistance (see Chapter 3), such as having acanthosis nigricans, polycystic ovary syndrome, high blood pressure, abnormal lipids, or excess fat in the liver (NAFLD or non-alcoholic fatty liver disease) (We discuss these conditions in Chapter 6.)

- Have impaired glucose tolerance (see Chapter 4)

- Use certain types of medicines (antipsychotics or atypical neuroleptics) used to treat psychiatric disease

Like children with type 1 diabetes, those with type 2 diabetes may be afraid of being stigmatized and so may neglect the health issue so he or she can be like everyone else when it comes to eating, watching television, and so forth.

The CDA target A1C (refer to Chapter 9) for most children with type 2 diabetes is no greater than 7. The first therapy for a child with type 2 diabetes is intensive lifestyle measures (diet, weight control, exercise), but pills (in particular, metformin; refer to Chapter 12) and insulin (Chapter 13) may be necessary. The metformin or insulin may be withdrawn once the benefits of lifestyle measures have taken effect.

You must help your obese child to lose weight. With the assistance of a dietitian, you can figure out the food that your child can eat to maintain growth and development without inappropriate weight gain. One of the most helpful techniques is to take the child into the supermarket and point out the difference between unhealthy foods (such as those rich in fat) and those that are nourishing. Another is never to use foods such as cake and candy as rewards. Finally, if you keep problem foods out of the house, your child is much less likely to eat them.

If your child with type 2 diabetes becomes unwell, you need to be sure that he or she is drinking enough liquids. Clear liquids (like caffeine-free teas and soft drinks) are usually best. As long as your child can hold down clear liquids, you can generally continue to take care of him or her — unless the blood glucose level is particularly high or your child is very unwell, in which case you will need to seek medical attention. If your child can't keep down even clear fluids — in which case dehydration becomes a real concern — you'll need to visit a hospital.

Your Child Has MODY

An unusual type of childhood diabetes goes by the name *MODY,* which stands for maturity-onset diabetes of the young. This is a genetic condition leading to diabetes that has some features of type 1 diabetes and some features of type 2 diabetes. For example, affected children aren't obese on the one hand, yet aren't prone to ketoacidosis on the other. MODY exists in several forms, and the treatment will depend on which of these types is present.

Although the term *MODY* remains in common use, it is being phased out to be replaced by the names of the specific genetic defects present in the various types (for example, *Chromosome 20, HNF-4alpha* is the new name for *MODY1*). *MODY* may be not be as scientifically precise, but it sure is a heck of a lot easier to say (and remember)!

Chapter 16

Diabetes and the Elderly

• •

In This Chapter
▶ Identifying diabetes in the elderly
▶ Coping with intellectual difficulties
▶ Dealing with dietary considerations
▶ Focusing on eye problems
▶ Addressing urinary and sexual problems
▶ Finding the best methods to control blood glucose

• •

*E*veryone wants to live a long time, but no one wants to get old. Nevertheless, as someone once said, getting old is better than the alternative! Woody Allen says the one advantage of dying is that you don't have to do jury duty. We think we'd rather do jury duty.

Defining *elderly* is the first problem. Although some medical studies have defined elderly as being as young as 60 (egads!), and although every year the definition seems to change, it's probably fair to say that about the age of 70 is the beginning of elderly. Using that definition, more than 20 percent of the Canadian population will be elderly by the year 2020. And one-fifth or more of that group will have developed diabetes.

Elderly people are hospitalized 70 percent more often than the general elderly population. Even without hospitalization, elderly people with diabetes have special problems. In this chapter, we look at those problems and the best ways to handle them.

Recognizing that every person — including every elderly person! — is unique, the Canadian Diabetes Association recommends that "otherwise healthy elderly people with diabetes should be treated to achieve the same (blood glucose), blood pressure and lipid targets as younger people with diabetes." On the other hand, if you are elderly *and* have poor health or limited life expectancy, such stringent targets would be inappropriate.

Bring a second set of ears with you when you see the doctor, pharmacist, diabetes educator, or, for that matter, any other member of your health care team. Diabetes and its management are complex, and having someone else listen in on the conversation will provide you with an additional resource later on.

Diagnosing Diabetes in the Elderly

Like so much else in the world of medicine, there is both debate and uncertainty (perhaps the one never exists without the other) about why diabetes becomes increasingly likely as we get older. Some experts have suggested that aging itself leads to diabetes, but the main factor that causes diabetes may not be the number of years people have under their belts but rather the number of inches under their belts. That, of course, is a very encouraging piece of news because it means that if you can keep your weight under control as you get older, you can help to protect yourself from developing diabetes.

Depending on their mental functioning, elderly people who have developed hyperglycemia may or may not recognize the onset of typical symptoms such as increased urination and greater thirst. Instead, their main symptoms may be loss of appetite, weight loss, confusion, incontinence of urine, or weakness and lethargy. Because symptoms like weakness and lethargy are so nonspecific, the cause can initially go unrecognized. And a doctor or patient may easily (and understandably) attribute urinary incontinence to prostate problems in elderly men or bladder problems in older women. (We have yet to see an elderly woman diagnosed as having an enlarged prostate!)

Evaluating Intellectual Functioning

Knowing the intellectual functioning of an elderly person with diabetes is extremely important because managing the disease requires a number of different skills. The patient has to follow a special diet, administer medications properly, and test the blood glucose. Studies have shown that elderly people with diabetes, for uncertain reasons, have a higher incidence of dementia (loss of mental functioning) than people without diabetes, making it much harder for them to perform those tasks. (We discuss this further in Chapter 6.)

If necessary, a physician can formally assess an elderly person's mental functioning by administering certain types of tests. When required, psychologists can conduct even more sophisticated testing. Testing makes it easier to tell whether the patient can be self-sufficient or will need help. Some people now living alone with no assistance are a danger to themselves and would benefit from an assisted-living situation. Elderly people are often fiercely independent and — as millions of members of the "sandwich" generation know — changing their living situation can be very difficult.

Dealing with Eye Problems

Elderly people with diabetes are more prone to eye problems that people without diabetes can also get, including cataracts, macular degeneration, and glaucoma. And they also are at risk of eye disease unique to diabetes: diabetic retinopathy. (See Chapter 6 for more information on these eye problems.)

Many elderly people don't receive the eye care they require. Everyone with diabetes — especially the elderly, who can have a whole variety of different eye problems — must see an eye specialist routinely. Removal of a cataract — a simple outpatient procedure nowadays — may make all the difference in the world.

Coping with Urinary and Sexual Problems

Urinary and sexual problems are very common in elderly people with diabetes and greatly affect quality of life. An older person with diabetes may have weakness of the bladder muscle involving retention of urine, followed by overflow incontinence when the bladder fills up. An older person may be unable to get to the bathroom fast enough. A chronically distended bladder can also lead to frequent urinary tract infections.

Almost 60 percent of men over the age of 70 have erectile dysfunction, and 50 percent have no libido (desire to have sex). The elderly take an average of seven medications daily, some of which may affect sexual function. Many elderly women with diabetes also experience sexual dysfunction. The causes for sexual dysfunction in both men and women are discussed in Chapter 7.

To have sex at any age, you need sexual desire and the physical ability to perform, you need a willing partner, and you need a safe, private place. For the elderly, any or all of these may be missing.

Treating sexual dysfunction isn't always necessary if you and your partner are okay with the situation as it is. If not, however, a number of effective therapies are available (see Chapter 7).

Regrettably, elderly people are sometimes seen as asexual — even by members of the medical profession who should know better. For this reason you may have to take the initiative and bring up the issue of your sexual difficulties when you visit your physician.

Considering Treatment for High Blood Glucose

Goals for a very elderly, debilitated person with diabetes and a short life expectancy will be different from those of a person with diabetes who is elderly but physiologically strong and could live for 15 or 20 more years. A person who has lived to age 65 has a life expectancy of at least 18 more years — plenty of time to develop complications of diabetes.

In a broad sense, blood glucose control in an elderly person has two main objectives. You can aim

- To maintain blood glucose levels in a range that will keep you free of symptoms of hyperglycemia (under 10 mmol/L or so). This is an appropriate target in an elderly person with a limited life expectancy and for whom any undue restrictions are inappropriate and, indeed, perhaps even cruel.

- For blood glucose levels that will minimize your risk of developing complications (4 to 7 mmol/L before meals; 5 to 10 mmol/L two hours after meals; see Chapter 9). This target is appropriate if life expectancy and life quality are good.

Every elderly person with diabetes can treat his or her blood glucose control successfully (even if not easily).

As important as good blood glucose control is, other essential aspects of your diabetes management must get the attention they deserve. When you're seeing your health care providers to review your diabetes management, make sure that you discuss your blood pressure and your lipids. We look at these issues in Chapter 6.

Nutrition therapy

Healthy nutrition is a cornerstone of good diabetes care for the elderly just as it is in the younger population.

In addition to the intellectual function required to understand and prepare proper meals, the elderly may have other problems when it comes to eating healthfully:

- ✔ They may have poor vision and be unable to see to read or cook.
- ✔ Their ability to taste and smell may be decreased, so they lose interest in food.
- ✔ They often have a loss of appetite, especially if they live alone after the loss of a spouse or if they're depressed.
- ✔ They may have arthritis that makes cooking more difficult.
- ✔ They may have poor teeth or a dry mouth, either of which make eating more difficult.
- ✔ They may have low income and be unable to purchase the foods that they require.

Any one of these problems may be enough to prevent proper eating, and as a result, nutrition and, ultimately, the general health of an elderly person are at risk.

As we say throughout this book, even when obstacles to good diabetes management are present, they're never insurmountable. If you're facing some of the hurdles mentioned in the above list and are unsure how to deal with them, we recommend you arrange a visit with the dietitian.

Because nutrition is often not sufficiently robust or complete in elderly individuals, unless you're sure you're eating very well (see Chapter 10), taking a daily multivitamin would be a good idea.

Exercise therapy

An elderly person who can exercise will derive many benefits from it, including improved blood glucose control, better blood pressure and lipids, and, importantly, a better sense of well-being. Because elderly patients have more coronary artery disease, arthritis, eye disease, neuropathy, and peripheral vascular disease, for some individuals exercise may not be possible or, at the least, may need to be very limited. Nonetheless, even if an elderly patient can't walk at all, he or she may still be able to do resistance exercises while sitting in a chair. (See Chapter 11 for more on exercise.)

Medication therapy

If lifestyle therapy with diet and exercise isn't controlling blood glucose levels, then oral hypoglycemic agents (see Chapter 12) or insulin (see Chapter 13) becomes necessary. Taking these medications is complicated by a number of considerations special to the elderly:

- The person may not be able to read the prescription label or dose to be dialed up on an insulin pen device.
- The person may be mentally unable to take the medicine properly.
- Physical limitations may prevent the person from taking medication, especially insulin.
- Older people often have decreased kidney function, making some drugs last longer or build up to excessive levels.
- Poor nutrition may make the person more prone to hypoglycemia.

For all these reasons, your physician must take great care in selecting the appropriate types and doses of your medicines. Also, your pharmacist will need to spend the extra required time to sit down with you and review your medications and how to take them.

When it comes to selecting the best medicine to reduce blood glucose levels for an elderly person, a variety of choices exist:

- For most people with type 2 diabetes — including elderly individuals — metformin is a good choice unless you have poor kidney function. (This is determined by a blood test.) Metformin does not cause hypoglycemia, which makes it particularly well suited to people at risk for this. We discuss metformin and the other medicines mentioned in this list in detail in Chapter 12.
- Sulfonylureas need to be used cautiously as they can cause hypoglycemia. If a sulfonylurea is used, it should be started with a low dose and the dose should be slowly increased. The preferred sulfonylureas are gliclazide and glimepiride — rather than glyburide — because they are less likely to cause low blood glucose.
- TZDs (Actos, Avandia) are helpful, but, because they can cause heart failure, need to be used cautiously and only if you have normal heart function.
- If you have irregular eating habits, a good choice is an oral hypoglycemic agent like GlucoNorm (repaglinide) that is taken only with meals and is short-acting and so isn't as likely to cause hypoglycemia as some longer-acting oral agents like glyburide.

> ✔ Insulin is often a very good choice. If insulin is used, the same basic principles apply to the elderly as they do to younger individuals. We discuss these in detail in Chapter 9.

A seven-day pill dispenser (organizer) is an invaluable tool for people who are taking a number of different medicines. We recommend you ask your pharmacist to prepare your medicines for you in these containers. Ian and Heather McDonald-Blumer discuss this and other related topics regarding safe and effective use of medications in *Understanding Prescription Drugs For Canadians For Dummies* (Wiley).

Before you leave the doctor's office, discuss your medicines with your doctor and, in particular, determine what side effects might occur. Having a similar discussion with your pharmacist is also wise.

Chapter 17

Diabetes in Aboriginal Peoples

· ·

In This Chapter

▶ Investigating the growing problem of diabetes in Aboriginal peoples

▶ Screening for diabetes in Aboriginal peoples

▶ Combatting diabetes in Aboriginal peoples

· ·

*A*boriginal peoples in Canada include First Nations, Inuit, and Métis populations. Although type 2 diabetes has become increasingly prevalent in all communities across Canada, the problem has reached truly epidemic proportions among Aboriginal peoples, with rates in some age groups as high as one out of every four people. Aboriginal leaders are tackling the challenge head-on, however, by developing and implementing strategies to deal with it. This chapter looks at the main elements of the problem and some of the solutions that Aboriginal leaders are pursuing.

Exploring Why Aboriginal Peoples Are More Prone to Diabetes

No one knows definitively why certain groups of people are more prone to develop diabetes, but that they are more prone isn't in question. Aboriginal communities throughout the world have been beset with rapidly rising rates of diabetes. Whether in Australia, South America, North America, or elsewhere, the trend has been the same. Given the widespread nature of the problem, clearly there must be a common thread. The leading proposal is what's termed the *thrifty gene hypothesis.*

As we discuss in Chapter 4, the thrifty gene hypothesis maintains that over the course of many generations, peoples that have lived without a consistent food supply may have genetically evolved a protective mechanism that enables them to use carbohydrates in a very efficient way metabolically. Thus, when food is scarce, they are protected. The unfortunate flip side to this is that when food is plentiful, their bodies end up readily storing the extra calories as fat, which, in turn, increases their risk of developing diabetes. Adding to the problem is that the Aboriginal diet has changed to one high in calories and saturated fat, and that, like their fellow Canadians, Aboriginal peoples have become much more sedentary. Obesity rates have progressively risen, and in some communities almost 50 percent of children are now obese.

Considering the Extent of the Problem

An estimated 12 percent of First Nations peoples living on reserves have diabetes, and 25 percent of those over the age of 45 are affected. These rates are far above those of the Canadian population as a whole (which has an average rate of 7.5 percent or so) and it is thought that the prevalence is going to increase further.

Inuit people actually have prevalence rates that are below average for the Canadian population, though even in this group, the number of people with diabetes is increasing.

Not only are diabetes prevalence rates high, but also there is evidence that the risk of the following complications (see Chapter 6) is greater amongst Aboriginal peoples:

- Coronary artery disease (heart disease)
- Diabetic retinopathy
- High blood pressure
- Kidney disease
- Peripheral vascular disease

A number of factors compound the combined one-two punch of greater risk of diabetes and greater risk of complications:

- Earlier age at onset
- Delay until a diagnosis is made
- Less access to diabetes education (Diabetes education is essential in helping you keep yourself healthy, yet less than 40 percent of First Nations with diabetes attend diabetes clinics.)
- Less access to other, important health care services such as dialysis (In some cases this necessitates travelling long distances to receive appropriate treatment and can require moving the entire family.)

Aboriginal children and adolescents are affected by type 2 diabetes at rates substantially greater than their non-Aboriginal counterparts. Also, Aboriginal women are more than twice as likely as non-Aboriginal women to develop gestational diabetes (see Chapter 7).

Screening for Diabetes for Aboriginal Peoples

Because of the high prevalence and early onset of diabetes in Aboriginal peoples, the Canadian Diabetes Association recommends early and frequent diabetes screening if one or more additional risk factors (we list these on the Cheat Sheet at the front of this book) are present. In this circumstance, the CDA recommends the following screening schedule:

- **For adults:** A fasting blood glucose test should be done every one to two years. (For adults with prediabetes, the CDA instead recommends a yearly glucose tolerance test; we discuss prediabetes and this test in Chapter 4.)

- **For children:** A fasting blood glucose test should be done every two years beginning at the age of 10 or puberty. (For children who are very obese, the CDA instead recommends a yearly glucose tolerance test.)

Looking at How Aboriginal Peoples Are Combatting the Problem

Having recognized the extent and severity of the problem, Aboriginal communities are now tackling the problem on a number of fronts. Among initiatives in place in some regions are the following:

- Teaching diabetes prevention programs in elementary schools

- Organizing field trips to the local grocery store to teach about food selection

- Introducing programs to increase physical fitness (For example, the Sandy Lake community in northern Ontario has built a well-used and highly successful 6.5-kilometre (4.5-mile) walking trail. See the sidebar.)

- Establishing health services programs geared specifically toward Aboriginal health issues and concerns

- Banning junk food from schools

- Getting local stores to promote healthy foods over snack foods

Clearly, non-Aboriginal communities would be well served by following the lead set by these Aboriginal communities and adopting similar healthy-living strategies.

The Sandy Lake Health and Diabetes Project

Sandy Lake, Ontario, has one of the highest rates of diabetes in the country, but the community is in the forefront in the battle to fight the problem. Deputy Chief Harry Meekis said in an interview with the *Toronto Star* in April 2000, "We did it for the children. We want to be known, not just as the community with the third highest diabetes rate, but as the community that did something about it." They set up the Sandy Lake Health and Diabetes Project (www.sandylake diabetes.com), a multi-faceted program aimed at preventing diabetes. Components include classroom teaching on healthy eating and physical exercise, regular discussions on the radio, a cooking club, and the promotion of healthy foods in local stores. As a result of this project, the community is stemming the rate of the rise of diabetes.

Aboriginal people living in larger urban areas can contact Native Friendship Centres (www.nafc-aboriginal.com), which can provide helpful advice regarding available treatment resources.

Chapter 18

Special Circumstances: Employment, Insurance, Safe Driving and Piloting, and Preparing for Disaster

. . . .

In This Chapter

▶ Dealing with the workplace

▶ Discovering insurance options

▶ Driving safely

▶ Piloting when you having diabetes

▶ Preparing for when disaster strikes

. . . .

After he found his very first job, one of Alan's young patients wrote to his mother, "Dear Mom, I'm working, even though my pancreas isn't."

And speaking of work, many of us drive to our place of employment; that is, when we're not driving our kids to hockey, soccer, or dance or having our kids drive *us* to distraction! Most of us, as adults, also require insurance, and this too can pose its own set of issues.

In this chapter we look at the challenges of employment, driving, piloting, and insurance as they pertain to diabetes. We also look at how you can prepare yourself if a disaster — natural or otherwise — should strike.

Employing Both You and Your Rights

As a person with diabetes, you may run into various forms of discrimination when you try to get a job. As you can imagine, there are a number of reasons for this. Part of it is a seldom-justified concern on the part of prospective employers regarding the safety of having a person with diabetes working for them. Part of it has to do with their lack of understanding the great strides that have been made in diabetes care, which mean that a person with diabetes often has a better record of coming to work than a person without diabetes. Like virtually all aspects of discrimination in society, discrimination against people with diabetes is based on ignorance.

Fighting for your rights

Canadians with diabetes have protections that citizens of other countries often do not. Section 15.1 of the Canadian Charter of Rights and Freedoms states:

> *Every individual is equal before and under the law and has the right to the equal protection and equal benefit of the law without discrimination and, in particular, without discrimination based on race, national or ethnic origin, colour, religion, sex, age or mental or physical disability.*

Although considering diabetes as being a disability isn't appealing, this designation does give you certain legal protections under the Charter.

Ian recently chatted with the mother of a 10-year-old boy with type 1 diabetes. An active, outgoing, athletic, and bright child, he had just read in a newspaper story that diabetes was a disability. He brought the article over to his mother and asked, "Mom, what's a disability?" His mother was speechless. Looking at her "I can do anything" child, she could only smile in wonder.

Other groups and organizations actively campaign for your rights, including the Canadian Medical Association, which has an official policy position that "previous blanket discrimination in the workplace . . . should now be replaced with a case-by-case review."

The Canadian Diabetes Association's position statement states that

- A person with diabetes should be eligible for employment in any occupation for which he or she is individually qualified.

- A person with diabetes has the right to be assessed for specific job duties on his or her own merits based on reasonable standards applied consistently.

> ✔ Employers have the duty to accommodate employees with diabetes unless the employer can show it to cause undue hardship to the organization.

Employers cannot say that *any* cost they incur is an undue hardship. This provision is not meant to be used as an excuse to avoid hiring people with diabetes. As you know, most people with diabetes — including yourself — require minimal accommodation on the part of their employer. Usually all that's necessary is the allowance of a few extra minutes per day for blood glucose testing and the taking of medicines, as well as appropriate breaks for snacks and meals.

When you're going for a job interview, you don't have to inform your prospective employer that you have diabetes, or, for that matter, tell him or her anything else about your health unless the health issues are directly related to a specific job requirement or you are applying for a "safety-sensitive" position such as working as a police officer or firefighter (see the next section). As well, after you're hired, you don't need to provide medical information unless your employer needs to know certain things in order to make appropriate accommodation to your specific needs.

The Canadian Human Rights Commission document, *A Place for All: A Guide to Creating an Inclusive Workplace* (`www.chrc-ccdp.ca/pdf/chrc_place_ for_all.pdf`), is designed to assist both employers and employees in understanding their legal rights and responsibilities in setting up an accommodating workplace.

Affecting your ability to work

In part because of the now established rights that people with diabetes have achieved, there are virtually no organizations that will issue an outright ban on hiring you just because you have diabetes. People with diabetes work just about anywhere and everywhere. And they function as effectively and efficiently as anybody else. Of course!

As we mention in the previous section, however, there are some (not many, mind you, but some) exceptions to your usual employment rights. If you're applying for a safety-sensitive position (such as firefighting or police work), the inherent unpredictability of these jobs (are fires or robberies ever predictable?) may work against your being hired. Nonetheless, no blanket or uniform policy across Canada exists, and each fire department and police force determines its own hiring practices.

We have many police officers, firefighters, and paramedics among our patients; however, most of these individuals were diagnosed after they had been hired. Would they have been hired anyway? Impossible to know. Will diabetes potentially jeopardize their jobs? That too is impossible to answer, although our personal observation is that a shift in job description is not unusual (for example, a firefighter being moved to a supervisory role).

In the end, the following factors, among others, may influence your ability to obtain and retain a safety-sensitive job:

- The policies of a given force
- Whether a force has set earlier precedents
- How knowledgeable and comfortable the health staff and administrators are about diabetes
- How well controlled your blood glucose levels are and, in particular, how often you have hypoglycemia (especially, severe hypoglycemia) and what your general state of health is
- How able you are to perform the required tasks

The last two items on this list seem far and away the most important to us. Each person is different. And that includes each person with diabetes.

If having hypoglycemia is, potentially, especially hazardous for your particular line of work, we strongly recommend you look at getting a continuous glucose monitoring system (CGMS). We discuss continuous glucose monitoring in detail in Chapter 9.

The Canadian Forces have the wise policy of making decisions on a case-by-case basis, which of course is as it should be. Their general policy, however, is that

- If you already have diabetes when you apply for a position with the Canadian Forces, they're unlikely to hire you.
- If you develop type 2 diabetes after you're already enrolled, you'll likely be "retained without career restrictions."
- If you develop type 1 diabetes after you are already enrolled, you'll "normally be released" or you "may be accommodated for a 3 year period, then released."

The most important point is that, with a few exceptions such as those described above, there is almost nothing you cannot do if you have diabetes. You can climb mountains — in both the literal and the figurative senses. And when it comes to employment, there are almost no jobs in Canada that you cannot both obtain and perform.

Exploring your avenues of recourse

If you feel you've been discriminated against, because of your diabetes, regarding employment or prospective employment, you have several avenues of recourse:

✔ If discrimination occurs in federal jurisdiction, you can file a human rights complaint with the Canadian Human Rights Commission. Information on this is available on their Web site (www.chrc-ccdp.ca).

✔ If discrimination occurs outside of federal jurisdiction, you can file a complaint with the human rights commission in the appropriate province or territory.

✔ The Canadian Diabetes Association (CDA) has a National Advocacy Council, composed of both volunteers and staff, mandated primarily to "act on broad policy matters which can have a positive impact for many people affected by diabetes." The Council "offers advice and guidance," but in general is looking at the "big picture," and unless your concern has national implications, given their limited resources, they may not be able to take on your particular case. If you have a concern you want addressed, start by contacting your local CDA branch and go from there.

Sometimes you can rectify a situation resulting from discrimination by lifting the veil of ignorance from your employer's eyes. You may find the quickest remedy to your concerns is to educate your employer. If you don't have success with your own efforts at teaching them about diabetes, you may wish to refer them to the CDA document *Diabetes in the Workplace: A Guide for Employers and Employees* (www.diabetes.ca/about-us/what/position-statements/discrimination/workplace).

Insuring Your Health

Most of this book is about doing your best to insure your good health. As hard as that can seem at times, obtaining the other type of insurance you may want is often the harder of the two.

Thankfully, Canadians have a publicly funded, universal health care program, so fundamental health care will be available to you regardless of your income. When it comes to life, disability, and travel insurance, things get more difficult. The protections offered to you by human rights laws that we talk about earlier in this chapter don't apply in the same way when it comes to insurance policies. Indeed, when you're applying for insurance, you can expect to be asked if you have diabetes, and you must tell the truth; otherwise, any policy you are granted may be subject to revocation or non-payment of benefits.

The Canadian Diabetes Association has partnered with Ingle International and Imagine Financial to make it easier for you to get insurance. You can find out more about the various available insurance offerings at www.diabetes.ca/about-diabetes/living/guidelines/insurance. A very helpful FAQ (Frequently Asked Questions) resource is available at www.diabetes.ca/files/FAQ-CDA.pdf.

Life insurance

Having diabetes does not automatically exclude you from obtaining life insurance, though it does make it more difficult. Of course, if you develop diabetes while you're already covered, you'll have an easier time than if you're applying for insurance (or an increase in your coverage) after you have been diagnosed (what insurance companies refer to as having a "pre-existing condition").

Insurance companies make their determination about your insurability on a case-by-case basis, meaning that they'll look at you as an individual and make their decision on more than the simple fact of your having diabetes. They'll look at what kind of therapy you're receiving, what kind of glucose control you have, whether you have complications from your diabetes, and so forth.

If you are approved for a policy, you'll likely find that your premiums are higher, for the same level of benefits, than those of a person without diabetes.

If you look after your health well, you may live longer (and be healthier) than a person without diabetes who doesn't look after him- or herself well. Hopefully, insurance companies will take into account all the rapidly accumulating data about how healthy people with diabetes can be. Can you imagine the surprise if insurance companies were ever to charge people with diabetes less than others because of their good habits?

Bear in mind that different insurance companies have different policies (so to speak), so if one place turns you down, try somewhere else. Another thing you can do is to go through a licensed insurance broker who can act on your behalf, deal with multiple insurers, and try to help you obtain an appropriate policy.

Disability insurance

Unless you had disability insurance before you were diagnosed as having diabetes, you will likely find it difficult (though not impossible) to find an insurance company that will offer you a policy. If you are otherwise in excellent health, your odds of successfully finding an insurer will be, as you might imagine, far greater.

Travel insurance

Travel insurance is much easier to obtain than disability insurance; however, you will need to carefully scrutinize any policy you are offered to see what is excluded from coverage. You may find that if you become ill with a diabetes-related condition, you won't be covered.

Driving When You Have Diabetes

Few adults in Canada get by without ever having to drive somewhere. (And of course if you are a teenager you have to drive *everywhere!*) We're so dependent on our cars to get us to work or the movies, grocery shopping or the hardware store, doctors' appointments or dentists' appointments, that for most people, losing their licence is not just inconvenient, it can be down-right devastating. In this section we take a look at the measures you can take to help preserve your licence, and, if you have lost it, what steps you can take to regain it.

ANECDOTE

A collision with hypoglycemia

The moment Juan entered Ian's office, Ian knew something was very wrong. For one thing, the usually easygoing teacher was visibly anxious and upset. For another, he was followed into the room by his wife — someone who had never come to a previous appointment. "What's the matter?" Ian asked.

"I could've killed someone," Juan replied. "You could've killed yourself," his wife quickly added. Juan went on to explain that, the day before, he had overslept. He took his rapid-acting breakfast-time insulin, but as he then sat down to eat, realized he was going to be late for work, so he tossed his barely eaten bagel in his briefcase, tossed the briefcase in the trunk of his car, and started driving to work.

He never made it. En route to work he developed severe hypoglycemia, crashed his car, and the next thing he knew he was in the emergency department of the local hospital. Fortunately he had not injured himself (or anyone else). After receiving some intravenous glucose he was quickly back to his normal self, but as Juan was about to leave the ER, the doctor advised him not to drive.

The doctor also told him that he had a legal obligation (see the sidebar "Your physician's duty to report") to notify the Ministry of Transportation of the event and that in all likelihood the ministry would suspend Juan's license. Juan was understandably devastated. Juan did, indeed, lose his licence, but, following the advice in this chapter, eventually regained it and learnt how to protect himself from ever having another disastrous episode of severe hypoglycemia whilst driving.

Determining if you're medically fit to drive

To most people it would seem self-evident that if you have diabetes you would be at much higher risk of having a car accident. Of course, at one time it was self-evident to most people that the world was flat, too. The truth of the matter is that medical studies do not show convincing evidence that having diabetes increases your risk; in fact, one study even showed that people with type 1 diabetes had a lower risk than drivers without diabetes who were under the age of 30. How about that! Nonetheless, provincial and territorial bodies have the important and appropriate task of ensuring that drivers are safe to operate motor vehicles, so you may have to overcome a number of hurdles.

Your ability to obtain and retain a licence will depend on a number of factors, including the means by which your diabetes is being treated. This section looks at those issues specific to your diabetes (of course, non-diabetes factors may also affect your fitness to drive). The recommendations in this section are based on those established by the Canadian Diabetes Association (www.diabetes.ca/about-diabetes/living/guidelines/commercial-driving). Note that these are recommendations, not legally binding rules or regulations.

Taking necessary precautions

The CDA recommendations include the following for *all* drivers with diabetes:

- Have your fitness to drive assessed based on your personal situation (that is, the decision about your suitability to drive should be made on a case-by-case basis).

- Have a periodic medical examination that pays special attention to whether you have any serious complications from your diabetes.

- Test your blood glucose level routinely and keep a log of your results.

- Ensure that you are up-to-date on how to avoid hypoglycemia and how to treat it if it occurs.

- Measure your blood glucose level immediately before and at least every four hours during long drives. If you have hypoglycemia unawareness (see Chapter 5) you should test more often. (We recommend testing hourly, even though that may seem like quite a hassle; trust us, it would be much more of a hassle if you got into an accident because of hypoglycemia.)

- Always have your hypoglycemia treatment nearby. (The trunk of your car isn't nearby!)

- Don't drive if your blood glucose level is less than 4 mmol/L. If your level is between 4.0 and 5.0, ingest some carbohydrate before you resume driving. (If you are a commercial driver, you should never drive if your blood glucose level is less than 6.0 mmol/L.)

x.

✔ Don't resume driving until at least 45 minutes have passed since you treated an episode of hypoglycemia.

Pull off the road and stop in a safe area if you think you may be hypoglycemic. Don't keep driving!

Applying for a commercial licence

As you might imagine, obtaining and maintaining a professional driver's licence is much trickier if you have diabetes, especially if you're taking insulin therapy. Nonetheless, your suitability to drive should be judged on a case-by-case basis, and indeed, licensing bodies increasingly recognize this, we're pleased to say.

When you first apply for a commercial licence, the appropriate government body will review your request and base its decisions on many different factors, including, importantly, your blood glucose control (especially whether or not you're having problems with hypoglycemia) and whether you have complications from your diabetes.

This section discusses commercial licence issues *in Canada*. As licensing requirements differ in the United States, if you will be driving a commercial vehicle into the U.S., we recommend you first look into their specific requirements, rules, and regulations.

CDA recommendations for commercial licence requirements

To assist both governments and individuals with diabetes, the CDA has developed recommendations. Like the CDA recommendations in the preceding section, these aren't legally binding rules or regulations. If you want to apply for a commercial licence, you should contact the appropriate licensing body to see what their specific requirements are, but it's a safe bet that they'll want you to do — as a minimum — the following things as suggested by the CDA:

✔ Complete a questionnaire that pays particular attention to both your risk of having hypoglycemia and how often you may have been experiencing hypoglycemia. (You can get a sample questionnaire from the CDA.)

✔ Have your diabetes specialist perform a full assessment of your health status.

✔ Have a full eye exam performed by your eye specialist.

✔ Obtain documentation from your diabetes education centre proving that you have attended their program.

✔ Have a recent A1C result.

✔ Have a record of your blood glucose measurements (taken at least twice daily) dating back six months (or less, of course, if you were diagnosed less than six months ago).

The licensing body will likely be more impressed with a downloaded log from your glucose meter than a handwritten record.

CDA exclusion criteria for maintenance of a commercial licence

The Canadian Diabetes Association's exclusion criteria (that is, those things that, if present, would prevent you from holding a commercial licence) include your having

✔ An episode of severe hypoglycemia within the past six months

✔ Ongoing hypoglycemia unawareness (see Chapter 5)

✔ Poorly controlled blood glucose levels (hyperglycemia or hypoglycemia)

✔ The recent introduction of insulin or, if you're already on insulin, a change in your type of insulin or the frequency that you give it

✔ Significant visual impairment

✔ Peripheral neuropathy or cardiovascular disease (see Chapter 6) that's severe enough that it could affect your ability to drive

✔ Inadequate frequency of blood glucose monitoring

✔ Inadequate knowledge of the causes, symptoms, and treatment of hypoglycemia (Don't worry, we have yet to see this determined by a quiz or essay! It's an impression that your health care providers would make based on your discussions. It is essential that you — and anyone with diabetes — know all about hypoglycemia anyway. If you don't, read Chapter 5 and, in addition, be sure to ask your health care team to review this crucial subject with you.)

Keeping your driver's licence

If you have diabetes and lose your licence, the most likely reason would be that you had an episode of hypoglycemia while you were driving that led either to a collision or to your being pulled over by police because of erratic driving. (This, of course, is one of the most important reasons for you to wear a medical alert, so that those who come to your aid can quickly recognize that you have diabetes and that you are not simply intoxicated.) Hypoglycemia bad enough to lead to this situation is usually only seen if you're treated with insulin (rather than oral hypoglycemic agents) and is much more likely to occur if you have type 1 diabetes.

Many things about having diabetes are unfair, but perhaps least fair of all is that the better your glucose control is, the more prone to hypoglycemia you'll be. Nonetheless, that's a fact of diabetes life and you have to work around it to protect you and your licence. Fortunately, most of the time you can avoid episodes of severe hypoglycemia while driving by taking a few relatively simple steps. (We list the measures recommended by the CDA earlier in this section.)

In our experience, these are the two most important measures you can undertake to avoid losing your licence:

- ✔ Never drive your vehicle unless you have checked your blood glucose level immediately before you're about to drive, to ensure that it's not low.

- ✔ Check your blood glucose levels very frequently. It may be a hassle to keep interrupting your driving, but if you test every hour, you substantially reduce your likelihood of running into problems. You would readily determine if your levels were dropping and could equally readily deal with it before it got out of hand. Of course there are exceptions, and your level could drop quickly even if you checked half an hour before, but for the majority of people, hourly testing is a good protective manoeuvre.

When you're driving, never assume your blood glucose levels are normal just because you do not feel low. You must test to be sure. And never say to yourself, "Oh, I think I might be getting low; if I start to feel worse I'll pull off the road." If you think your levels are low, get off the road immediately! Your licence may depend on it. More importantly, your life (and the lives of others) may depend on it.

Regaining your driver's licence

Though each area of the country has its own policies, if you lose your licence because of an incident that occurred when you were hypoglycemic, in our experience the following are the two most important things the licensing body will look for in considering your request for reinstatement of your licence:

Your physician's duty to report

Physicians are trained always to look out for the best interests of their patients. And that is as it should be. Physicians are also bound — quite rightly — by rules of confidentiality. There are, however, exceptions to the way that physicians normally practise. Indeed, in most areas of Canada it is the law that doctors have to report (to the appropriate licensing body) a patient that the physician feels is unsafe to operate a motor vehicle. This is a terribly difficult position for physicians to be in, as the person being reported is invariably and understandably very upset. Even worse, it's often emergency room physicians who have to make this report, and they don't have the benefit of a previous relationship with the patient. Reporting patients is one of the most difficult and unpleasant tasks that doctors face.

✔ Evidence of satisfactory blood glucose control as reflected by a carefully kept and accurate log of your readings for the preceding few months, with this record revealing an absence of frequent or severe hypoglycemia. (***Note:*** Hyperglycemia is not as dangerous when it comes to the safety of your driving.)

✔ A letter from your diabetes specialist or a copy of your diabetes specialist's records that reflect your ongoing co-involvement in your management (remember, you're a part of your health care team; see Chapter 8) and your adherence to therapy.

Flying High with Diabetes

Certainly one of the most remarkable examples of how prejudices are diminishing when it comes to diabetes is the fairly recent change in the rules governing the suitability of pilots to maintain a licence after they develop diabetes. These changes, however, have not come easily or quickly, as Stephen Steele's story (see the sidebar, "Regaining his wings") demonstrates.

Your success in being allowed to pilot an aircraft will depend on a number of factors, including your blood glucose control and the nature of your diabetes therapy. We discuss these issues in the following sections.

Piloting with non-insulin treated diabetes

Although the Aviation Medicine Review Board now decides each individual's case on its own merits, Transport Canada Civil Aviation guidelines (www.tc.gc.ca/CivilAviation/Cam/TP13312-2/diabetes/menu.htm) include statements to the effect that

✔ If you're able to control your blood glucose levels with diet alone, you may be considered fit to have a licence so long as you don't have other, serious health problems that could interfere with your ability to perform your duties.

✔ If you require oral hypoglycemic agents to control your blood glucose levels, you may be considered for medical certification as long as

• You have not experienced any recent severe hypoglycemia.

• Your oral agent has not recently changed in type or dose.

• You have stable blood glucose control.

• You don't have any serious complications from diabetes.

ANECDOTE

Regaining his wings

Stephen Steele vividly remembers the day back in May 1986 when his life turned upside down. At the time he was a successful pilot with a major Canadian airline with over 14 years of safe flying under his belt. Then, in the spring of 1986, he recognized worrisome symptoms and was soon diagnosed as having type 1 diabetes. His career instantly evaporated as he was immediately and permanently grounded from flying. No country in the world would permit a person with insulin-treated diabetes to pilot an aircraft. Stephen's career was over.

Or was it?

In 1992, Transport Canada's Civil Aviation Medicine Branch initiated a review of the implications of diabetes on piloting in the context of modern diabetes therapy. The branch created new guidelines wherein people with insulin-treated diabetes could be considered for medical certification based on their individual situation. This gave new hope to Stephen and he set his sights on regaining the pilot's seat he had been forced to relinquish. Driven by passion and conviction, he poured his energies into upgrading his skills to meet the needs of contemporary aircraft, all the while paying meticulous attention to his health. This was no flight of fancy; this was a mission.

Stephen did everything within his power to rule his diabetes. He monitored his blood glucose readings numerous times per day, he exercised regularly, he avoided in his diet those things that could unfavourably affect his blood glucose control, and he made it a practice to adjust his insulin to suit his needs.

After 15 long years, in November 2001, Stephen Steele regained his Airline Transport pilot's certification. His unfailing efforts had finally paid off in what was both a personal victory and a victory for all people with diabetes.

Piloting with insulin-treated diabetes

Each individual's case will be treated on its own merits; however, the most important element in determining your ability to pilot an aircraft is whether you meet Transport Canada's definition of "low risk" for hypoglycemia. Low-risk criteria include the following:

- ✔ No history of severe hypoglycemia
- ✔ Stable blood glucose control
- ✔ No problems with hypoglycemia unawareness

Because hypoglycemia is the single greatest concern for pilots with diabetes, pilots must maintain higher blood glucose levels than is generally considered best in terms of preventing long-term damage to the body. As such, the pilot with insulin-treated diabetes is obliged to make the uncomfortable trade-off between optimal blood glucose control and job preservation.

Preparing for When Disaster Strikes

Of all the horrors (and there were so many) associated with Hurricane Katrina, one we found particularly gut-wrenching was the story of people with diabetes who risked death because they had run out of insulin and, isolated in their flood-ravaged homes, were unable to obtain more. In Canada we may not be at high risk of a hurricane (although Juan's — and, more remotely, Hazel's — devastating legacy does live on), but we do have more than passing familiarity with extended power outages, tornadoes, and, of course, blizzards. These and other forms of disaster require that you, as a person with diabetes, take special precautions to protect yourself in the event of a calamity.

These are the things you should have on hand so that you're prepared if disaster strikes:

- ✔ An up-to-date list of all your health conditions and all the medicines — including the doses — you're taking. (During a disaster your health records — including your doctor's files and your pharmacist's data — may be unavailable.)

- ✔ At least a few days' supply of non-perishable, diabetes-friendly foods.

- ✔ At least a three-day supply of bottled water.

- ✔ A source of carbohydrate to treat hypoglycemia. (Refer to Chapter 5.)

- ✔ At least a two to four weeks' supply of your diabetes medications (including your oral hypoglycemic agents and insulin) and testing supplies (including lancets, test strips, a meter — or even two — and an extra battery). This means making sure you have these extra quantities of these essential items with you as, for example, you head up to the cottage for that winter getaway in snow country.

- ✔ An insulated container for storing your insulin to keep it from being exposed to temperature extremes.

- ✔ A glucagon emergency kit (if you're taking a medicine — such as glyburide or insulin — that can cause hypoglycemia). (For more about glucagon, refer to Chapter 5.)

- ✔ A first-aid kit that contains bandages, dressings, and topical medications (such as an antibiotic cream or ointment) to treat cuts, abrasions, and so on.

In a disaster, you should never walk barefoot (as is the case in all circumstances anyhow).

Part V
The Part of Tens

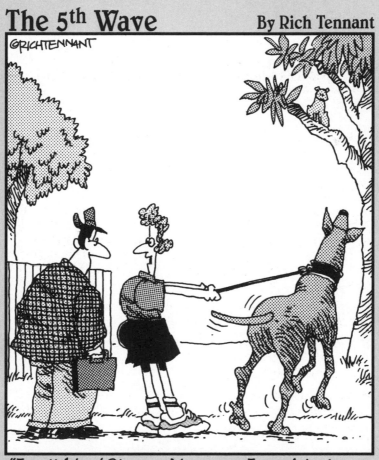

The 5th Wave   By Rich Tennant

GRICHTENNANT

"I call him 'Glucose,' because I need to keep him under control every day."

In this part . . .

Just ahead, a potpourri of tips that will help you achieve and maintain good health and steer your way through the health care system. We also look at frequently asked questions posed by people with diabetes.

Chapter 19

Ten Ways to Stay Healthy and Avoid Complications

*W*e're thrilled you're reading this chapter because here we discuss the top ten things you need to know to stay healthy with your diabetes. If we were given a podium high enough and a speaker loud enough, these are the key messages we would shout out for all to hear.

If you don't have diabetes yourself and are reading this book on behalf of someone you love who does (which many of our readers tell us is the case), even if your loved one elects not to read this book in its entirety, please insist he or she looks at this chapter. Blame us for your insistence.

Following the advice on these pages could be the difference between disability and early death or a long and healthy life. More than two-thirds of diabetes complications are avoidable if the ten points we discuss in this chapter are followed. We consider it a tragedy, one that frustrates us and saddens us to the point of tears, that people are getting sick and even dying because they don't know the information in this chapter. We wrote this book — and particularly this chapter — to change things.

The ten points we discuss in this chapter are, indeed, the ten most important ways that you can stay healthy and lead a full and active life with your diabetes. And these measures are readily available to each and every person with diabetes. But — and this is a very big but — remember one other crucial point: Even if you follow just a portion of the recommendations in this chapter, you're still making headway. Even if you don't meet all your targets for weight control, blood glucose, blood pressure, and so forth, that doesn't mean you've failed and it doesn't mean it was all for naught. Any improvement in your weight or exercise or blood pressure or glucose levels or any of the other items we list here will help you reduce your likelihood of developing complications. So be proud of your work and your successes and, for those things lagging behind, well, it's always good to have additional goals to strive for.

Learn for Life

Every day, the two of us read professional journals or attend lectures or go to conferences, all with the express purpose of educating ourselves about how best to look after people with diabetes. And the family physicians we work with do the same. As do the diabetes nurse educators and dietitians. As do the podiatrists and the pharmacists and all the other professionals whose mission is to help you stay healthy. Your whole diabetes team is always learning. You, too, are a part of your diabetes team. So that means you also have to do your share of leaning.

The more you know, the better your odds are of being healthy. Ian's motto — present on the home page of his Web site (www.ourdiabetes. com) and guiding his professional life — is the saying, "Rule your diabetes; don't let it rule you!" Your continued education is the single most important factor in allowing you to do this. Don't be in the dark. Know what you should eat. Know how you should exercise. Know what your blood pressure is and what it should be, what your lipids are and what you are aiming for. Know what the best medicines are and how to safely and effectively use them. Whoever said "Ignorance is bliss" surely didn't have diabetes. Or, if they did, they likely came to rue the day they said it.

Don't be a passive partner in your diabetes care; be actively involved. You can learn from the other members of your health care team (especially from your diabetes nurse educator and dietitian). You can learn by reading this book, reviewing (reputable) Web sites such as that of the Canadian Diabetes Association (www.diabetes.ca), and attending meetings of your local CDA branch. Until there is a cure for diabetes, learning needs to be a part of your life. It's as simple as that.

Remember that you'll find a lot of misinformation on the Web, so you must be careful to check out a recommendation before you start to follow it. Even information on reliable sites may not be right for your particular problem.

Eat Earnestly

The most important point about a "diabetic diet" is that it is a healthy diet for anyone, with diabetes or without. You shouldn't feel like a social outcast because you're eating the right foods. And you shouldn't feel guilty if occasionally you eat the wrong foods either, for that matter. ***Remember:*** There is no such thing as cheating. A healthy diabetes meal plan is not a crash diet, a high-protein diet, a grapefruit diet, or any other fad diet. A diabetes meal plan is a lifelong program of healthy, well-balanced eating.

You can follow a diabetic diet wherever you are, not just at home. Every menu has something on it that's appropriate for you. If you're invited to someone's home, let them know you have diabetes and that you can eat only a limited amount of carbohydrate and fat. If that fails, then limit the amount that you eat. And if that's somehow not possible, then accept the fact that your diet won't always be perfect (and whose is?) and go on from there.

Follow a healthy diet designed by both you and your dietitian and you'll have an excellent foundation in your plan for good health. Ignore proper nutrition and you'll be destined to have poor glucose control; indeed, both the pills and the insulins we use to control blood glucose are much less effective in the absence of a proper diet. Your destiny is in your hands — and in your mouth.

See Chapter 10 for more on your diet.

Exercise Enthusiastically

If we were to tell you that we had a treatment for you to take that would cost you nothing; that would only have to be taken once per day; that could help keep your blood glucose levels under control, reduce your blood pressure, improve your lipids, reduce your stress level, and help prevent heart attacks; and that could lower your risk of dying over the next ten years by one-half, you would not only be wanting it, you would be demanding it! Okay then, it's yours. Exercise.

Preferably daily (or at least most days of the week). Preferably for at least 25 minutes per day. Make exercise as much a part of your life as breathing. The key to success with exercise? Finding the type you like and sticking with it. There is no need to run the Boston Marathon or swim across Lake Ontario (though you are welcome to if you want); something as simple (and inexpensive) as a daily walk is highly therapeutic.

See Chapter 11 for more on exercise.

Give the Heave-Ho to Harmful Habits

You win a lottery . . . but lose your ticket. You buy a brand-new car . . . and minutes later, lock your keys inside. You have a breakaway . . . and mishandle the puck. We all have our missteps — golden opportunities that we manage to make a mess of. But most of these are small miscues or, at worst, temporary setbacks. Having diabetes may be no piece of cake (well, actually, you can have a piece of cake, but that's another story), but with careful management you can lead a full, active, and long life. What a shame that smoking can wreck all that.

Smoking is bad enough for a person without diabetes, but if you have diabetes, smoking makes almost every complication more likely to occur. In essence, smoking rots your arteries. You place yourself at enormous risk of a heart attack or a stroke, blindness, or amputations; the list goes on and on. But you can change the odds. Quit smoking now and you can markedly improve your likelihood of avoiding these complications. Some things in life are beyond our control. Smoking isn't one of them. Millions of Canadians have quit smoking. So can you.

Does it seem unfair that once you were diagnosed as having diabetes, all those well-meaning people (family, friends, doctors, nurses, dietitians, . . .) asked you to change your diet, your exercise, your weight, and, if you smoke, your tobacco use too? Well, if you think so, then you may also think it unfair that we will now ask you to moderate your drinking. No more than one (for women) or two (for men) a day. Tops. Your health is our raison d'être. No apologies for that.

See Chapter 6 for tips on quitting smoking. See Chapter 10 for more on alcohol and diabetes.

Controlling Your Numbers: Optimizing Your Blood Glucose, Blood Pressure, Cholesterol, and Kidney Function

You can rest assured that your doctor knows your average blood glucose (as reflected by your A1C level), your blood pressure, your cholesterol, and your kidney function. Yet despite this, most Canadians with diabetes don't have all these levels under control and as a result are developing what are often avoidable complications. Clearly something's wrong with this picture.

We won't go into all the many factors here, but will point out one particularly important and easily correctable one: Most people with diabetes don't know their own numbers, and as a result don't know when they are above target (we discuss targets in the following sections; also, they are listed on the Cheat Sheet at the front of this book), and thus, also don't know when corrective action needs to be taken.

"If it ain't broke, don't fix it," some people say. Okay, we'll go along with that. But what if you don't know that it's broke? What then? Your blood glucose, blood pressure, cholesterol, and kidney function tests all belong to *you*. Indeed, they're part of you. And you need to know them. Period.

Now that we've hopefully convinced you (perhaps you didn't need convincing), let's look at the numbers you should be targeting and what to do if they are being exceeded.

Blood glucose levels

High blood glucose is a toxin to your body. It can lead to blindness, kidney failure, and nerve damage. But you're clearly not just waiting around for bad things to happen; if you were, you wouldn't be reading this book right now. To prevent high blood glucose from damaging your body, be sure to test your blood glucose regularly. (Refer to Chapter 9.) Your blood glucose target is 4 to 7 mmol/L before meals, 5 to 10 mmol/L two hours after meals. Your A1C target is no more than 7. If your A1C is above 7 despite good before-meal readings, then your two-hour, after-meal target is 5 to 8 mmol/L. (These are the targets for the great majority of people with diabetes. As we discuss in other chapters, target values are different for children, pregnant women, and some elderly individuals.)

If your blood glucose levels are too high, speak to your health care team (particularly your diabetes nurse educator, dietitian, family doctor, and, if you have one, your diabetes specialist) about what changes can be made to your treatment plan to help get your blood glucose control where it should be.

Lipids (cholesterol and triglycerides)

High LDL cholesterol, low HDL cholesterol, high triglycerides, and a high total cholesterol/HDL ratio are bad things. Low LDL, high HDL, low triglycerides, and a low total cholesterol/HDL ratio are good things. Now, which package do you want for your birthday? Got the wrong gift? So trade it in. Don't accept poor lipids. Optimal lipids will reduce your risk of cardiovascular disease, so optimal lipids are what we're after. The CDA target is for the LDL level to be less than or equal to 2 mmol/L and the total cholesterol/HDL ratio to be less than 4. These are the priorities. Be sure to know your own levels, and, if they are above target, speak to your physician to discuss how to make things better. She may recommend a visit to the dietitian, a change to your exercise program, or medication. We discuss lipids further in Chapter 6.

Blood pressure

Among the nasty things that high blood pressure causes are strokes, eye damage, heart attacks, and kidney failure. Quick: What was your blood pressure the last time your doctor checked it? And was that within the CDA target? If you know these two answers, congratulations. If you don't, then we're again thrilled that you're reading this. Your blood pressure should be less than 130/80. If your value is higher than this, speak to your doctor about how you can bring it into target. We discuss blood pressure in detail in Chapter 6.

See Your Eye Doctor

You may have 20/20 vision; heck, you may be able to see a speck of dust on the back of a gnat on the tail of a bird on the top of a tree on the peak of a mountain — but what you can't see is the back of your eyes. Only a skilled eye professional can determine the true health of your eyes. Don't be misled into thinking that your visual acuity (as reflected by your need for — and the strength of — prescription lenses) has anything to do with the health of your eyes. It doesn't. See your eye doctor regularly so you can, well, continue to see your eye doctor.

See Chapter 6 for more on eye care.

Fuss Over Your Feet

We walk, on average, about 184,000 kilometres in our lifetime. That's over four trips around the equator (well, okay, we realize that those darn oceans would keep getting in the way, but you know what we mean). So if you want to keep those lovely lower appendages of yours up to this task, you gotta look after 'em. Having diabetes means that your feet are at risk of damage including ulcerations, infections, and even frank gangrene and, potentially, amputation. But these devastating complications are largely avoidable. Show your feet you care by looking after them with all the helpful measures we discuss in Chapter 6. Go ahead, love your feet. It's okay; really. In fact, it's essential.

Master Your Medicines

You may have noticed that your success with diabetes is based on a combination of things, including knowledge, lifestyle treatment, and medicine use. Although no one wants to take medicines, you cannot underestimate their importance. Indeed, with each passing year, physicians are asking people with diabetes to take more and more pills. The reason is simple: These medicines can keep you healthy and even save your life. Most people with diabetes need to take medicines to accomplish one or more of the following:

- **Optimize blood glucose:** If you have type 2 diabetes, this usually requires metformin, often with one or two other blood-glucose-lowering medicines. (See Chapter 12.)

- **Optimize blood pressure:** This usually requires an ACE inhibitor or ARB along with one, two, or even three other types of medicine. (See Chapter 6.)

- **Optimize lipids:** This usually requires a statin and sometimes another medicine as well. (See Chapter 6.)

- **Prevent heart attacks and strokes:** If you're at high risk of cardiovascular disease, you should be taking either an ACE inhibitor or an ARB. (See Chapter 6.)

- **Prevent kidney failure:** If you have any evidence of diabetes-related kidney malfunction, you should be taking an ACE inhibitor or ARB. (See Chapter 6.)

- **Prevent pneumonia:** (At least this isn't a pill you have to remember to take!) Many people with diabetes fall ill each year from pneumonia. But you can markedly reduce your risk for developing influenza pneumonia by the simplest of measures: Have an annual flu shot. You should also have a vaccination to protect you against a different form of pneumonia called pneumococcal pneumonia (revaccination is sometimes given five years after the initial vaccination).

More controversial is whether or not people with diabetes should routinely take ASA to prevent blood clots. We discuss this in Chapter 6.

"My goodness!" you might (and should) say. "That could be seven or more different types of medicine to take every day." No one should tell you that's not a big deal. It *is* a big deal. But lying in a hospital bed with a stroke or an amputation or a dialysis machine at your side is, by far, a bigger deal. We have the means to keep you healthy and to help you live a long, full life. And those means include medicines. Don't think of the pills you need to swallow each day as an anchor dragging you down. Think of them as a life preserver lifting you up!

Help Your Doctor Help You

Your family doctor went through four years of undergraduate university then four years of medical school then two or more years of further training for one simple reason: Your doctor is a glutton for punishment. (Please don't tell your doctor we said that! We really, really didn't mean it.)

Your doctor did all this training because he wanted to be suitably equipped to help you stay healthy. But without your help, all that training is largely wasted. Having diabetes is not like having appendicitis. If you have appendicitis, all you have to do is lie on an operating table while the anesthetist puts you to sleep and the surgeon takes out your diseased organ. If you have diabetes, on the other hand, you have to be an active and keen partner, working with your doctor by regularly attending appointments, sharing with your doctor how you are doing with your nutrition program and your exercise, what your blood glucose levels are, what your blood pressure is (when, for example, using a machine at a drug store), if you are missing doses of your medicines or believe you're having side effects from them, and if you're experiencing symptoms such as chest pain or shortness of breath, erectile dysfunction or vaginal discharge, numbness or burning in your feet, and so on.

Your doctor relies on you to work with her for the common goal of keeping you healthy. Without your help, your doctor may just as well take those diplomas down off the wall and burn them. And that we do truly mean.

Don't Try to Do It Alone

In the previous section we discuss how you and your doctor can successfully work together. And, as we discuss in Chapter 8, many other health care professionals, including diabetes nurse educators and dietitians, podiatrists, eye specialists, pharmacists, and others, are not only available to help you, but are keen to help you. Also, never underestimate the importance of your *family's* involvement on your health care team. If someone else in the home does the cooking, take him or her with you when you meet with the dietitian. Have family members learn how to help you if your blood glucose level is low. If you can't inspect your own feet, ask a loved one to look for you. And if, at times, you're feeling frustrated or even fed up with the hassles of living with diabetes from day to day (we'd never deny that having diabetes can be a hassle), seeking the comfort of a loved one is often the best medicine of all.

Chapter 20

Ten Frequently Asked Questions

*T*hough every person with diabetes is unique — and needs to be treated as such — some questions do come up remarkably often. Sometimes it's because the answer isn't obvious (for instance, why in the world blood glucose levels would go up overnight even if you haven't been eating), and sometimes it's because the answer isn't easy to find (for example, how to get your doctor to be a more effective communicator). This chapter looks at the ten most commonly asked questions that we hear in our offices. (And we even supply the answers!)

Why Are My Blood Glucose Levels Higher When I Get Up in the Morning than When I Go to Bed?

Those higher blood glucose levels in the morning can seem like quite a conundrum. Did you take an unremembered stroll to the fridge at 3 a.m.? Not likely, unless you're one very hungry sleepwalker. Was it an overly big snack at bedtime that made your readings go up? Improbable, unless your snack was so huge that it would make Dagwood Bumstead proud. No, the answer lies within your body, not within your fridge or pantry.

Beginning about 3 a.m., your body starts to increase production of hormones such as cortisol and growth hormone, which are important for normal metabolism but which can, in a person with diabetes, lead to the release of glucose from the liver. This is called the *dawn phenomenon*.

Although this is a common problem, it's not one we take, ahem, lying down. The most successful strategy to fight the dawn phenomenon is to take a dose of intermediate- (NPH) or long-acting (Lantus, Levemir) insulin at bedtime. (Sometimes Lantus and Levemir are given at other times.) Suppertime doses of some oral hypoglycemic agents such as metformin or glyburide can also help but are often less effective.

If you're having this problem despite already taking bedtime insulin, then a simple solution may be to increase your insulin dose. Be sure to discuss this possibility with your physician or diabetes educator.

We discuss insulin issues in detail in Chapter 13.

Why Are My Blood Glucose Levels All Over the Place?

If you're like most people with diabetes (especially type 1 diabetes), you will have experienced times when, despite your best efforts, your glucose control seemed a mess. High one minute, low the next. High for a couple of days, low for the next two. Up and down, down and up, for no apparent rhyme or reason.

But of course there's a reason; there's *always* a reason. It's just a matter of detective work to figure out what that reason is. Sometimes doctors and patients naively think that all we have to worry about in terms of glucose control is what you eat, how you exercise, and what medicines you take. Although these are the most important factors, many other things can influence blood glucose control, including your stress level, your stomach and bowel function, your menstrual cycle, and more.

We discuss these issues in detail in Chapter 9.

Why Are My Blood Glucose Levels Getting Worse as Time Goes By?

Few things are as frustrating to a person with type 2 diabetes as finding that, despite following a proper diet (with occasional indiscretion — which is perfectly fine, by the way), taking more and more pills, and exercising regularly (okay, maybe irregularly, but doing some anyhow), his or her blood glucose levels are progressively worsening. If you have been in this situation, you probably asked yourself, "What am I doing wrong?"

The answer is, you are probably doing nothing wrong.

The problem is that diabetes is a progressive disease. We wish it wasn't, but it is. Which means that despite your (and our) best efforts, your pancreas is going to have a hard time keeping up. In fact, the day your type 2 diabetes was diagnosed, your pancreas was already running at only half normal function, and with each passing year it's likely to lose more and more of its ability to produce insulin. The net result is that, with all likelihood, you're going to require more and more medicine to control your glucose levels as time goes by. Worsening pancreas function is also the reason that the majority of people with type 2 diabetes will eventually require insulin therapy. That's not a sign that *you* have failed; it's a sign that *your pancreas* has. And that, of course, is not your fault.

It's theoretically possible that certain types of medicine will help slow down (or even stop) this deterioration in pancreas function. We have some evidence that TZD drugs may help preserve the pancreas's function, but if so, it's only to a limited extent. Newer incretin-based therapies (see Chapter 12 for a discussion on TZDs and incretins) also may help to protect the pancreas, but this is not yet proven. Stay tuned. . . .

What's the Difference between an A1C Level and a Blood Glucose Level?

One of the most important tests in assessing overall glucose control is also one of the least understood. Your A1C (hemoglobin A1C) helps us know what your average blood glucose level has been over the preceding three months. It's measured in percentage (unlike blood glucose, which is measured in mmol/L), and the result represents the proportion of your hemoglobin (the substance in your red blood cells that carries oxygen) that's permanently attached to glucose. The higher your average glucose readings over the preceding few months, the more glucose your hemoglobin is exposed to and the higher your A1C will be. Because it's an entirely different test from the one for blood glucose level, an A1C of 7 percent, for example, does not mean that your average blood glucose level is 7 mmol/L, but, rather, indicates your average blood glucose is 8.6 mmol/L. Fortunately, on the near horizon we will likely abandon discussing average blood glucose in terms of A1C levels and instead will simply use the same units (mmol/L) that you measure when doing your blood glucose meter tests. This will surely make life easier for both people with diabetes and health care professionals alike.

We discuss this in detail — and provide a table comparing average blood glucose to A1C — in Chapter 9.

I Used to Be on Pills, but Now I'm on Insulin. Does that Mean I've Developed Type 1 Diabetes?

No, you still have type 2 diabetes. We can say that you have *insulin-treated* diabetes, but that's not the same as having type 1 diabetes, where you would be absolutely dependent on insulin to stay alive, not just to maintain good blood glucose control.

Once You're on Insulin You're on It Forever, Right?

If you have type 1 diabetes, then yes, you need to be on insulin, and for all intents and purposes it will be forever (or until we have a cure).

If you have type 2 diabetes and, despite appropriate lifestyle and oral hypoglycemic agent therapy, your blood glucose control is still not what it should be, then yes, you really need to be on insulin, and yes, it will likely be forever. But if you're starting out with much to improve in your lifestyle, then there is a significant chance that with diet, exercise, and weight loss, oral hypoglycemic agent therapy will start to work better and, sometimes, effectively enough that you may end up being able to come off insulin.

I'm Watching My Diet, So Why Is My Cholesterol Level High?

Some people can eat a bacon double cheeseburger and have normal cholesterol levels. And other people could order a veggie burger and have abnormal cholesterol levels. The difference? Genetics. Some people are simply genetically programmed to have livers that manufacture excess cholesterol. Indeed, all of us produce the bulk of our cholesterol within our bodies. If you have a body that tends to over-produce cholesterol, you can combat this by following a proper diet, exercising, and getting your blood glucose control in order — but often this is not sufficient. Our genes are very strong. Often that helps us. Sometimes it doesn't.

We discuss cholesterol levels in detail in Chapter 6.

Why Do I Need Blood Pressure Pills If My Blood Pressure Is Good?

There are two reasons for taking blood pressure medication even when your blood pressure is good:

✔ Good blood pressure is seldom good enough.

✔ Certain types of blood pressure pills also have other important roles to play that are separate from and independent of their blood pressure–lowering function.

If you have diabetes, then your risk of cardiovascular, kidney, and eye disease is high enough that your blood pressure can't just be good or okay. It has to be perfect. Great. Excellent. Spectacular. Marvellous. Stupendous. . . . Optimal blood pressure will go a lot farther in keeping you healthy than will good blood pressure. And to achieve optimal blood pressure (less than 130/80), high blood pressure medicines are often required.

ACE inhibitors and ARBs are commonly called *blood pressure pills;* however, studies have shown that these medicines do more than just lower blood pressure. Indeed, even if your blood pressure is within target to begin with, these medicines can lower your risk of a heart attack (if you're at high risk) and help prevent deterioration in your kidney function (if you have evidence of kidney damage). We discuss these topics in detail in Chapter 6.

How Can I Get My Doctor to Be More Communicative?

Congratulations. That you have asked this question tells us that you want to be an active participant in your health care. You aren't content to assume that everything must be okay because your doctor hasn't told you otherwise. You want to know your blood pressure and your cholesterol levels. You want to know your last A1C and whether your eye doctor observed any retinopathy.

Even if he or she does not necessarily always show it, you can be quite confident that your doctor is absolutely thrilled that you're interested enough in your health that you want to be actively involved in your diabetes management. Nonetheless, there are some doctors who, at times, are not particularly good communicators.

If you're feeling in the dark, you can follow several steps to obtain more information. We suggest trying these in the order they are listed, proceeding to the next step if the earlier one didn't meet with success:

1. **Let your doctor know you're interested:** Perhaps your doctor simply doesn't realize that you want to know the specifics of your results. Your first step should always be to simply let your physician know that you are keenly interested in your health and would like to know as much as possible about how you're doing. He or she will likely be overjoyed.

2. **Ask specific questions:** "Doctor, what is my blood pressure?" is more likely to get you a specific number than is asking "Doctor, how's my pressure?" which would likely be met with "It's fine."

3. **Ask for copies of your lab results:** You are fully entitled to knowing what your lab results are (heck, it's your blood and urine after all!), and you are similarly entitled to having a copy of them provided to you. Usually, simply discussing your results with your doctor is sufficient; however, if you feel that this isn't providing you with enough in the way of specifics, then ask your doctor for a photocopy of your results. When you ask for these, make sure you word your request in a non-threatening way; otherwise, your doctor may feel that you are second guessing his or her judgment (which you may be, but there's no benefit to you if your doctor feels defensive). Try something like "Doctor, I like to keep tabs on my lab results. May I please have a photocopy for my records?"

4. **Ask other members of your health care team:** If none of the previous steps has succeeded, try asking other members of your health care team. It may well be that if one of your physicians (say, for example, your diabetes specialist) is not readily forthcoming, another one may be (for example, your family physician). Your diabetes educator is another person to try, because he or she may have received copies of lab results or consultation letters from your physician(s).

Will I Always Have Diabetes?

We're sure you can tell why we saved this question for last; it is far and away the most difficult question we ever have to answer. The quick answer is a simple "we don't know" — and, of course, we don't. The more complicated answer is (and this is our personal and highly subjective guess) the following:

✔ If you have type 1 diabetes, you're unlikely to have it forever. It's only a matter of time before a cure is found (perhaps islet cell transplants will get perfected, perhaps gene therapy will be refined, perhaps stem cell research will find an answer, . . .). Sure, you may have heard this prophecy year after year and may be frustrated by the eternal wait. (And who could blame you?) Nonetheless, we can tell you that we would never have used the word *cure* ten years ago, but in the new millennium we dare to mention it. When will a cure be found? That we cannot say. But that there will be one, we have no doubt.

✔ If you have type 2 diabetes, the situation is much trickier, and we suspect that there won't be a cure in the foreseeable future. The factors leading to type 2 diabetes are complex and far from completely understood. It's highly unlikely that we're dealing with a single cause for which there will be a single cure. On the other hand, more and better treatment options are rapidly emerging. Even if we can't undo your diabetes, it's likely that we'll be able to offer such effective therapy that your diabetes will become less and less difficult for you to deal with.

As diabetes specialists, we're always full of hope. Every day, research comes out revealing new insights into the condition. And the pace at which new and better therapies are emerging is simply astounding. The single greatest advantage to you in having a disease that's rapidly becoming more common is that this stimulates research scientists to put tremendous resources into finding ways to help you.

When we look back at our careers and see what medical science knows now that it did not when we first began our practices, we can only marvel at the progress we've made in our quest to keep people with diabetes healthy. Some people with diabetes, alas, tell us they do not feel that scientists are really looking for a cure. We find this comment so sad, for it is so untrue. Thousands of scientists — people who have dedicated their entire careers to this cause — are looking for a cure. Not just finding a new, expensive drug to control diabetes, but an honest-to-goodness cure. How can we be so certain? Because we read their research papers, and hear them speak, and meet them all the time.

Chapter 21

Ten Ways to Get the Best Possible Health Care

In This Chapter

▶ Preparing for your visit to your doctor

▶ Getting ready for a hospital stay

▶ Knowing key things about your drugs

▶ Staying current

*I*n medical school you learn lots about anatomy and physiology. You learn lots about pathology and statistics. And you learn lots about diseases and how to treat them. But one thing that you don't learn is how to help your patients get the most out of their visits to their health care providers and from the health care system in general. In this chapter we share with you some key tips that we have learned over the years — tips that will help you when you see your health care team, help save you time and aggravation, and help you stay healthy.

Prepare for Your Visit

If you were going to be travelling to the Caribbean for a holiday, you would make sure you packed the right things and dressed appropriately for your destination. Well, when you are going to be seeing a member of your health care team it's a good idea to be similarly prepared. The evening before your appointment is a good time to make sure everything is ready. Let's say, for example, you're going to see your diabetes specialist. Here's what you'd be wise to do:

- ✔ **Make sure your glucose logbook is ready.** (And don't leave it behind on the kitchen counter!) If you don't usually write down your readings — and, by the way, we think you should — transcribe them from your meter's memory into your book or, if you have the appropriate software and cable, download them to your computer and print them. Providing readings for your doctor to review will make giving advice regarding your blood glucose control a lot easier and a lot more effective.

- ✔ **Take your medicines with you.** Put all your medicines in a bag and take them with you to your appointment. Your doctor will likely want to review them with you. Simply taking a list isn't nearly as good, but if you do opt to take a list, ensure that it's up-to-date and includes, for each drug, the name, the dose, and how often you take it. If you're taking alternative or complementary therapies (see Chapter 14), take those with you too.

- ✔ **Check to see if you'll be needing any prescription renewals.** Some doctors will renew prescriptions only while the patient is with them in their office. If that's true of your doctor, save yourself the hassle of a return visit just to get a prescription: Ask your doctor for one while you're there.

- ✔ **Dress for the occasion.** It's much easier to be a diabetes specialist in Canada in mid-July than in mid-January. In summer, shirts having replaced sweaters and shoes having replaced boots, it's a piece of cake to check a blood pressure or examine a foot or assess some other part of the anatomy. But alas, in Canada summer lasts about two weeks (okay, maybe longer in Victoria and, perhaps, even Vancouver). Still, there's no reason for you not to get the physical examination you require just because it's –30 degrees Celsius outside. When you're getting dressed, make sure that you wear clothes that will allow:

  - Your neck to be readily exposed so that your thyroid can be examined.

  - Your arm to be easily accessed to allow for a blood pressure measurement. Avoid wearing sleeves that can't be rolled up easily.

  - Your feet to be readily exposed for checking. Pantyhose, for example, may help keep you warm, but they may prevent your feet from being examined. (A simple yet highly effective way to make sure that your feet get examined is to remove your shoes and socks while you are waiting for your doctor to come in the examining room.)

- ✔ **Think ahead about what questions you want to ask.** If you have been waiting to ask your doctor about certain things, write them down and bring the paper with you. Otherwise, you may forget your questions, only to remember them after you have left the office. And that can be very frustrating!

✔ **Plan to bring two sets of ears.** If you feel that you want the support of a friend or family member, or, equally important, the benefit of two memories, then plan on bringing someone with you to your doctor's appointment.

If you're going to bring someone with you to your appointment, make sure you ask your doctor if it's okay to have them join you before your companion walks, unannounced, into the examining room. Otherwise, you may severely regret bringing your teenage daughter with you when your doctor asks you whether you're experiencing erectile dysfunction. (Reversing generations — and perhaps more disconcerting to you — your teenage daughter with diabetes may be far less likely to talk to her doctor about her need for birth control if you're sitting there.)

If you'll be seeing your dietitian and if you aren't the person in charge of food preparation in your house, both you and the person who cooks should go. Oh, by the way, don't announce to the dietitian that you don't have to know the information because you don't do the cooking. It's unlikely that you'll be eating 100 percent of your meals at home, and besides, the food will be going in your mouth — don't you want to know why?

Plan for Your Next Visit

Your diabetes specialist and ophthalmologist likely have their appointment schedule drawn up many months in advance. Indeed, some specialists are fully booked for well over six months. So if you realize on April 1 that, say, you haven't seen your eye doctor for a year and you want an appointment for the next day, the receptionist will likely tell you that you sure are in the spirit of April Fool's Day and wasn't that a good joke you just made.

A much better idea is to book your *next* appointment before you leave the *present* one, even if the next appointment won't be for another year. If you're asked to call later to book an appointment because they don't know what the doctor's office hours will be that far in advance, ask when you should call and then mark the date on your calendar so that you don't forget.

Tired of waiting an hour or more in your doctor's waiting room? Try booking your next visit for the first appointment of the day.

A Requisition for Success

If you have diabetes, you and your forearm are no stranger to the local laboratory. Typically, your doctor will give you a requisition as you leave his or her office, ask you to go to the lab, and tell you that you'll be contacted if there's a problem. Well, we can tell you we immediately see a problem! The problem is that you will have missed out on a golden opportunity to review your test results face-to-face with your doctor. And if you won't be seeing your doctor again for six months, that's a long time to be in the dark.

A much better system is to get a requisition as you're leaving your doctor's office, not for tests that you need then, but for the tests you will need later (that is, at the time of your next appointment). Go for the tests two weeks or so before your next visit and, that way, when you arrive for your appointment, your doctor will already have the results and you can review them together.

Healthy Numbers

You will get a lot more out of your visit to your doctor — and work more effectively with him or her — if you are familiar with what your numbers are. The Cheat Sheet at the front of this book summarizes these for you. Here are the key numbers to know:

- Blood pressure
- A1C
- Blood glucose levels
- Lipids (most important of these are your LDL cholesterol and your total cholesterol/HDL cholesterol ratio)
- Urine albumin/creatinine ratio (ACR)

Remember that knowing what your numbers are is of little value unless you know what your targets are supposed to be. Additionally, it's crucial that if your numbers aren't within target, you and your health care team undertake measures to achieve your goals.

Has It Really Been That Long?

Okay, quick — we're going to have a little quiz. Tell us the following:

- When was the last time you saw your family physician and when does he or she want to see you next?

- ✔ When was the last time you saw your diabetes specialist and when does he or she want to see you next?

- ✔ When was the last time you saw your diabetes nurse educator and when does he or she want to see you next?

- ✔ When was the last time you saw your dietitian and when does he or she want to see you next?

- ✔ When was the last time you saw your eye doctor, podiatrist, and the rest of your health care team and when do they want to see you next?

We're easy markers, so we'll consider a pass to be 40 percent. So, did you get the necessary two questions right? If you did, congratulations! If you didn't, try this test again in a few weeks. Because the average member of your health care team looks after several thousand people, whereas you look after just you (and, of course, you may well be looking after your loved ones), no one is in a better position than you to keep track of when you're supposed to see a health care team member. If your health care provider hasn't told you when you're to return, ask.

Not every member of your health care team is necessarily involved in your ongoing health care. Your diabetes specialist, for example, may have seen you a few times, given you and your family physician a suggested treatment program, and then handed your care back to your family doctor. Nonetheless, if you feel you'd like to see your specialist again, feel free to discuss this with your family physician. This becomes especially important if, despite your and your family physician's best efforts, you aren't reaching your targets (Canadian Diabetes Association recommended targets are listed on the Cheat Sheet at the front of this book).

Know Who Does What

Having read the previous tip, you have now arranged all the necessary follow-up appointments you need with the various members of your health care team. As we discuss in Chapter 8, each of them has a special role to play; however, sometimes it can be confusing for the person with diabetes to know who is going to be doing what and when. Indeed, sometimes (thankfully, not often) the various members of the team mistakenly assume that another member of the team is going to be doing something, and as a result no one does it. You can avoid this by having a look at the Cheat Sheet at the front of this book, where we note how often different parts of you (such as your eyes and your feet) need to be examined and how often certain laboratory tests should be performed. If you're due for one of these procedures but you're unclear who will be arranging things, ask your health team members. They may well appreciate the reminder.

No News Is Good News. Not!

If your doctor tells you that you'll be called if your test results come back abnormal, you can rest assured that he or she will. Unless, of course, the lab report gets sent to the wrong doctor, or gets lost in the filing, or gets accidentally discarded, or the lab did the wrong test, or the lab didn't do the test at all, or the lab did the right test on the wrong patient, or . . .

If you're sent for a test, make sure that if you don't hear back from your physician's office with the result, you contact the office to double-check that everything was all right. You don't need to speak directly to the doctor; simply ask the receptionist to check for you. The receptionist may well tell you, "We would have called you if there was a problem." In which case you can tell him or her that you read this book by Drs. Blumer and Rubin called *Diabetes For Canadians For Dummies* and they said to call. Blame us; we can handle it.

Here's a far better way to avoid the uncertainty of waiting for a call about your results. Have your tests done — when feasible — in advance of your appointment. That way, the results are available for review at the time of your doctor's appointment (see "A Requisition for Success" earlier in this chapter).

Staying in the Loop When You're Hospitalized

We can assure you that if you have severe ketoacidosis or hyperosmolar hyperglycemic state (both of which we discuss in Chapter 5), there is no better place for you to be than in the hospital. Indeed, your life could depend on it.

On the other hand, if you're hospitalized with a problem not directly related to your diabetes, your diabetes may not get the same degree of attention as the condition that landed you in hospital. Although this is understandable, it remains important that your diabetes get the attention it requires.

The following tips will help when you are hospitalized:

✔ If you're in hospital with a major illness (such as a heart attack), make sure your glucose readings are tested regularly and that your control is maintained at a good level.

✔ If you're well enough to use them, bring your diabetes supplies (including your blood glucose meter, insulin administration devices, and even your insulin) with you to hospital. Nurses in hospitals are terribly overworked and may find it a huge relief to know that you're able to assist with looking after your own basic diabetes needs. (You'll likely need to get permission from your attending doctor in hospital to be allowed to do this.)

✔ Most of the people looking after you will be very knowledgeable and helpful when it comes to your diabetes. Recognize, however, that you may encounter certain health care providers who aren't quite so familiar with diabetes issues, and you may have to spend some time explaining your diabetes management to them. This is especially true if you are using an insulin pump (see Chapter 13) and/or a continuous glucose monitoring system (Chapter 9).

The following tips will help you if you're having outpatient surgery:

✔ Ask for your case to be scheduled for "first case of the day," as this will make it easier for you to get promptly back on your usual insulin or oral hypoglycemic agent schedule.

✔ Ask your doctor what to do with your insulin (or oral hypoglycemic agents) the night before your surgery, the morning of your surgery, as well as later on that day. If it's anticipated that you may not be eating properly for a few days (such as after dental surgery), check with your physician (or your diabetes educators) about how to adjust your diet and your insulin (or oral agents) for those few days.

Often, what works well in preparation for outpatient surgery is to take one-half of your usual bedtime intermediate- or long-acting insulin the night before your surgery. When you arrive at the hospital in the morning, check your blood glucose and, depending on the result, give yourself anywhere from no insulin to a full dose of your rapid-acting or regular insulin. It's essential that you do *not* do any of this without first checking with your physician.

Know Your Drugs

Anytime you are handed a prescription, you're being given a medicine that is supposed to enhance your health. But as you likely know (perhaps all too well), medicines can have their downsides too. Sulfonylureas (such as glyburide), for example, can help bring down high blood glucose but can also lead to low glucose. ACE inhibitors are great at protecting the kidneys, but can also lead to bothersome coughing. Statins can prevent heart attacks, but can cause muscle aching. We could go on and on. Fortunately, the numbers of people who benefit from these and other drugs are vastly greater than the numbers of people who have serious adverse effects.

Here are some important things you should know about any medicine you are prescribed:

- ✔ How often you are to take it
- ✔ Whether it needs to be taken with food or on an empty stomach
- ✔ Whether you can consume alcohol if you are taking it
- ✔ What you should do if you forget a dose
- ✔ What the most common side effects are
- ✔ What the most serious side effects are
- ✔ What the likelihood of you experiencing a side effect is
- ✔ What you should do if you believe you are experiencing a side effect
- ✔ What laboratory tests (if any) are to be done to monitor for toxicity (Some drugs require periodic testing of, for example, your liver.)
- ✔ Whether one of your drugs can interact adversely with another of your drugs
- ✔ Whether you are to repeat your prescription after the initial supply has run out

A commonly made — and potentially dangerous — error is to assume you're finished with a drug after the pill bottle is finished. You'll need to take most medicines used to treat diabetes (including those for glucose control, high blood pressure, and high cholesterol) on an ongoing basis.

It's not only unhelpful, it's downright counterproductive for you to simply be given a long list of all the possible side effects that a particular drug can cause. Such lists do little more than frighten or intimidate people — or else they're simply ignored. What you want to know are the key things to look for.

Remember that your alternative or complementary therapies may have their own set of risks, including the way they interact with your prescription drugs. Be as informed about your alternative and complementary therapies as you are about your prescription drugs.

Know How to Stay "In the Know"

As we mention elsewhere in this book, you'll no longer have to stay current about diabetes treatment when you no longer have diabetes. Until that day comes, it will be crucial for you to stay abreast of new developments and, in particular, new therapies that will help you stay healthy.

The simplest and often most effective way for you to stay "in the know" is to be in regular contact with your health care team. In addition, reading the publications (such as *Diabetes Dialogue*) of the Canadian Diabetes Association is very helpful, as is having a look from time to time at high-quality, well-maintained Web sites (see Appendix C).

Even if you don't need routine contact with a diabetes specialist, it's often a good idea to see one from time to time. Doing so is particularly helpful if you've heard about (or if your diabetes educator has told you about) some new therapy that has come out and you're wondering if it may be appropriate for you. Your family physician may be knowledgeable about it and be able to guide you, but if not, he or she would likely be happy to send you back to see your specialist.

Part VI
Appendixes

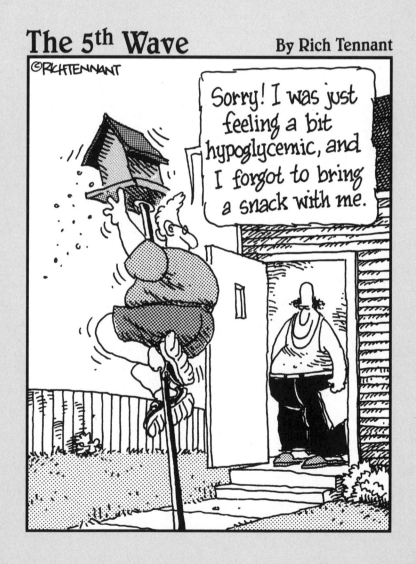

The 5th Wave   By Rich Tennant

Sorry! I was just feeling a bit hypoglycemic, and I forgot to bring a snack with me.

In this part . . .

Although your body may have but one appendix, *Diabetes For Canadians For Dummies* has three! In the first appendix we look at the food group system. After you have digested that (or before, if you prefer), you can quench your appetite for even more information by having a look at Appendix B where we list some particularly satisfying Web sites. Lastly, Appendix C provides a quick reference glossary so you can look up the meaning of those words — both obscure and not so obscure — that you may be uncertain about.

Appendix A

The Food Group System

*1*n this appendix, you discover the method that dietitians in Canada are using to help their patients eat the right number of calories from the correct energy sources while permitting them to vary their foods. Although many thousands of different foods are available, each one can be broken down on the basis of the energy source (carbohydrate, protein, or fat) that is most prevalent. This basic feature underlies nutrition planning, as you will see.

Here we look at the general principles of meal planning (and snacks, too!); you will need to see a dietitian to create a nutrition program that fits with your specific needs. We discuss the role of dietitians as part of your health care team in Chapter 8.

To assist people with diabetes in choosing healthy foods for their meals and snacks, the Canadian Diabetes Association has developed *Beyond the Basics: Meal Planning for Healthy Eating, Diabetes Prevention and Management*. In this system, foods are divided into seven groups according to the amount of carbohydrate, protein, and fat they contain. Here are the groups:

✔ Grains and Starches

✔ Fruits

✔ Milk and Alternatives

✔ Other Choices (sweet foods and snacks)

✔ Vegetables

✔ Meat and Alternatives

✔ Fats

Each group includes many different food choices. The amount specified beside each food in the tables that follow represents one choice from that group and can be interchanged with any other choice in the same group. This system is highly effective, as long as you're keeping track of the amounts you're eating from the different groups.

Listing all food sources in this space isn't possible, but you can obtain a list of just about all the foods you might eat by ordering *Beyond the Basics* from the Canadian Diabetes Association (www.diabetes.ca or 800-226-8464). You can learn more about this publication at www.diabetes.ca/about-diabetes/nutrition/meal-planning.

In the United States they use a similar concept, but they use the word *exchanges* rather than choices.

In the remainder of this appendix we look at each of the seven food groups. We then discuss a sample nutrition plan.

Grains and Starches

Grains and Starches food choices are listed in Table A-1. Each choice contains about 15 grams of carbohydrate, 2 grams of protein, and 68 calories. *Beyond the Basics* recommends high-fibre starch choices. On food labels, look for 4 grams or more of fibre per serving.

Table A-1	Grains and Starches Food Choices
Food	*Serving*
Cereals, Grains, Pasta	
Bran cereals	125 mL (½ cup)
Cooked cereals	175 mL (¾ cup)
Shredded wheat biscuit	1
Wild rice (cooked)	75 mL (⅓ cup)
Pasta (cooked)	125 mL (½ cup)
Puffed wheat	375 mL (1½ cup)
Rice (cooked)	75 mL (⅓ cup)
Shredded wheat (bite size)	125 mL (½ cup)

Food	Serving
Bread	
Bagel small	½
Breadsticks	2
English muffin	½
Wiener	½, bun
Hamburger	½ bun
Pita	15 cm (6"), ½
Raisin bread	1 slice
Tortilla	15 cm (6"), 1 round
White or whole wheat bread	1 slice
Crackers/Snacks	
Soda crackers	7
Graham crackers	3
Matzoh	15 cm (6"), 1
Melba toast	7 slices
Triscuits	5
Rusks	2
Starchy Vegetables	
Corn (kernel)	125 mL (½ cup)
Corn on the cob	½ medium
Potato (baked or broiled)	½ medium
Plantain	75 mL (⅓ cup)
Starchy Foods with Fats	
Waffle	1
Tea biscuit	1
French fries	10
Pancake	10 cm (4"), 1
Croissant	1 small
Mashed potatoes	125 mL (½ cup)

Fruits

All fresh, frozen, and canned fruits as well as unsweetened juices are in this group. Choose whole fruit and eat the edible skins as much as possible for the benefit of fibre, vitamins, and minerals. Each Fruits choice (see Table A-2) contains about 15 grams of carbohydrate, 1 gram of protein, and 64 calories of energy.

Table A-2	Fruit Choices
Food	*Serving*
Fresh and Canned Fruit	
Apple	1 medium
Applesauce, unsweetened	125 mL (½ cup)
Apricots	4
Banana	1 small
Blackberries	500 mL (2 cups)
Blueberries	250 mL (1 cup)
Cantaloupe	250 mL (1 cup)
Cherries	15
Cherries (canned)	125 mL (½ cup)
Figs, fresh	2 small
Fruit cocktail	125 mL (½ cup)
Grapefruit	1 small
Grapes	250 mL (1 cup) or 15
Honeydew	250mL (1 cup)
Kiwi	2 medium
Mango	125 mL (½ cup)
Nectarine	250mL (1 cup)
Orange	1 medium
Papaya	250 mL (1 cup)
Peach	1 large
Peaches (canned in light syrup)	125 mL (½ cup)
Pear	1 medium

Food	Serving
Pears halves (canned, in light syrup)	125 mL (½ cup)
Persimmon	½
Pineapple, fresh	175 mL (¾ cup)
Pineapple (canned in light syrup)	125 mL (½ cup) or 2 rings
Plum	2 medium
Raspberries	500 mL (2 cups)
Strawberries	500 mL (2 cups)
Tangerine	2 medium
Watermelon	250 mL (1 cup)
Dried Fruit	
Apple	4 rings
Apricots	8 halves
Dates	2
Pear	½
Prunes	3
Raisins	25 mL (2 tbsp.)
Fruit Juice	
Apple	125 mL (½ cup)
Grape	75 mL (⅓ cup)
Grapefruit	125 mL (½ cup)
Orange	125 mL (½ cup)
Pineapple	125 mL (½ cup)
Prune	75 mL (⅓ cup)

Milk and Alternatives

The different kinds of milk vary only in their fat content. The carbohydrate and protein content remain the same. One Milk and Alternatives choice (see Table A-3) contains about 15 grams of carbohydrate, 8 grams of protein, and from trace to 8 grams of fat (skim milk, trace grams fat and 80 calories; 1 percent milk, 2 grams fat and 98 calories; 2 percent milk, 5 grams fat and 125 calories; homogenized milk, 8 grams fat and 152 calories).

Table A-3	Milk and Alternatives Choices
Food	**Serving**
Milk (skim, 1%, 2%, or homo)	250 mL (1 cup)
Chocolate milk	125 mL (½ cup)
Evaporated milk	125 mL (½ cup)
Powdered milk, skim	50 mL (4 tbsp.)
Plain or artificially sweetened yogurt	175 mL (¾ cup)

Other Choices (sweet foods and snacks)

Sugar and food with added sugar such as candy, Popsicles, and regular jam can be part of a healthy meal plan. This group consists of common snack foods and treats. Choose these foods in moderation as many lack fibre, vitamins, and minerals and may contain a lot of fat. Current recommendations suggest no more than 10 percent of the total calories you consume be supplied by sugar. For example, if you are on a 2,000-calorie-per-day meal plan, your recommended amount of carbohydrate in the form of sugar would be 50 grams. Each choice in this group (see Table A-4) contains 15 grams of carbohydrate, generally very small amounts of protein (except for milk-based items), and from 0 to 12 grams of fat. Calorie values vary from approximately 77 to 164.

Table A-4	Other Choices
Food	**Serving**
Popcorn, air popped, low fat	750mL (3 cups)
Honey/molasses/corn/maple syrup/white or brown sugar	15 mL (1 tbsp.)
Milk pudding, skim, no added sugar	125 mL (½ cup)
Regular jam, jelly, or marmalade	15 mL (1 tbsp.)
Hard candy	5 small
Popsicles	1 bar
Ice cream	125mL (½ cup)
Oatmeal granola bar	1 bar (28 grams)
Muffin, small	1
Potato chips	10
Chocolate chip cookies	2

Vegetables

Vegetables are rich in nutrients, contain no fat, contain typically small, but variable, amounts of protein (depending on the particular vegetable), and, with the exception of those that are richer in carbohydrates (parsnips, sweet peas, squash, and beets, which should be limited to half-cup portions at a meal), can be eaten in unlimited quantities in a healthy diet. Potatoes and corn are included in the Grains and Starches group due to their carbohydrate content.

These are examples of vegetables that can be eaten in unlimited quantities:

- ✔ Asparagus
- ✔ Beans, string, green, or yellow
- ✔ Bok choy
- ✔ Broccoli
- ✔ Brussels sprouts
- ✔ Cabbage
- ✔ Carrots
- ✔ Cauliflower
- ✔ Celery
- ✔ Cucumber
- ✔ Frozen mixed vegetables
- ✔ Lettuce
- ✔ Mushrooms
- ✔ Okra
- ✔ Onion
- ✔ Peppers, green, red, and yellow
- ✔ Spinach
- ✔ Tomato (tomato is, technically, a fruit, but since it fits best here, we're sneaking it into this list)
- ✔ Zucchini

Meat and Alternatives

One choice of Meat and Alternatives (see Table A-5) contains no carbohydrate (except for legumes; that is, beans and lentils), about 7 grams of protein, 3 grams of fat, and 55 calories of energy. Legumes are low in fat and high in fibre and are excellent protein sources. Each half-cup portion will provide 15 grams of carbohydrate.

Only lean Meat and Alternatives choices are listed here. All foods listed are cooked.

Table A-5	Meat and Alternatives Choices
Food	*Serving*
Meat and poultry	
Beef: round, sirloin, flank, tenderloin, ground	30 grams (1 oz.)
Pork: fresh, canned, cured, or boiled ham, ground	30 grams (1 oz.)
Veal: all cuts except for cutlets	30 grams (1 oz.)
Poultry: chicken, turkey	30 grams (1 oz.)
Fish and shellfish	
All fish, fresh and frozen	30 grams (1 oz.)
Crab, lobster	50 mL (¼ cup)
Oysters	3 medium
Canned in water (tuna or salmon)	50 mL (¼ cup)
Canned sardines	3 small
Fresh shrimp	5 large
Cheese	
Low fat (about 7% milk fat)	1 slice, 30 grams (1 oz.)
Cottage cheese	50 mL (¼ cup)
Ricotta cheese	50 mL (¼ cup)
Alternatives	
Egg, large	1
Legumes: beans and lentils	125 mL (½ cup)
Hummus	75 mL (⅓ cup)
Vegetarian patty/wiener	1
Peanut butter	25 mL (2 tbsp.)

The following Meat and Alternatives choices are high in saturated fat (choose them less often):

- Bologna: 1 slice
- Canned luncheon meat: 1 slice
- Sausage: 1 link
- Weiner, hot dog: 1
- Salami: 1 slice
- Regular cheese (greater than 20 percent milk fat): 1 slice, 30 grams (1 oz.)

Fats

These foods (see Table A-6) have 5 grams of fat and little or no protein or carbohydrate per portion. Therefore, each choice contains 45 calories. The important thing in this category is to notice the foods that are high in cholesterol and saturated fats — and avoid them.

Table A-6	Fat Choices
Food	*Serving*
Unsaturated Fats	
Avocado	⅛ medium
Salad dressing, regular	5 mL (1 tsp.)
Margarine, regular, non-hydrogenated	5 mL (1 tsp.)
Salad dressing, low fat	25 mL (2 tbsp.)
Margarine, light, non-hydrogenated	15 mL (1 tbsp.)
Mayonnaise, regular	5 mL (1 tsp.)
Almonds	8
Cashews	5
Pecans	5 halves
Peanuts	10
Walnuts	2 whole
Sunflower seeds	15 mL (1 tbsp.)
Pumpkin seeds	20 mL (4 tsp.)
Oil (corn, olive, soybean, sunflower, peanut)	5 mL (1 tsp.)

(continued)

Table A-6 *(continued)*

Food	Serving
Olives, small	10
Saturated Fats	
Butter	5 mL (1 tsp.)
Bacon	1 slice
Coconut milk, canned	25 mL (2 tbsp.)
Cream, half and half	45 mL (3 tbsp.)
Cream, sour, regular	25 mL (2 tbsp.)
Cream, heavy	15 mL (1 tbsp.)
Cream cheese	15 mL (1 tbsp.)
Gravy	25 mL (2 tbsp.)
Lard	5 mL (1 tsp.)
Pâté, liverwurst	15 mL (1 tbsp.)
Shortening	5 mL (1 tsp.)

Free Foods

These foods do not contain a significant amount of calories, so you can eat as much of them as you want without worrying about serving size (though, of course, if you eat a pound of chili powder you may regret it for other reasons!).

- **Drinks:** Bouillon, sugar-free drinks, club soda, coffee, and tea

- **Condiments:** Horseradish, mustard, pickles (unsweetened), and vinegar

- **Seasonings:** Basil, lemon juice, celery seeds, lime, cinnamon, mint, chili powder, onion powder, chives, oregano, curry, paprika, dill, pepper, salt, flavouring extracts (vanilla, for example), pimiento, garlic, spices, garlic powder, ginger, soy sauce, herbs, wine (used in cooking), lemon, and Worcestershire sauce

As we discuss in Chapter 10, a number of types of sugar-free candy, sugar-free gum, sugar-free jam or jelly, and sugar substitutes can, depending on their contents, be consumed fairly liberally. However, bear in mind that sugar alcohols vary in the degree to which they are absorbed into the body, and, in high doses, they can cause unpleasant gastrointestinal symptoms such as abdominal cramping and diarrhea.

Using "Beyond the Basics" to Create a Nutrition Plan

Having different foods in each group that can be interchanged makes it easy to create a nutrition plan with great variation. The following menus show the amounts for diets of 1,500 (Table A-7) and 1,800 (Table A-9) calories.

Table A-7	1,500 Calories		
Breakfast	*Lunch*	*Dinner*	*Snack*
2 Grains and Starches choices	2 Grains and Starches choices	2 Grains and Starches choices	1 Grains and Starches choice
1 Fruits choice	1 Fruits choice	1 Fruits choice	1 Milk (1%) and Alternatives choice
1 Milk (1%) and Alternatives choice	2 Meat and Alternatives choices	3 Meat and Alternatives choices	
1 Meat and Alternatives choice	1 Fats choice	2 Fats choices	
2 Fats choices	Vegetables as desired	Vegetables as desired	

This menu provides 180 grams of carbohydrate, 82 grams of protein, and 49 grams of fat, keeping it in line with 50 percent of energy from carbohydrate, 20 percent of energy from protein, and 30 percent of energy from fat.

Translating this into food, you can have the menu in Table A-8 on one day.

Table A-8		A Sample Menu	
Breakfast	**Lunch**	**Dinner**	**Bedtime Snack**
2 slices toast	2 slices bread	1 medium potato	1 shredded wheat biscuit
1 pear	1 large peach	15 grapes	250 mL (1 cup) 1% milk
250 mL (1 cup) 1% milk	1 slice cheese (low-fat) & 1 slice ham	90g (3 oz.) lean beef	
1 egg	5 mL (1 tsp) margarine	10 mL (2 tsp.) regular salad dressing	
2 tsp., non-hydrogenated margarine	Vegetables (such as lettuce, cucumber for sandwich)	Salad , as desired, and 125 mL(½ cup) peas	

For a 1,800-calorie diet, you could have the menu in Table A-9.

Table A-9		1,800-Calorie Sample Menu	
Breakfast	**Lunch**	**Dinner**	**Bedtime Snack**
2 Grains and Starches choices	3 Grains and Starches choices	3 Grains and Starches choices	1 Grains and Starches choice
1 Fruits choice	1 Fruits choice	2 Fruits choices	1 Milk (2%) and Alternative choice
1 Milk (2%) and Alternatives choices	2 Meat and Alternatives choices	3 Meat and Alternatives choices	
2 Meat and Alternatives choices	2 Fats choices	2 Fats choices	
2 Fats choices	Vegetables as desired	Vegetables as desired	

This diet provides 225 grams of carbohydrate, 96 grams of protein, and 61 grams of fat, again maintaining the 50:20:30 division of calories. Using the example of the 1,500-calorie diet, go ahead and try to make up an 1,800-calorie diet at this point.

Appendix B

Straight Goods on a Tangled Web: Diabetes Web Sites Worth Visiting

- -

In This Appendix

▶ Starting at the authors' Web sites

▶ Checking general sites about diabetes

▶ Investigating scientific sites

▶ Exploring sites that address Aboriginal issues

▶ Discovering sites about children and diabetes

▶ Finding sites for the visually impaired

▶ Sniffing out Web sites with recipes for people with diabetes

▶ Looking at companies that make diabetes products

▶ Searching Web pages in French

▶ Getting the lowdown on diabetes in dogs and cats

- -

*T*he World Wide Web can be a great resource for just about anything, but, of course, as any Web surfer knows, with the good comes the bad. One minute you're looking at a high-quality, reputable, well-maintained site like that of the Canadian or American diabetes associations, and the next click you're looking at Uncle Bob's Instant Diabetes Cure. The problem is not that great information isn't out there; the problem is trying to figure out which sites have it and which just pretend to.

In this appendix, we discuss sites that we have found particularly useful. You should be able to get answers to just about any questions that you have. However, you must be cautious. A Web site is offering information to many people; it doesn't know you and your unique needs. Therefore, you shouldn't make any major changes in your diabetes care without first checking with your health care team. Remember also that the Web is constantly changing and growing, so the Web addresses we mention — and the information they contain — may change.

If you want to stay abreast of new, worthwhile sites, one helpful way to do this is to periodically check the "links" pages of sites that you have come to know and trust.

Ian's and Alan's Web Sites

Start your search at our Web pages:

- www.ourdiabetes.com
- www.drrubin.com

You can find general information and advice about diabetes, tips, new developments, and answers to questions.

Ian's site has a list of all the Web sites listed in this appendix, so you need only click on them to see them for yourself.

General Sites

All-encompassing sites such as the following will tell you about diabetes from A to Z. In keeping with that, we list them alphabetically:

- **The American Diabetes Association(ADA):** This helpful site, www. diabetes.org, offers loads of information, but as you can imagine, it uses American units (for glucose, cholesterol, and so on), which can make it confusing for those of us north of the 49th parallel. Also, it uses American guidelines, which at times can be quite different from Canadian ones.

- **Ask NOAH About Diabetes:** This site, www.noah-health.org, provides a large amount of information in both English and Spanish. It comes from the New York Online Access to Health, a partnership of New York institutions.

- **The Canadian Diabetes Association (CDA):** The CDA site, www. diabetes.ca, is particularly helpful because it looks at diabetes issues from a Canadian perspective. Canadian guidelines are the backbone of the supplied information, and, of course, this site uses Canadian (international, actually) units. Particularly helpful is the listing of resources (including addresses and phone numbers) available in your province or territory and even within your community. Note that the CDA Web site underwent a major overhaul in 2008, so if you have previously bookmarked links to certain of that site's pages, you may have to hunt around to find the new location for the information you seek.

- ✔ **Diabetic Exercise and Sports Association:** This site, www.diabetes-exercise.org, is a place where you can find out about many different kinds of exercises and how they fit with your diabetes. You will also find others who share your interests.

- ✔ **The Diabetes Monitor:** This site, www.diabetesmonitor.com, is the creation of diabetes specialist Dr. William Quick. He discusses every aspect of diabetes, including the latest discoveries.

- ✔ **MEDLINEplus Drug Information:** You'll find excellent information at this site, www.nlm.nih.gov/medlineplus/druginformation.html. It provides clear and well-presented information on virtually any drug you're likely to be prescribed. It also provides detailed information on complementary and alternative medicines. Highly recommended.

- ✔ **Online Diabetes Resources by Rick Mendosa:** On his site, www.mendosa.com/diabetes.htm, Rick Mendosa has catalogued a vast amount of information on the Web concerning diabetes. Also available are some excellent articles that he's written on various topics in diabetes.

Scientific Sites

These sites are geared toward health care professionals; however, if you have a good understanding of diabetes and can put up with the medicalese, you'll be able to find very useful information here:

- ✔ **CenterWatch Clinical Trials Listing Service:** Whether you are a layperson or a physician, you may find it very difficult to keep tabs on what research studies are underway. Even the Internet is only partially helpful, because no one site lists all the studies that are going on at any given time. Also, many studies are run on a small scale and/or are industry-sponsored, and these studies are often not noted on the Web.

  CenterWatch Clinical Trials Listing Service, www.centerwatch.com, lists many studies that are looking for participants. If you think you're interested in being part of research (some of which is truly cutting edge), have a look at this site.

- ✔ **Google Scholar:** This site, http://scholar.google.ca, is just one of the increasingly diverse resources available through the Google behemoth. This resource allows you to search the world's scientific literature on the topic of your choice. You'll need to be pretty specific in your search, though, otherwise you'll find yourself smothered in more information than you could possibly sift through. For example, type in the word *diabetes* and you'll be rewarded (or, depending on how you view it, punished) by getting over 4 million hits!

✔ **Medscape Diabetes and Endocrinology:** This site, `www.medscape.com/diabetes-endocrinology`, is particularly helpful for finding what's in the news on the topic of diabetes: new drugs, new safety information, new industry developments, and so forth.

✔ **PubMed Search Service of the National Library of Medicine:** Surf on over to this site, `www.ncbi.nlm.nih.gov/PubMed`. It's easy to use and gives you (for free) a large number of the latest scientific papers on any medical topic of interest. Bear in mind that these are academic references and are written for health care professionals.

Sites about Diabetes and Aboriginal Populations

Addressing the needs and interests of Aboriginal peoples, the following sites provide helpful and interesting information:

✔ **Canadian Diabetes Association (CDA):** The CDA site, `www.diabetes.ca`, has excellent information on Aboriginal issues and has links to a number of additional Aboriginal diabetes sites.

✔ **Diabetes Close to Home:** Though this site, `www.diabetes.kcdc.ca`, focuses on awareness and prevention of diabetes in northern Saskatchewan, the well-presented information is widely applicable.

✔ **Sandy Lake Health and Diabetes Project:** Read here, `www.sandylakediabetes.com`, about the innovative project that the Sandy Lake community has developed to combat diabetes.

Sites about Diabetes and Children

Many of the general information Web sites listed earlier in this appendix provide abundant, helpful information to help you learn more about diabetes in children. Other sites are specifically geared toward providing information on this topic. Particularly good ones are

✔ **Children with Diabetes:** This site, `www.childrenwithdiabetes.com`, is the creation of a father of a child with diabetes and has an enormous database of information for the parents of children with diabetes.

✔ **Juvenile Diabetes Research Foundation of Canada (JDRF):** The JDRF appropriately prides itself on its contribution to research in diabetes, and this site, `www.jdrf.ca`, reflects that. You can find what you want to know about the latest government programs that emphasize finding a cure for diabetes.

Sites for the Visually Impaired

Some excellent sites are geared specifically to the issue of visual impairment:

- ✔ **American Foundation for the Blind:** This site, www.afb.org, has resources, information, reports, talking books, and limitless other facts and wisdom about dealing with visual impairment.

- ✔ **Blindness Resource Center:** This site, www.nyise.org/blind.htm, points you in the right direction for information on every aspect of blindness. It is a guide to other sites about visual impairment.

- ✔ **The Canadian Council of the Blind:** This site, www.ccbnational.net, is the online home of an advocacy group for visually impaired people, run by visually impaired people.

- ✔ **The Canadian National Institute for the Blind (CNIB):** The CNIB is a well-known organization that serves to assist people with visual impairment. Their well-organized site, www.cnib.ca, details the different services they have to offer.

Recipe Web Sites for People with Diabetes

You can find a number of excellent recipes on World Wide Web sites. Particularly good ones are noted here:

- ✔ **The American Diabetes Association (ADA):** The ADA site, www.diabetes.org, has an extensive list of recipes — enough to keep you full for ages.

- ✔ **The Canadian Diabetes Association (CDA):** Not as extensive as the ADA's list, but still food for thought, is the CDA's list of recipes at www.diabetes.ca.

- ✔ **Children with Diabetes:** At www.childrenwithdiabetes.com you'll find a huge collection of recipes including many submitted by their readers (which is good in that they come personally recommended; however, it also means the recipes may not have been evaluated by a registered dietitian).

- ✔ **Diabetic Gourmet Magazine:** In this online magazine, www.diabeticgourmet.com, you'll find many recipes and even a rating system — you can vote thumbs up or down on last night's dinner. Of course, your kids will already have voiced their opinion without the computer.

Sites of Companies That Make Diabetes Products

Are you looking for information from the companies that make the products you need to control your diabetes? If you have questions about the proper use of a drug or a device, you can usually find it answered here:

- ✔ Insulin

  - Eli Lilly: www.lilly.ca

  - Novo Nordisk: www.novonordisk.ca

  - Sanofi-Aventis: www.sanofi-aventis.ca

- ✔ Insulin pumps

  - Animas Canada: www.animas.ca

  - Disetronic Medical Systems: www.disetronic-ca.com

  - Medtronic Diabetes of Canada.: www.minimed.ca

  - Smiths Medical Canada Ltd.: www.cozmore.com

- ✔ Glucose meters

  - Abbott Diabetes Care: www.abbottdiabetescare.ca

  - Auto Control Medical: www.autocontrol.com

  - Bayer Healthcare: www.bayerdiabetes.ca

  - Lifescan Canada: www.lifescancanada.com

  - Roche Diagnostics: www.accu-chek.ca

- ✔ Pens and pen needles

  - Auto Control Medical: www.autocontrol.com

  - Becton-Dickson: www.bddiabetes.com

  - Eli Lilly: www.lilly.ca

  - Novo Nordisk: www.novonordisk.ca

  - Sanofi-Aventis: www.lantus.com/solostar/solostar_insulin_pen.aspx

- ✔ Lancing devices and lancets

  - Abbott Diabetes Care: www.abbottdiabetescare.ca

  - Auto Control Medical: www.autocontrol.com

  - Bayer: www.bayerdiabetes.ca

- Becton-Dickson: www.bddiabetes.com
- Lifescan: www.lifescancanada.com
- Roche: www.accu-chek.ca

✔ Syringes

- Becton-Dickson: www.bddiabetes.com

✔ Urine test strips

- Bayer: www.bayerdiabetes.ca
- Roche: www.accu-chek.ca

Sites in French

Not nearly as many sites are available in French as in English, but the following are particularly helpful:

✔ **Association Canadienne du diabète:** www.diabetes.ca

✔ **Association diabète Québec:** www.diabete.qc.ca

✔ **Section Diabète, site de Santé Canada:** http://www.hc-sc.gc.ca/dc-ma/diabete/index-fra.php

✔ **Dr. Samuel:** http://drsamuel.cyberquebec.com

Animals with Diabetes

Yes, your dog and cat and many other animals can get diabetes. Here's a site for your beloved pet: www.petdiabetes.com.

Appendix C

Glossary

A1C: A measurement of overall blood glucose control for approximately the last three months (also referred to as the hemoglobin A1C or HbA1C).

Acarbose: An oral hypoglycemic agent that lowers blood glucose by slowing the rate of absorption of glucose from the small intestine into the blood.

ACE inhibitor: A class of drug that lowers blood pressure, protects the kidneys, and reduces the risk of heart attack in people with diabetes. (An example of an ACE inhibitor is ramipril.)

Actos: See *pioglitazone*.

Amaryl: See *glimepiride*.

Amino acids: Compounds that link together to form proteins.

Antibodies: A type of protein formed — as part of the immune system — when the body detects something foreign such as bacteria.

Apidra: See *aspart*.

Aspart: A type of rapid-acting insulin.

Atherosclerosis: Narrowing of arteries due to deposits of cholesterol and other substances.

Autoimmune disorder: Disease such as type 1 diabetes and Hashimoto's thyroiditis in which the body's immune system mistakenly attacks its own tissues.

Autonomic neuropathy: Diseases of nerves that affect organs not under conscious control, such as the heart, lungs, and intestine.

Avandia: See *rosiglitazone*.

Basal insulin: The low level of insulin present in the body, around the clock, in people taking intermediate- or long-acting insulin or on insulin pumps. Basal insulin is generally used in combination with bolus (mealtime) insulin.

Basal-bolus insulin therapy: Therapy that combines use of both basal and bolus insulin.

Beta cell: The insulin-producing cells of the pancreas.

Blood glucose meter: A small, portable machine that allows for moment-to-moment measurement of your blood glucose level.

Body mass index: A measure of whether or not you're at a healthy weight for your height.

Bolus insulin: Rapid-acting (or regular) insulin given with meals or snacks to quickly raise the blood insulin levels to reduce blood glucose.

Brittle diabetes: A condition of erratic blood glucose control in people with type 1 diabetes, often leading to hospitalizations with ketoacidosis or hypoglycemia. With optimal diabetes management, brittle diabetes is seldom encountered.

Byetta: See *exenatide*.

Carbohydrate: One of the three major energy sources; usually found in grain, fruits, and vegetables, and most responsible for raising the blood glucose.

Carbohydrate counting: Estimating the amount of carbohydrate in food in order to determine bolus insulin requirements.

Cataract: A clouding of the lens of the eye often found earlier and more commonly in people with diabetes.

Cholesterol: A fat-like substance that is needed in the body (for example, for the production of certain hormones), but if present in excess levels can contribute to the development of atherosclerosis. See also *high-density lipoprotein (HDL)* and *low-density lipoprotein (LDL)*.

Creatinine: A substance in blood that reflects the approximate level of kidney function. Used to calculate the creatinine clearance (or estimated GFR; eGFR), which is a more precise measure of how efficiently your kidneys are able to purify your blood.

Dawn phenomenon: The tendency for blood glucose to rise in the early morning due to secretion of hormones that counteract insulin.

Detemir: A long-acting, basal insulin.

Diabeta: See *glyburide*.

Diabetes: A disease in which there is too much glucose in the blood due to insufficient or ineffective insulin.

Diabetologist: A physician who specializes in diabetes treatment.

Dialysis: Artificial cleaning of the blood when the kidneys aren't working.

Diamicron: See *gliclazide*.

DPP-4 inhibitors: A class of glucose-lowering agent that works by multiple mechanisms including promoting insulin release from the pancreas.

Dyslipidemia: Abnormal cholesterol and triglyceride levels in the blood.

Endocrinologist: A physician who specializes in diseases of the glands, including the adrenal glands, the thyroid, the pituitary, the parathyroid glands, the ovaries, the testicles, and the pancreas.

Exenatide: A type of *GLP-1 analogue*.

Fats: The most concentrated source of calories of the three major energy sources. Some fats come from animals and some from plants. Excess levels of certain types of fats can increase the risk of atherosclerosis.

Fibre: A substance in plants that can lower fat and blood glucose and can help prevent constipation.

Food Group System: A system — designed to facilitate diabetes meal planning — that divides foods into seven groups according to the amount of carbohydrate, protein, and fat they contain.

Fructose: The sugar found in fruits, vegetables, and honey.

Gastroparesis: A form of autonomic neuropathy involving nerves to the stomach that results in a slowing of the rate that the stomach expels food into the small intestine.

Gestational diabetes: Diabetes that develops during pregnancy and goes away once pregnancy ends, but that indicates you are at increased risk of later developing type 2 diabetes.

Glargine: A long-acting, basal insulin.

Gliclazide: An oral hypoglycemic agent that lowers glucose by stimulating insulin release from the pancreas.

Glimepiride: An oral hypoglycemic agent that lowers glucose by stimulating insulin release from the pancreas.

GLP-1 analogues: A class of glucose-lowering medicine that is injected under the skin and works by multiple mechanisms including promoting insulin release from the pancreas.

Glucobay: See *acarbose.*

GlucoNorm: See *repaglinide.*

Glucose: A form of sugar that is the body's main source of energy.

Glucose tolerance test: A test where you consume a sugar-rich drink and your glucose levels are measured several times to establish if you have diabetes.

Glumetza: A once-a-day formulation of metformin.

Glyburide: An oral hypoglycemic agent that lowers glucose by stimulating insulin release from the pancreas.

Glycemic index: The extent to which a given food raises blood glucose.

Glycogen: The storage form of glucose in the liver and muscles.

Health care team: The group of people who work together to keep you healthy. You, the person with diabetes, are the most important member of the team. Other members include your family doctor, your diabetes specialist, your diabetes educator, your dietitian, your eye doctor, your pharmacist, and, when necessary, other specialists (such as a social worker, podiatrist, dentist, cardiologist, kidney specialist, neurologist, emergency room physician, and so forth).

Hemoglobin A1C: See *A1C.*

High-density lipoprotein (HDL): A good form of cholesterol that helps to protect you from atherosclerosis.

Honeymoon phase: A period of variable duration, usually no more than a few months, after the onset of type 1 diabetes when the need for injections of insulin is temporarily reduced or eliminated.

Humalog insulin: See *Lispro insulin*.

Hyperglycemia: Higher than normal blood glucose levels.

Hyperosmolar hyperglycemic state: A dangerous condition in type 2 diabetes of very high blood glucose associated with severe dehydration.

Hypoglycemia: Lower than normal blood glucose levels.

Impaired fasting glucose (IFG): A condition in which fasting blood glucose levels are higher than normal, but not high enough to establish a diagnosis of diabetes. See *prediabetes*.

Impaired glucose tolerance (IGT): A condition in which the blood glucose level is higher than normal — but not high enough to establish a diagnosis of diabetes — during the post-drink phase of a glucose tolerance test. Also see *prediabetes*.

Incretins: Hormones, made by the intestine, that are important in regulating blood glucose control.

Insulin: The key hormone, made by the islet cells of the pancreas, that permits glucose to enter cells.

Insulin pump: A device that delivers insulin into the body through a small catheter under the skin.

Insulin reaction: Hypoglycemia as a consequence of injected insulin.

Insulin resistance: A condition in which the body does not properly respond to insulin. This is typically present in people with type 2 diabetes.

Intensive diabetes management: The term typically applied to people with type 1 diabetes who are on three or more insulin injections per day or are using an insulin pump. (This term is, however, more appropriately used to refer to all people with diabetes, regardless of the type of treatment they are on, as long as the treatment is aimed at achieving optimal blood glucose control.)

Islet cells: The cells in the pancreas that make insulin, glucagon, and other hormones.

Januvia: See *sitagliptin*.

Ketoacidosis: An acute loss of control of diabetes with high blood glucose levels and breakdown of fat leading to acid production. Much more common in type 1 than type 2 diabetes.

Ketone: A breakdown product of fat formed when fat, rather than glucose, is being used for energy.

Ketonuria: Ketones in the urine.

Lancet: A sharp needle to prick the skin for a blood glucose test.

Lantus: See *glargine*.

Laser treatment: Using a device that burns small areas at the back of the eye to prevent worsening of retinopathy.

Levemir: See *detemir*.

Lipohypertrophy: Area of fatty deposit under the skin from overuse of an insulin injection site.

Lispro insulin: A type of rapid-acting insulin.

Low-density lipoprotein (LDL): A bad form of cholesterol that contributes to the development of atherosclerosis.

Macrosomia: An overly big baby.

Macrovascular complications: Damage to the heart, brain, or legs due to blockage of large blood vessels.

Metabolic syndrome: A combination of several conditions, typically including an overweight state, abnormal lipids, elevated blood pressure, and increased blood glucose that puts you at increased risk of diabetes and cardiovascular disease.

Metabolism: The body's use of energy and nutrients to maintain good health.

Metformin: An oral hypoglycemic agent for diabetes that lowers blood glucose by blocking release of glucose from the liver.

Microalbuminuria: Abnormal loss of a specific type of protein, called albumin, from the body into the urine.

Microvascular complications: Damage to the retina, nerves, or kidneys due to blockage of small blood vessels.

Monounsaturated fat: A form of fat from certain vegetable sources that does not raise cholesterol.

Nateglinide: An oral hypoglycemic agent that lowers blood glucose by stimulating insulin release from the pancreas.

Neovascularization: Formation within the eyes of abnormal, fragile blood vessels that are prone to bleeding.

Nephropathy: Damage to the kidneys.

Neuropathy: Damage to parts of the nervous system.

NovoRapid: See *aspart*.

NPH insulin: A type of intermediate-acting insulin.

Omega-3 fatty acids: A type of fat, found in certain fish, that may protect against the development of atherosclerosis.

Ophthalmologist: A medical doctor who specializes in diseases of the eyes.

Oral hypoglycemic agent: A glucose-lowering drug taken by mouth.

Pancreas: The organ behind the stomach that is actively involved in digestion and metabolism and contains the insulin-producing islet cells.

Peripheral neuropathy: Damaged nerve fibres, typically in the feet, that cause pain and numbness.

Pioglitazone: An oral hypoglycemic agent that lowers glucose by reducing insulin resistance.

Podiatrist: A type of health care professional who specializes in treating diseases of the feet.

Polydipsia: Excessive intake of water.

Polyunsaturated fat: A form of fat from certain vegetable sources that may lower HDL.

Polyuria: Excessive urination.

Post-prandial: After eating.

Prediabetes: A term that includes *impaired fasting glucose* and *impaired glucose tolerance*. Having prediabetes puts you at much greater risk of later developing diabetes.

Pre-prandial: Before eating.

Protein: One of the three major energy sources, the one usually found in meat, fish, poultry, and beans. Protein is necessary for the body to maintain healthy tissues.

Proteinuria: Abnormal loss of protein from the body into the urine.

Regular insulin: A type of fast-acting insulin.

Repaglinide: An oral hypoglycemic agent that lowers glucose by stimulating insulin release from the pancreas.

Retina: The part of the eye that senses light.

Retinopathy: Disease of the retina.

Rosiglitazone: An oral hypoglycemic agent that lowers glucose by reducing insulin resistance.

Saturated fat: A form of fat from animals that raises cholesterol.

Sitagliptin: A type of DPP-4 inhibitor.

Somogyi phenomenon (effect): A rapid increase in blood glucose to a high level in response to hypoglycemia occurring during the night. Recent scientific evidence suggests that this seldom happens.

Starlix: See *nateglinide*.

Sulfonylureas: A class of glucose-lowering agents, which work by stimulating insulin secretion from the pancreas.

Thiazolidinedione: A class of glucose-lowering agents, which works by reducing insulin resistance, thereby helping glucose enter into fat and muscle cells.

Trans fatty acids: A type of fat, formed during food processing, that may worsen cholesterol levels and contribute to the development of atherosclerosis.

Triglycerides: The main form of fat in animals.

Index

The Discovery of Insulin (Bliss), 32
discrimination, job, 296–299
disposal, sharps, 148, 250
dizziness, 59
DKA (diabetic ketoacidosis). *See* ketoacidosis
doctor appointments. *See* appointments
domperidone, 100
dot hemorrhages, 79
double diabetes, 31
D-phenylalanine derivatives, 61, 221–222
DPP-4 inhibitors, 218, 225, 361
drinks, 61–62, 348
driving, 57, 301–305
drowsiness, 59, 68
Drucker, Dan, 128
drug therapy. *See* medications; *specific drug*
dry mouth, 72
duty to report, physician's, 301, 305
dysesthesiae, 96
dyslipidemia
  defined, 361
  genetic susceptibility, 92, 323
  in metabolic syndrome, 48
  overview, 90–93
  as risk factor for heart attack, 85
  screening for, 91, 278
  as symptom of insulin resistance, 280
  treatment, 92, 317

• E •

eAG (estimated average glucose), 167–168
eating disorders, 163, 196, 276
Eating Well with Canada's Food Guide, 176
ED (erectile dysfunction), 110–112, 285
elderly, 24, 38, 73, 286–289
Eli Lilly, 235, 254, 356
emergency assistance, 23, 63, 84
emergency preparedness, 308
emotions, 11–15
employment rights, 296–299
endocrinologist, 136, 361
endoscopy, 101
environmental triggers, 37
epinephrine (adrenaline), 56, 58, 163
erectile dysfunction (ED), 110–112, 285
estimated average glucose (eAG), 167–168

estrogen, vaginal, 113
exenatide, 226, 361
exercise
  adherence to, 313
  amount of, 204–206
  benefits, 43, 192, 198, 200
  calories burned during, 203
  by children, 273
  effect on blood glucose levels, 163, 200
  by elderly, 287
  for gestational diabetes, 116
  overview, 197
  precautions, 64, 165, 199–201, 204, 212–213
  types of, 202
exercise stress test, 200
expiration dates, 63, 164, 249
extra-ocular muscle palsy, 98
Exubera, 258
eye disease, 78–83, 285. *See also* retinopathy; vision changes; *specific disorder*
eye examinations
  children, 278
  elderly, 285
  importance of, 140, 316
  pregestational diabetes, 123, 125
  recommended schedule, 80–81
eye specialists, 81, 140, 285, 316
ezetimibe, 92
Ezetrol. *See* ezetimibe

• F •

family involvement, 14, 62, 74, 142–143, 284, 318, 329
family physician, 135, 136–137
fast-acting carbohydrates, 61–62
fast-acting insulin. *See* regular insulin
fasting blood glucose, 18, 47, 293
fat. *See* body fat; dietary fats
fatigue, 21, 35, 41, 60, 68, 72
fatty acids, 29, 184, 365, 366
fatty liver, 100
fears, 120, 233, 241–243, 322
fenugreek, 262
fibre, dietary, 181, 190, 254, 361
fight-or-flight situations, 58
first-aid kit, 308

iodine, 186
iron, 50, 186
islet cell, 27, 363
islet cell antibodies, 36
islet cell transplantation, 325

• J •

Januvia. *See* sitagliptin
Jarvis, Chris (athlete), 10
jet injectors, 244
job discrimination, 296–299
juvenile-onset diabetes. *See* type 1 diabetes

• K •

ketoacidosis
 in children, 277
 defined, 34–35, 363
 development of, 23, 35, 67–68
 overview, 67–71
 with uncontrolled glucose levels, 23
ketones
 defined, 118, 364
 testing, 68, 69, 118, 125, 155
ketonuria, 364
kidney disease, 93–95. *See also* nephropathy
kidney failure, 93
kidney function tests, 93, 123, 220, 278

• L •

labour, 125–127
LADA (Latent Auto-immune Diabetes of Adults), 46–47
lancet, 148, 150, 256, 356–357, 364
lancet holder, 148
lancing devices, 148, 149, 356–357
Lantus. *See* glargine
Lantus Compassionate Care Program, 235
Latent Auto-immune Diabetes of Adults (LADA), 46–47
laughter, 265
LDL (low-density lipoprotein), 85, 90, 91, 184, 315, 364
legal issues, 296–297, 301, 305
Levemir. *See* detemir

Levitra, 111
life insurance, 300
Lifescan Canada, 156, 356, 357
lifestyle therapy. *See also* exercise; nutrition therapy; weight loss
 adherence to, 132, 241, 313
 after gestational diabetes, 119
 blood glucose testing while on, 150–151
 for children, 280
 components, 22–23
 as diabetes prevention, 43
 for dyslipidemia, 92
 for elderly, 287
 for gestational diabetes, 116
 as key component of treatment, 227–228
 medication compared to, 43–44, 192, 199, 218, 241
 success of, 42
Lilly Canada Cares Insulin Assistance Program, 235
Lilly Diabetes Journey Awards, 254
lipids. *See* cholesterol; dyslipidemia; triglycerides
Lipitor. *See* atorvastatin
lipohypertrophy, 104–105, 164, 250, 364
liraglutide, 226
lispro insulin, 234, 236, 364
liver
 effect of diabetes on, 31, 100–101
 functions, 27–29, 92, 183, 323
liver function tests, 101
logbook, 147, 155–159, 328
long-acting insulin, 234, 238–239
long-term complications, 76–78, 311–318. *See also specific complications*
loss of consciousness, 59, 72
low-density lipoprotein (LDL), 85, 90, 91, 184, 315, 364
Lyrica. *See* pregabalin

• M •

Macleod, John (scientist), 32, 231
macrosomia, 118–119, 364
macrovascular complications, 77, 78, 84, 364. *See also specific complications*
macular degeneration, 285
macular edema, 78, 79

• *U* •

• *V* •

BUSINESS & PERSONAL FINANCE

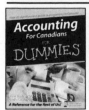
978-0-470-83878-5

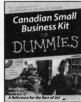
978-0-40-83818-1

Also available:
- Buying and Selling a Home For Canadians For Dummies 978-0-470-83740-5
- Investing For Canadians For Dummies 978-0-470-83361-2
- Managing For Dummies 978-0-7645-1771-6
- Money Management All-in-One Desk Reference For Canadians For Dummies 978-0-470-15428-1

- Negotiating For Dummies 978-0-470-04522-0
- Personal Finance For Canadians For Dummies 978-0-470-83768-9
- Small Business Marketing For Dummies 978-0-7645-7839-7
- Starting an eBay Business For Canadians For Dummies 978-0-470-83946-1
- Stock Investing For Canadians For Dummies 978-0-470-83925-6

EDUCATION, HISTORY & REFERENCE

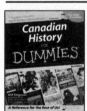
978-0-470-83656-9

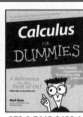
978-0-7645-2498-1

Also available:
- Algebra For Dummies 978-0-7645-5325-7
- Art History For Dummies 978-0-470-09910-0
- Chemistry For Dummies 978-0-7645-5430-8
- French For Dummies 978-0-7645-5193-2

- Math Word Problems For Dummies 978-0-470-14660-6
- Spanish For Dummies 978-0-7645-5194-9
- Statistics For Dummies 978-0-7645-5423-0
- World War II For Dummies 978-0-7645-5352-3

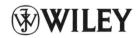

FOOD, HOME, GARDEN, & MUSIC

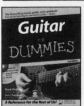

978-0-7645-9904-0

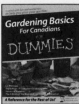

978-0-470-15491-5

Also available:
- ✔ 30-Minute Meals For Dummies
  978-0-7645-2589-6
- ✔ Bartending For Dummies
  978-0-470-05056-9
- ✔ Brain Games For Dummies
  978-0-470-37378-1
- ✔ Gluten-Free Cooking For Dummies
  978-0-470-17810-2

- ✔ Home Improvement All-in-One
  Desk Reference For Dummies
  978-0-7645-5680-7
- ✔ Violin For Dummies
  978-0-470-83838-9
- ✔ Wine For Dummies
  978-0-470-04579-4

GREEN/SUSTAINABLE

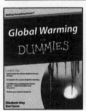

978-0-470-84098-6

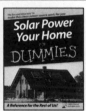

978-0-470-17569-9

Also available:
- ✔ Alternative Energy For Dummies
  978-0-470-43062-0
- ✔ Energy Efficient Homes For
  Dummies 978-0-470-37602-7
- ✔ Green Building & Remodeling
  For Dummies 978-0-470-17559-0

- ✔ Green Business Practices
  For Dummies 978-0-470-39339-0
- ✔ Green Cleaning For Dummies
  978-0-470-39106-8
- ✔ Green Your Home All-in-One
  For Dummies 978-0-470-40778-3
- ✔ Sustainable Landscaping
  For Dummies 978-0-470-41149-0

HEALTH & SELF-HELP

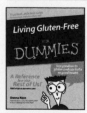

978-0-471-77383-2

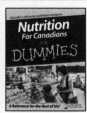

978-0-470-15307-9

Also available:
- ✔ Breast Cancer For Dummies
  978-0-7645-2482-0
- ✔ Depression For Dummies
  978-0-7645-3900-8
- ✔ Healthy Aging For Dummies
  978-0-470-14975-1

- ✔ Improving Your Memory
  For Dummies 978-0-7645-5435-3
- ✔ Neuro-linguistic Programming
  For Dummies 978-0-7645-7028-5
- ✔ Pregnancy For Canadians
  For Dummies 978-0-470-83945-4
- ✔ Understanding Autism
  For Dummies 978-0-7645-2547-6

HOBBIES & CRAFTS

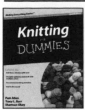

978-0-470-28747-7

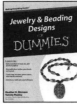

978-0-470-29112-2

Also available:
- Crochet Patterns For Dummies
  978-0-470-04555-8
- Digital Scrapbooking For Dummies
  978-0-7645-8419-0
- Home Decorating For Dummies
  978-0-7645-4156-8
- Knitting Patterns For Dummies
  978-0-470-04556-5

- Oil Painting For Dummies
  978-0-470-18230-7
- Origami Kit For Dummies
  978-0-470-75857-1
- Quilting For Dummies
  978-0-7645-9799-2
- Sewing For Dummies
  978-0-7645-6847-3

HOME & BUSINESS COMPUTER BASICS

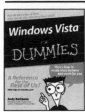

978-0-471-75421-3

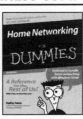

978-0-470-11806-1

Also available:
- Blogging For Dummies
  978-0-471-77084-8
- Excel 2007 For Dummies
  978-0-470-03737-9
- Office 2007 All-in-One Desk
  Reference For Dummies
  978-0-471-78279-7

- PCs For Dummies
  978-0-7645-8958-4
- Web Analytics For Dummies
  9780-470-09824-0

INTERNET & DIGITAL MEDIA

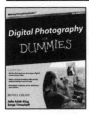

978-0-470-25074-7

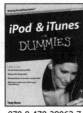

978-0-470-39062-7

Also available:
- eBay For Canadians For Dummies
  978-0-470-15348-2
- MySpace For Dummies
  978-0-470-09529-4
- Pay Per Click Search Engine
  Marketing For Dummies
  978-0-471-75494-7

- Search Engine Marketing
  For Dummies 978-0-471-97998-2
- The Internet For Dummies
  978-0-470-12174-0
- YouTube For Dummies
  978-0-470-14925-6

MACINTOSH

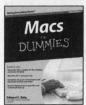

978-0-470-27817-8

978-0-470-05434-5

Also available:

- iMac For Dummies
  978-0-470-13386-6
- iPhone For Dummies
  978-0-470-42342-4
- iPod & iTunes For Dummies
  978-0-470-39062-7
- MacBook For Dummies
  978-0-470-27816-1

- Mac OS X Leopard For Dummies
  978-0-470-05433-8
- Office 2008 For Mac For Dummies
  978-0-470-27032-5
- Switching to a Mac For Dummies
  978-0-470-14076-5
- Upgrading & Fixing Macs & iMacs
  For Dummies 978-0-7645-0644-4

PETS

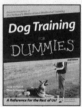

978-0-7645-8418-3

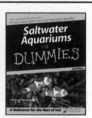

978-0-470-06805-2

Also available:

- Birds For Dummies
  9780764551390
- Boxers For Dummies
  9780764552854
- Cockatiels For Dummies
  9780764553110
- Ferrets For Dummies
  9780470127230
- Golden Retrievers For Dummies
  9780764552670

- Horses For Dummies
  9780764597978
- Puppies For Dummies
  9780470037171

SPORTS & FITNESS

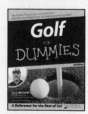

978-0-471-76871-5

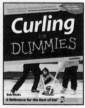

978-0-470-83828-0

Also available:

- Exercise Balls For Dummies
  978-0-7645-5623-4
- Coaching Hockey For Dummies
  978-0-470-83685-9
- Fitness For Dummies
  978-0-7645-7851-9

- Rugby For Dummies
  978-0-470-15327-7
- Ten Minute Tone-Ups
  For Dummies 978-0-7645-7207-4
- Yoga with Weights For Dummies
  978-0-471-74937-0